Heart Failure

Algorithms in **Heart Failure**

Editors

Alan S Maisel MD
Professor of Medicine
Director, CCU and HF Program
Department of Medicine and Cardiology
VA Medical Center, University of California
San Diego, California, USA

Gerasimos S Filippatos MD FESC FHFA
Professor of Cardiology
Heart Failure Unit, Department of Cardiology
Attikon University Hospital
University of Athens, School of Medicine
Athens, Greece

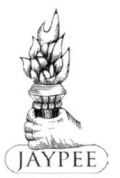

The Health Sciences Publisher

New Delhi | London | Philadelphia | Panama

Jaypee Brothers Medical Publishers (P) Ltd

Headquarters

Jaypee Brothers Medical Publishers (P) Ltd
4838/24, Ansari Road, Daryaganj
New Delhi 110 002, India
Phone: +91-11-43574357
Fax: +91-11-43574314
Email: jaypee@jaypeebrothers.com

Overseas Offices

J.P. Medical Ltd
83 Victoria Street, London
SW1H 0HW (UK)
Phone: +44 20 3170 8910
Fax: +44 (0)20 3008 6180
Email: info@jpmedpub.com

Jaypee-Highlights Medical Publishers Inc
City of Knowledge, Bld. 237, Clayton
Panama City, Panama
Phone: +1 507-301-0496
Fax: +1 507-301-0499
Email: cservice@jphmedical.com

Jaypee Medical Inc
325 Chestnul Street
Suite 412, Philadelphia, PA 19106, USA
Phone: +1 267-519-9789
Email: support@jpmedus.com

Jaypee Brothers Medical Publishers (P) Ltd
17/1-B Babar Road, Block-B, Shaymali
Mohammadpur, Dhaka-1207
Bangladesh
Mobile: +08801912003485
Email: jaypeedhaka@gmail.com

Jaypee Brothers Medical Publishers (P) Ltd
Bhotahity, Kathmandu, Nepal
Phone: +977-9741283608
Email: kathmandu@jaypeebrothers.com

Website: www.jaypeebrothers.com
Website: www.jaypeedigital.com

© 2016, Jaypee Brothers Medical Publishers

The views and opinions expressed in this book are solely those of the original contributor(s)/author(s) and do not necessarily represent those of editor(s) of the book.

All rights reserved. No part of this publication may be reproduced, stored or transmitted in any form or by any means, electronic, mechanical, photocopying, recording or otherwise, without the prior permission in writing of the publishers.

All brand names and product names used in this book are trade names, service marks, trademarks or registered trademarks of their respective owners. The publisher is not associated with any product or vendor mentioned in this book.

Medical knowledge and practice change constantly. This book is designed to provide accurate, authoritative information about the subject matter in question. However, readers are advised to check the most current information available on procedures included and check information from the manufacturer of each product to be administered, to verify the recommended dose, formula, method and duration of administration, adverse effects and contraindications. It is the responsibility of the practitioner to take all appropriate safety precautions. Neither the publisher nor the author(s)/editor(s) assume any liability for any injury and/or damage to persons or property arising from or related to use of material in this book.

This book is sold on the understanding that the publisher is not engaged in providing professional medical services. If such advice or services are required, the services of a competent medical professional should be sought.

Every effort has been made where necessary to contact holders of copyright to obtain permission to reproduce copyright material. If any have been inadvertently overlooked, the publisher will be pleased to make the necessary arrangements at the first opportunity.

Inquiries for bulk sales may be solicited at: jaypee@jaypeebrothers.com

Algorithms in Heart Failure

First Edition: **2016**

ISBN: 978-93-85999-64-2

Printed at Sanat Printers

Contributors

EDITORS

Alan S Maisel MD
Professor of Medicine
Director, CCU and HF Program
Department of Medicine and Cardiology
VA Medical Center, University of California
San Diego, California, USA

Gerasimos S Filippatos MD FESC FHFA
Professor of Cardiology
Heart Failure Unit, Department of Cardiology
Attikon University Hospital
University of Athens, School of Medicine
Athens, Greece

CONTRIBUTING AUTHORS

Eric Adler MD
Associate Professor of Medicine
Driector of Advanced Heart Failure
and Cardiac Transplantation
Department of Medicine
University of California
San Diego, California, USA

Nancy M Albert PhD CCNS CHFN CCRN NE-BC FAHA FCCM FAAN
Associate Chief Nursing Officer
Nursing Research and Innovation
Clinical Nurse Specialist
Kaufman Center for Heart
Failure, Heart and Vascular
Institute, Cleveland Clinic
Cleveland, Ohio, USA

Khwaja S Alim MD
Practicing Internal Medicine
St. Martin Dominican Hospital
Las Vegas, Nevada, USA

Hermineh Aramin
Medical Doctor
VA Medical Center
Department of Cardiology
San Diego, California, USA

Boris Arbit MD
Cardiology Fellow
Department of Medicine
University of California
San Diego, California, USA

Kimberly C Atianzar MD
Fellow, Advanced Cardiovascular Imaging
Department of Internal Medicine
University of California
San Diego, California, USA

Vasiliki Bistola MD
Consultant Cardiologist
Department of Cardiology
Attikon University Hospital
Athens, Greece

Daniel G Blanchard MD FACC FAHA FASE
Professor of Medicine
Department of Cardiovascular Medicine
UC San Diego Cardiovascular Center
San Diego, California, USA

Rudolf A de Boer MD PhD FESC FHFA
Professor of Translational Cardiology
Department of Cardiology
University Medical Center Groningen
Groningen, Netherlands

Jeffrey Chan MD
Resident Physician
Department of Anesthesiology
University of Washington
Seattle, Washington, USA

Anthony J Choi ABIM
Cardiologist
Department of Cardiology
Naval Medical Center
San Diego, California, USA

Lori B Daniels MD MAS FACC
Professor of Medicine
Director, Coronary Care Unit
University of California
San Diego, California, USA

Jason M Duran MD PhD
Practicing Physician
Kaiser Permanente
San Diego, California, USA

Jeremy Egnatios
Medical Student
Department of Medicine
University of California
San Diego, California, USA

Lothar Faber MD FESC FAHA FACC
Professor
Department for Cardiology
Heart and Diabetes Center NRW
Bad Oeynhausen, North Rhine-Westphalia, Germany

Luna Gargani MD PhD
Cardiologist and Researcher
Institute of Clinical Physiology
National Research Council
Pisa, Italy

Erik A Green
Medical Student
Tulane University School of Medicine
New Orleans, Louisiana, USA

Meghana G Halkar MD FACP
Cardiology Hospitalist
Department of Cardiovascular Medicine
MedStar/Cleveland Clinic Heart and Vascular Institute
Washington, DC, USA

Contributors

JT Heywood MD
Director, Advanced Heart Failure, Mechanical Circulatory Support Program
Department of Cardiology
Scripps Clinic
San Diego, California, USA

Affan B Irfan MD PhD
Clinical Cardiology Fellow
Department of General Cardiology and Department of Physiology
University of Louisville
Louisville, Kentucky, USA

Shiro Ishihara MD
Research Associate
Department of Cardiology
Nippon Medical School Musashi-Kosugi Hospitals
Kanagawa, Japan
Biomarkers and Heart Diseases, UMR-942, Institut National de la Santé et de la Recherche Médicale (INSERM)
Paris, France

Tiny Jaarsma PhD RN
Professor in Nursing
Department of Social and Welfare Studies
Linköping University
Linköping, Sweden

Allan S Jaffe FAHA FACC FESC
Professor
Department of Cardiology and Laboratory Medicine and Pathology
Mayo Clinic and Medical School
Rochester, Minnesota, USA

Brian E Jaski MD
Medical Director, Advanced Heart Failure and Cardiac Transplant Program
Sharp Memorial Hospital
Director of Clinical Research
San Diego Cardiac Center
San Diego, California, USA

Corrine Y Jurgens PhD RN ANP FAHA FAAN
Associate Professor and Director of Cardiovascular Research
School of Nursing, Stony Brook University
Stony Brook, New York, USA

Matt M Kawahara BA
Staff Research Associate
VA San Diego Healthcare System
San Diego, California, USA

Benjamin A Kipper BS MD
Medical Student
School of Medicine
Oakland University William Beaumont School of Medicine
Rochester, Michigan, USA

David E Krummen MD FACC FHRS
Associate Professor
Department of Medicine
University of California
Director of Electrophysiology
VA San Diego Healthcare System
San Diego, California, USA

Vijaya A Kumar MD MPH
Assistant Professor
Department of Emergency Medicine, Wayne State University
Detroit, Michigan, USA

Algorithms in Heart Failure

Gautam G Lalani MD
Physician
Department of Cardiology and
Cardiac Electrophysiology
Kaiser Permanente San Diego
San Diego, California, USA

Elizabeth Lee BS
Research Coordinator
Maisel Cardiology Research Lab
Saratoga, California, USA

Phillip D Levy MD MPH
Associate Professor of Emergency
Medicine
Assistant Director of Clinical
Research, Cardiovascular Research
Institute
Associate Director of Clinical
Research, Department of
Emergency Medicine
Director, Clinical Research Center
Wayne State University School of
Medicine
Detroit, Michigan, USA

Alexander R Lyon MA BM BCh PhD FRCP
BHF Senior Lecturer and Honorary
Consultant Cardiologist
NIHR Cardiovascular Biomedical
Research Unit
Royal Brompton and Harefield
NHS Foundation Trust and
National Heart and Lung Institute,
Imperial College London
London, England, UK

Nicholas A Marston MD
Chief Medical Resident
Department of Internal Medicine
University of California
San Diego, California, USA

Josep Masip MD PhD FESC
Director
Department of Intensive Care
Department Consorci Sanitari
Integral
Head
Department of Cardiology
Hospital Sanitas CIMA
Associate Professor
Department of Cardiology
University of Barcelona
Barcelona, Spain

Patrick McCann MD
Director of Heart Failure and
Mechanical Circulatory Support
Department of Cardiology
Palmetto Health
Columbia, South Carolina, USA

Alexandre Mebazaa MD PhD
Professor
Department of Anesthesiology
and Critical Care Medicine
Biomarkers and Heart Diseases,
UMR-942, Institut National de la
Santé et de la Recherche
Médicale (INSERM)
Department of Anesthesiology
and Intensive Care
Lariboisière-Saint-Louis
University Hospital
Assistance Publique–Hôpitaux de
Paris, Université Paris
Diderot, Paris, France

Hirsch S Mehta MD FACC
Associate Director
San Diego Cardiac Center and
Sharp Memorial Hospital
San Diego, California, USA

Contributors

Wouter C Meijers MD
Professor
Department of Cardiology
University Medical Center Groningen
University of Groningen
Groningen, Netherlands

Wayne Miller FAHA FACC
Professor
Department of Cardiology
Mayo Clinic and Medical School
Rochester, Minnesota, USA

Rajeev C Mohan MD
Advanced Heart Failure and Transplant Cardiology Fellow
Department of Cardiology
Cedars-Sinai Medical Center
Los Angeles, California, USA

Andrew C Morley-Smith MB BChir MRCP
BHF Clinical Research Fellow
NIHR Cardiovascular Biomedical Research Unit, Royal Brompton and Harefield NHS
Foundation Trust and National Heart and Lung Institute, Imperial College London
London, England, UK

Silvia Navarin MD
Resident in Emergency Medicine
Department of Emergency Medicine, Sapienza University
Sant'Andrea Hospital
Rome, Italy

Keshav R Nayak MD FACC FSCAI
Director, Cardiac Cathlabs
Department of Cardiology
Naval Medical Center San Diego
San Diego, California, USA

Michel Noutsias FESC
Assistant Medical Director
Department of Cardiology
University Hospital of Jena
Jena, Thuringia, Germany

Minal V Patel BSc
Research Coordinator
Department of Medicine, Cardiology
University of California at San Diego
VA San Diego Healthcare System
San Diego, California, USA

John Parissis MD
Associate Professor of Cardiology
Department of Cardiology
Attikon University Hospital
Athens, Greece

W Frank Peacock MD FACEP
Professor
Department of Emergency Medicine
Baylor College of Medicine
Houston, Texas, USA

Kenneth Planas MD
Staff Physician
Department of Intensive Care
Consorci Sanitari Integral
Barcelona, Spain

Christian Prinz MD FESC
Cardiologist
Private Office for Cardiology
Sögel, Niedersachsen, Germany

Sonal Sarkariya MD
Internal Medicine
St. Joesephs Hospital
Orange County, California, USA

Amir A Schricker MD MS FACC
Assistant Professor
Department of Medicine
University of California
San Diego, California, USA

Kevin S Shah MD
Fellow, Department of Cardiology
University of California
Los Angeles, California, USA

Salvatore Di Somma MD PhD
Professor of Medicine
Director Emergency Medicine
Chairman Postgraduate School of
Emergency Medicine
Department of Medical-Surgery
Sciences and Translational
Medicine, Sapienza University
Sant'Andrea Hospital
Rome, Italy

Anna Strömberg PhD RN FAAN
NFESC
Professor, Department of Medical
and Health Sciences
Linköping University
Linköping, Sweden

Wai Hong W Tang MD
Professor of Medicine
Cardiovascular Medicine, Heart
and Vascular Institute
Cleveland Clinic
Cleveland, Ohio, USA

Rogier Van der Velde MD
Resident
Department of Cardiology
Isala Klinieken
Zwolle, Netherlands

Joel R Wilson MD
Assistant Professor of Medicine
and Radiology
Director, Advanced Cardiovascular
Imaging
Department of Internal Medicine
and Radiology
University of California
San Diego, California, USA

Yang Xue MD
Cardiologist
Department of Cardiology
Kaiser Permanente
Harbor City, California, USA

Preface

It is clear to every healthcare practitioner that heart failure has become a worldwide epidemic. The scourge of obesity and heart disease and the aging of the population have certainly contributed to this phenomenon, as has the longer survival following therapeutic interventions for acute myocardial infarction and cardiac disease in general. Thus, with the increasing prevalence of heart failure, it is important to examine the newest data as well as the latest treatment paradigms. Our first book, *Heart Failure: The Expert's Approach*, provided timely and useful information. This new book, is a shorter, hands-on version, replete with useful algorithms and flowcharts that can be immediately utilized by the practicing physicians.

As in the textbook, Professor Pang from Northwestern University handled section 1 on the emergency department. In this section, we have covered the spectrum of what one would see and do in the emergency. From the early evaluation of the dyspneic patient to the diagnostic techniques, including biomarkers, echocardiography, and impedance to appropriate triage, risk stratification, and treatment of the patient, we offer practical suggestions to simplify diagnosis and management in this urgent care setting.

Section 2 deals with heart failure in the hospital, which includes the use of biomarkers, the latest medical treatments, and the associated comorbidities such as hyponatremia, coronary artery disease, and cardiorenal syndromes.

Section 3 deals with how to take care of chronic heart failure patients in the outpatient setting. There are chapters on monitoring with echocardiography and biomarkers, as well as strategic chapters on preserved ejection fraction, atrial fibrillation, and issues with anticoagulation.

Section 4 deals with special issues in heart failure. This includes, age, gender, sex, and ethnic issues, along with heart failure in other countries as well as the veterans systems. We also deal with heart failure in the nursing home setting and get a good nursing perspective.

Section 5 deals with the approach to end-stage heart failure, and the final section deals with practical recommendations for diagnosis and management of cardiomyopathies.

We hope the readers, whether they be primary care physicians, house officers, practicing cardiologists, or nurses, will both learn and enjoy the contents of this book.

Alan S Maisel

Gerasimos S Filippatos

Acknowledgments

I would like to first acknowledge the now deceased Dr Ralph Shabetai, who as my first chief of cardiology gave me his time and advice and turned my interests towards challenges of the heart failure patient. Never have I met a more selfless and giving man than Ralph. Second, I would like to thank my laboratory personnel without whose help and support I would never have been productive. A special thanks to my lab director, Steve Carter, for 25 years of unwavering loyalty. I would like to thank the publishers M/s Jaypee Brothers Medical Publishers (P) Ltd. for being incredibly supportive to this long endeavor, in particular, Dr Neeraj Choudhary for his friendship and advice. Finally, I would be completely remiss if I did not thank my five children who, lost their mother several years ago and on a daily basis remind me of why God put me on earth. And Fran, my lovely wife, thanks for putting up with my long hours, extensive travel, and crazy sense of humor.

Alan S Maisel

Acknowledgments

I would like to acknowledge the help and support of my parents Spyridon and Angeliki. Till the end of their life, they were close to me, ready to help in any initiative, any new project that I started. I also owe much to Professor George Baltopoulos, who trained me in critical care and helped me from my first steps in research to my doctoral degree, more than 25 years ago. I am grateful to Professor Lambros Anthopoulos, former Chair of the Department of Cardiology at Evangelismos Hospital, who gave me the opportunity to develop and direct the Heart Failure Unit and the Intensive Cardiac Care Unit at Evangelismos Hospital in the mid-1990s; and to Professor Dimitrios Kremastinos, who asked me 10 years ago to organize and run the Heart Failure Unit at Attikon University Hospital. However, my biggest supporters are my wife Maria and my daughter Angela. It is difficult to make space for a life away from work. This becomes impossible if you are trying to find time to write a book on the top of the other activities. Thank you for your support.

Gerasimos S Filippatos

Contents

Section 1: The Emergency Department

1. **How to Evaluate Dyspnea in the Emergency Department?** 3
   W Frank Peacock

2. **Acute Heart Failure Disposition** 12
   Phillip D Levy, Vijaya A Kumar

3. **Using Natriuretic Peptides in the Emergency Department** 21
   Yang Xue, Elizabeth Lee, Jeffrey Chan, Sonal Sarkariya, Erik A Green, Alan S Maisel

4. **Role of Ultrasound in the Management of Acute Heart Failure** 32
   Luna Gargani

5. **Use of Bioelectrical Impedance Vector Analysis in the Dyspneic Patient** 41
   Salvatore Di Somma, Silvia Navarin

6. **Mechanical Ventilation in Acute Heart Failure: The Role of Noninvasive Ventilation** 50
   Josep Masip, Kenneth Planas

7. **When to Employ Cardiac Magnetic Resonance Imaging and Cardiac Computed Tomography in the Evaluation of Heart Failure?** 62
   Kimberly C Atianzar, Joel R Wilson

8. **When to Discharge the Heart Failure Patient?** 78
   Benjamin A Kipper

Section 2: Heart Failure in the Hospital

9. **Approach to Diuretics in the Hospital** — 89
   Meghana G Halkar, Wai Hong W Tang

10. **Vasodilators in Acute Heart Failure** — 103
    Shiro Ishihara, Alexandre Mebazaa

11. **When and How to Use Inotropes?** — 108
    John Parissis, Vasiliki Bistola

12. **Practical Approach to Hyponatremia in Heart Failure** — 119
    Rajeev C Mohan, Hirsch S Mehta, JT Heywood

13. **Heart Failure and Acute Coronary Syndrome** — 131
    Kevin S Shah

Section 3: Chronic Heart Failure Patients in the Outpatient Setting

14. **Echocardiography: Getting It Right** — 143
    Nicholas A Marston, Daniel G Blanchard, Jeremy Egnatios

15. **Initiation of Angiotensin Converting Enzyme Inhibitors and Beta-blockers in Heart Failure: Putting Evidence into Practice** — 153
    Boris Arbit, Alan S Maisel

16. **Atrial Fibrillation Done Right** — 160
    Amir A Schricker, David E Krummen

17. **Ventricular Tachycardia Done Right** — 172
    Gautam G Lalani, David E Krummen

18. **Management of the Patient with Heart Failure with Preserved Ejection Fraction** — 181
    Alan S Maisel, Gerasimos S Filippatos, Kevin S Shah, Jeffrey Chan

19. **Implantable Cardioverter Defibrillator and Cardiac Resynchronization Therapy in Heart Failure Patients: How to Choose the Right Device?** — 192
    Khwaja S Alim, Erik A Green

20. **Clinical Decision-making in the Outpatient Setting: the Use of Galectin-3** — 199
   Rogier van der Velde, Wouter C Meijers, Rudolf A de Boer

21. **ST2: How to Really Do It Right?** — 208
   Jason M Duran, Lori B Daniels

22. **Use of Cardiac Troponin to Assist in the Management of Patients with Congestive Heart Failure: A Practical Guide** — 217
   Affan B Irfan, Wayne Miller, Allan S Jaffe

Section 4: Special Issues in Heart Failure

23. **Heart Failure in the Nursing Home Setting** — 231
   Corrine Y Jurgens

24. **Heart Failure from the Nursing Perspective** — 241
   Nancy M Albert

Section 5: Advanced Heart Failure

25. **Left Ventricular Assist Device Versus Transplantation: How to Decide?** — 277
   Patrick McCann, Eric Adler

26. **Approach to Left Ventricular Assist Devices and Follow-up in Advanced Congestive Heart Failure** — 284
   Anthony J Choi, Keshav R Nayak, Brian E Jaski

27. **How to Approach Palliative and End-of-life Care?** — 296
   Tiny Jaarsma, Anna Strömberg

Section 6: Cardiomyopathies: Practical Recommendations to Diagnosis and Management

28. **Hypertrophic Cardiomyopathy** — 305
   Christian Prinz, Lothar Faber, Alan S Maisel

29. **Takotsubo Syndrome** — 315
   Andrew C Morley-Smith, Alexander R Lyon

30. **Myocarditis** — 323
   Michel Noutsias

31. **Acquired Immune Deficiency Syndrome Induced Cardiac Abnormalities and Heart Failure** 348
Khwaja S Alim, Hermineh Aramin, Minal V Patel, Elizabeth Lee

32. **New Onset Cardiomyopathy: Biopsy or Magnetic Resonance Imaging and Other Imaging Modalities** 353
Khwaja S Alim, Matt M Kawahara

Index *361*

SECTION 1

The Emergency Department

CHAPTER 1

How to Evaluate Dyspnea in the Emergency Department?

W Frank Peacock

INTRODUCTION

Dyspnea is unique in its universal significance. No activity may be continued in the face of mounting dyspnea, and ultimately nothing is more important than not being able to breathe. When asked "what would make you go to the emergency department?", the surprisingly short list is either dyspnea or pain. But dyspnea is dominant and is the reason that it is one of the most common presentations to the emergency department.

Like pain, dyspnea is subjective. And like pain, precise measures to accurately and objectively determine its severity simply do not exist. Therefore, to evaluate the effect of treatment on its relief, recording the patient's perception of their symptoms may provide utility. A common technique to rate and track dyspnea is the Visual Analog Scale (VAS). This is performed by having a patient indicates their degree of discomfort by drawing an indicator on a 0–100 mm line (Fig. 1). Although not validated for dyspnea, data from the

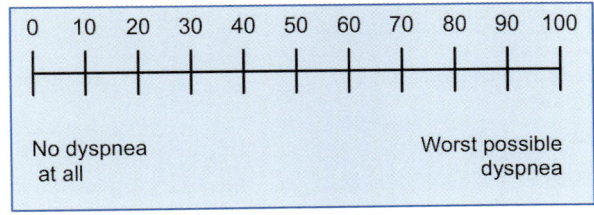

FIG. 1: Visual Analog Scale

pain literature data suggests that a clinically relevant change should be more than 13 mm. This method records the patient's perception of dyspnea at the moment the scale is administered. Alternatively, a second technique is commonly used that evaluates temporally relative dyspnea changes. This is performed by asking the patient, "compared to a prior time (e.g., emergency department presentation), how have your symptoms changed". Box 1 demonstrates potential responses. It should be noted that, while it is still useful to evaluate therapeutic impact, relative scales cannot evaluate dyspnea at presentation and are limited as they tend to be less sensitive for smaller dyspnea changes than VAS scoring.

Although dyspnea may be the result of normal physiologic processes (e.g., strenuous activity), it is also the final common symptom of many potentially fatal events (Table 1). Irrespective of its cause, failure to ventilate or oxygenate sufficiently to meet the metabolic needs of the corpus results in dyspnea. Because the list of causes is long, overlapping, and complicated, it is the emergency physician's challenge to rapidly identify and reverse the primary cause of dyspnea. To further increase the complexity of the task, relatively harmless mimics, such as anxiety, can present with profound dyspnea. This last caveat represents a serious diagnostic

Box 1: Relative dyspnea score

- Markedly better
- Moderately better
- Minimally better
- Unchanged
- Minimally improved
- Moderately improved
- Markedly improved

TABLE 1: Categorical examples of the causes of dyspnea

Mechanical	Metabolic	Hemodynamic
Foreign body/anaphylaxis	Acidosis (e.g., DKA)	HF/AMI
Asthma/COPD	Anemia	Septic shock
Trauma (e.g., pneumothorax, rib fx)	Toxin (e.g., cyanide)	Hemorrhagic shock
Airspace pus (pneumonia) or blood (trauma)		Cardiogenic shock
Pulmonary embolism		Shunts
Neurologic (ALS)		

AMI, acute myocardial infarction; ALS, amyotrophic lateral sclerosis; COPD, chronic obstructive pulmonary disease; DKA, diabetic ketoacidosis; HF, heart failure; Fx, fracture.

challenge, especially when a patient is older and at risk for potential fatal comorbidities that are likely to be present.

VITAL SIGNS

Vital signs are vital, and must be measured as soon as feasible after presentation. They represent the earliest objective measure of the extent of distress. While extremely insensitive when near normal, increasing deviations are associated with a logarithmically increased risk of a serious underlying event. When evaluating respiratory status, extremely slow respiratory rates (e.g., <6 respirations/min) represent a premorbid condition, with immediate therapeutic intervention necessary (e.g., endotracheal intubation, naloxone, etc.) to obviate a fatality. An algorithmic approach to etiologic considerations in the nonapneic patient is shown in figure 3.

Conversely, while very high respiratory rates (>30 respirations/min) can be tolerated initially, they cannot be maintained for long periods and will ultimately lead to respiratory failure if prompt intervention does not correct the underlying pathology. When respiratory rates are near normal, pulse oximetry may aide in providing objective measures of the oxygen transport capability. However, oxygen delivery must be considered in context of hemoglobin concentration, as tissue hypoxia may exist in the setting of low hemoglobin. Ultimately, any oxygen saturation below 90% should prompt an immediate evaluation and corrective interventions.

Pulse oximetry is a rapid, noninvasive, inexpensive, objective measure of the total function of the body's oxygen delivery system and it suffers from several caveats. Abnormalities of hemoglobin from some toxins (e.g., cyanide and carbon monoxide) may present as having normal oxygen transport capability when in fact tissue oxygen delivery is distinctly impaired. Further, the presence of adequate oxygenation does not reflect on ventilatory status, which must be considered independently.

Measurement of the blood pressure can be extremely useful in determining the underlying etiology in a patient presenting with dyspnea. Hypertension, associated with jugular venous distention (JVD) and rales, is highly suggestive of acute pulmonary edema, and treatment to rapidly lower the blood pressure may be highly effective at resolving dyspnea. This is true regardless of the type of heart failure (HF) (reduced or preserved ejection fraction), even with blood pressures as low as 140 mmHg. In patients with lower blood pressures, few signs volume overload, and with

Algorithms in Heart Failure

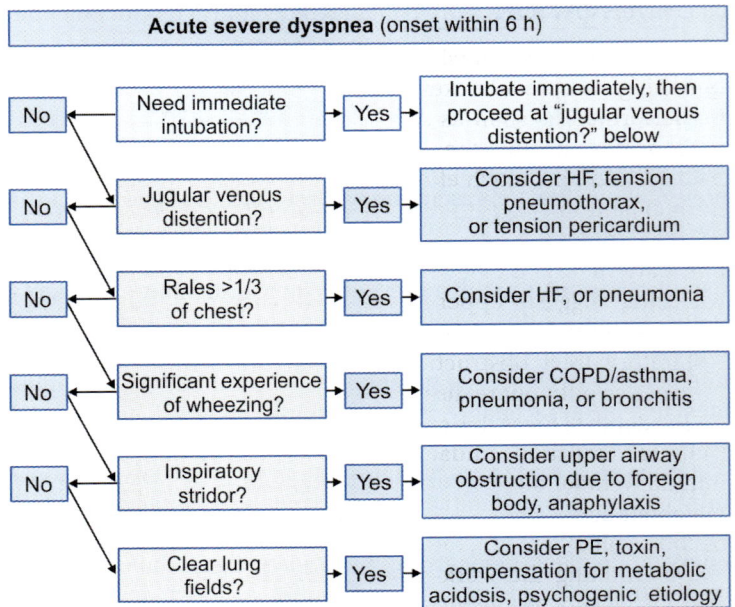

The decision to intubate a patient with severe dyspnea is not determined by the results of any objective testing. Rather, it is a clinical decision based solely on the physicians' impression that the patient is either currently, or imminently will, suffer acute respiratory failure. In co-operative, but distressed patients, a limited trial of bilevel positive airway pressure or continuous positive airway pressure may allow enough time for immediate therapeutic interventions to take effect, thus avoiding the need for more invasive measures. However, noninvasive ventilatory measures are not definitive airway management and should be considered as short-term temporary adjuncts. If improvement in clinical status is not seen relatively quick after their implementation, endotracheal intubation should be considered.

HF, heart failure; COPD, chronic obstructive disease; PE, pulmonary embolism.

FIG. 3: An approach to the patient presenting with acute severe dyspnea. The patient's process of breathing should be observed for several respiratory cycles. If afterward the physician is assured at least a modicum of time is available before immediate endotracheal intubation is required, the algorithm may be considered. While it is presented in a stepwise fashion, the entire process is performed in less than 15 seconds, while listening to the lung sounds

wheezing on auscultation, chronic obstructive pulmonary disease is a more likely diagnosis. Finally, if the blood pressure is very low (e.g., <90 mmHg) in the setting of HF, immediate intervention is required, as the mortality rate in this patient phenotype approximates 70%.

OBSERVATION

When patients present with dyspnea, watching the mechanics of breathing can provide extremely useful information and should be performed as soon as possible after arrival. The parameters to consider include the depth of inhalation, the respiratory pattern, and how much effort the patient is expending. While the normal pattern of breathing is an apparently effortless inhalation or exhalation with a timing relationship of 1:3, alterations of this pattern can provide an early diagnosis. While inhalation wheezing suggests upper airway pathology (e.g., foreign body and anaphylaxis), prolonged expiration is consistent with lower respiratory tract obstruction secondary to asthma or chronic obstructive pulmonary disease.

The depth of breathing can suggest changes in minute ventilation (minute ventilation = tidal volume × breaths/minute). Increased minute ventilation can occur as respiratory compensation for metabolic acidosis from any cause, is also seen with anemia, or may be the result of severe anxiety.

Determining the work of breathing is important as extreme exertion will not be tolerated for prolonged periods. The presence of accessory muscle use, sitting in an upright position, and concurrent abdominal muscle use are each consistent with increased breathing effort, as is the number of words that the patients may speak between breaths. If diaphoresis is present secondary to the effort of breathing, the patient is likely to tire quickly and must be rapidly addressed. Finally, nonpulmonary observations may suggest the cause of dyspnea, e.g., persistent JVD is consistent with HF, tension pneumothorax, or pericardial tamponade.

Physical Examination

As the physical examination provides very useful diagnostic information, after the vital signs have been measured and the respiratory status observed, if immediate treatment (e.g., endotracheal intubation) is not required, it should be performed. This begins by noting odors (e.g., spearmint suggests severe metabolic acidosis from aspirin poisoning with an oil of wintergreen ingestion) and touching the skin to determine the presence of fever (as may occur with pneumonia or sepsis), or if the patients is cold and wet from compensatory peripheral vasoconstriction (as may occur with acute pulmonary edema or in the setting of shock).

Pulmonary auscultation is useful to assist in determining the etiology for dyspnea. Asymmetric findings are consistent with asymmetric pathology (e.g., pneumonia, pneumothorax and pleural effusion). Although the detection of basilar rales is not diagnostic of a specific pathology, their extent may be related to the severity of the presentation. Finally, thoracic percussion may diagnose a pleural effusion when breath sounds are distant or absent.

Finally, inspection of the naked patient may also suggest a diagnosis. Notation of the presence or absence of JVD, abdominal distention (consistent with ascites), or peripheral edema (and its symmetry) can suggest the underlying cause of dyspnea.

INVESTIGATIONS

Laboratory Investigation

While laboratory investigations can be extremely useful, in the severely ill patient, the focus should be on the obtainable history and physical exam. Even point of care labs take some amount of time to perform and usually only confirm a suspected diagnosis. In the acutely ill patient, treatment should not be delayed pending lab results. In those with less acute severity at presentation, and an intervention can be postponed without harming the patient, specific labs may be helpful. These may consist of measuring troponin, natriuretic peptides, or D-dimer in selected cases. Chemistry analysis may aid in risk stratification and impact diagnostic strategies (e.g., an elevated creatinine may preclude a computed tomographic angiogram), as well as identify iatrogenic complications of outpatient therapy (e.g., hypokalemia and digoxin toxicity).

Finally, while arterial blood gas may determine acid-base status and guide ventilator parameters, they are rarely of diagnostic assistance in the acute setting. They should not be used to evaluate the airway or the need for intubation at the acute presentation. Although they may be helpful later in the patient's clinical course, at presentation the time used obtaining an arterial blood gas sample is better spent performing the clinical assessment and initial interventions.

Bioimpedance Vector Analysis

Bioimpedance vector analysis is a technology for determining total body water by the measuring the electrical conductive properties of the body. It provides rapid, noninvasive, inexpensive, reproducible, and objective results that correlate with total body water, diuretic therapy need, and the likelihood of the necessity for hospitalization from the emergency department. Although knowledge of total body water volume is not diagnostic in itself (as many pathologies are associated with increased total body water), when it is considered in combination with other bedside and lab findings, it has been shown to improve diagnostic accuracy.

Radiology

Chest X-rays are a very useful investigation, although they do suffer from a number of limitations (e.g., their findings may be delayed relative to the patient's presentation, they can be insensitive when done using a portable technique, they require radiation exposure, and are relatively more expensive than other procedures). Their significant advantage is that they can be performed rapidly and at the bedside. A normal chest radiograph in the setting of acute dyspnea should result in a marked change the differential diagnosis, if acute heart failure was initially suspected.

Lastly, the pulmonary computed tomography angiogram has become routine for evaluating suspected pulmonary embolism. It is very helpful in the acutely dyspneic patient, if the clinical diagnosis is likely acute pulmonary embolism. However, the pretest probability of the presence of a pulmonary embolism should be considered by using the Well's criteria (Table 2). Patients with higher scores should undergo scanning, while those a low score (<3) and a negative qualitative D-dimer test do not require further pulmonary embolism work up. Patients who are severely ill, hemodynamically unstable, and too dyspneic to lay flat are not computed tomography

TABLE 2: Well's Criteria

Clinical Findings	Points
Clinical signs and symptoms of deep vein thrombosis?	+3
Pulmonary embolism more likely diagnosis or equally likely	+3
Heart rate >100?	+1.5
Immobilization at least 3 days, or surgery in the previous 4 weeks	+1.5
Previous, objectively diagnosed pulmonary embolism or deep vein thrombosis?	+1.5
Hemoptysis?	+1
Malignancy with treatment within 6 months, or palliative?	+1

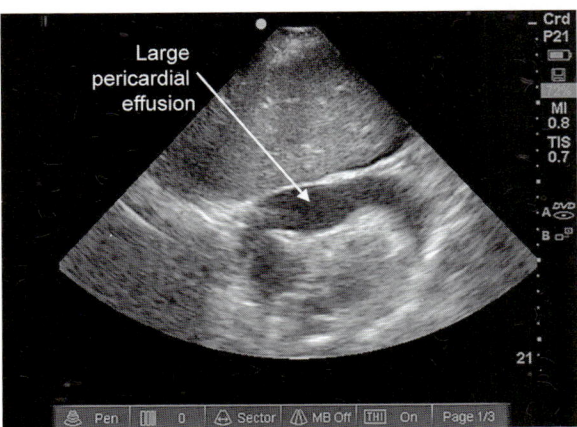

FIG. 2: Subxiphoid view of a pericardial effusion

evaluation candidates and may best be served initially by empiric treatment.

ULTRASOUND

When performed at the bedside by the emergency physician, ultrasound is a rapid, noninvasive and inexpensive measure to aid in determining the cause of dyspnea. It can evaluate for a possible pneumothorax, inform about cardiac contractility, and diagnose a pericardial effusion (Fig. 2). Lung ultrasound can help differentiate HF and chronic obstructive pulmonary disease by identifying B-lines, and it can detect volume overload by direct lung imaging or by observing the failure of vena cava diameter changes that normally occur during the respiratory cycle.

CONCLUSION

Dyspnea, the most common reason for patients with acute heart failure to present to the hospital, is the final common pathway for a large number of potentially fatal pathologies. Determining if an immediate airway intervention is necessary is defined by the acuity of the presentation and the diagnostic certainty of the practitioner. When severe, initial clinical decisions may be entirely based upon vital signs, the physical exam, and patient distress. However, if the patient is more stable and can tolerate investigations before therapy is initiated, then selected tests, bioimpedance measures, ultrasound, or radiographic testing may be considered to assist in limiting the differential diagnosis and increase diagnostic certainty.

KEY POINTS

- Hypertension, associated with jugular venous distention and rales, is highly suggestive of acute pulmonary edema
- Watching the mechanics of breathing can provide extremely useful diagnostic information
- Lung ultrasound can rapidly help differentiate heart failure and chronic obstructive pulmonary disease.

SUGGESTED READINGS

1. Dyspnea. Wikipedia website [online]. Available from: http://en.wikipedia.org/wiki/Dyspnea [Accessed Jan, 2016].
2. Todd KH, Funk KG, Funk JP, Bonacci R. Clinical significance of reported changes in pain severity. Ann Emerg Med. 1996;27:485-9.
3. Medline Plus. (2015). Vital signs. [online]. Available from: www.nlm.nih.gov/medlineplus/ency/article/002341.htm. [Accessed December, 2015].
4. Wells PS, Anderson DR, Rodger M, Stiell I, Dreyer JF, Barnes D, et al. Excluding pulmonary embolism at the bedside without diagnostic imaging: management of patients with suspected pulmonary embolism presenting to the emergency department by using a simple clinical model and d-dimer. Ann Inten Med. 2001;135(2):98-107.
5. Wolf SJ, McCubbin Tr, Feldhaus KM, Faragher JP, Adcock DM. Prospective validation of Wells Criteria in the evaluation of patients with suspected pulmonary embolism. Ann Emerg Med. 2003;44(5):503-10.

2 CHAPTER

Acute Heart Failure Disposition

Phillip D Levy, Vijaya A Kumar

INTRODUCTION

Appropriate disposition of the emergency department (ED) patient with acute heart failure (AHF) is a clinical challenge. While few who present to the ED with AHF are severely ill and many respond well to initial therapeutic intervention, nearly 85% end up being admitted to the hospital. Much of this is driven by a generally low threshold among ED physicians for postdischarge adverse events and fear associated with the implications of perceived negligence. Such perspectives are compounded by the relative lack of outcome data and an absence of validated, evidence based decision support tools derived specifically from ED patients. While the Heart Failure Society of America did propose criterion upon which hospitalization is either recommended or should be considered (Box 1) in their 2010 Comprehensive Practice Guidelines, the selected variables are loosely defined and based entirely on expert consensus (strength of evidence = C). Despite this, features such as those defined by the Society of Cardiovascular Patient Care (SCPC) are associated with risk of poor outcome for AHF patients (Table 1). By combining these with important clinical variables and psychosocial considerations (Box 2) into a single algorithm (algorithm 1), a more streamlined approach to AHF patient disposition may be achievable.

Acute Heart Failure Disposition

Box 1: Heart Failure Society of America Admission criteria

- Hospitalization recommended
  - Evidence of severe ADHF, including:
    - Hypotension
    - Worsening renal function
    - Altered mentation
  - Dyspnea at rest, as evidenced by:
    - Resting tachypnea
    - Oxygen saturation <90%
  - Hemodynamically significant arrhythmia
    - Including new onset of rapid atrial fibrillation
  - Acute coronary syndromes
- Hospitalization should be considered
  - Worsened congestion
    - With or without dyspnea
  - Signs and symptoms of pulmonary or systemic congestion
    - With or without weight gain
  - Major electrolyte disturbance
  - Associated comorbid conditions
    - Pneumonia
    - Pulmonary embolus
    - Diabetic ketoacidosis
    - Cerebrovascular disease
  - Repeated ICD firings
  - New onset heart failure

ADHF, acute decompensated heart failure; ICD, implanted cardioverter-defibrillator.

TABLE 1: Evidence based markers of acute heart failure risk

Marker	Threshold for increased risk
Systolic blood pressure	<100 mmHg
Respiratory rate	>32 breaths/min
Electrocardiography	New ischemic changes
Renal function	
BUN	>40 mg/dL
Creatinine	>3.0 mg/dL
Serum sodium	<135 mmol/L
Cardiac-specific troponin	Any value >99th percentile (varies by assay)
Natriuretic peptides	
BNP	>1,000 pg/mL
NT-pro BNP	>5,000 pg/mL

BUN, blood urea nitrogen; BNP, brain natriuretic peptide; NT-proBNP, N-terminal of the prohormone brain natriuretic peptide.

> **Box 2: Psychosocial considerations and potential barriers to effective disease self-management for acute heart failure patients**
> - Low health literacy and/or numeracy
> - Poor disease specific knowledge
> - Low patient activation
> - Underinsured or lack of insurance
> - Limited access to transportation resources
> - Absence of caregivers and lack of social support
> - Limited access to healthful foods
> - Limited access to primary and/or specialty care
> - Presence of comorbidities especially cognitive deficits and depression or other psychiatric disorders

STEP 1: ASSESS INITIAL SEVERITY

Assessment of initial severity for those who present to the ED with AHF is a critical first step that can be used to decide which patients should be directed toward early hospital admission, most often in a monitored setting. As shown in the algorithm, this primarily involves an evaluation of respiratory and hemodynamic status on arrival with incorporation of immediate, resuscitative interventions in the decision-making process. While further workup and additional therapy will certainly be needed for those who are critically ill, the need for accessory ventilatory support or vasoactive infusions will undoubtedly require admission to an intensive care setting. Patients with concerning features at presentation who do not require such high level treatment may respond well to more conventional therapy and the disposition decision can await reevaluation.

In stark contrast, a number of patients will be at the other end of the severity spectrum, with completely stable vital signs and no evidence of respiratory difficulty at rest. Such individuals have often been recently admitted for AHF and their ED visit represents a failure of effective transitional care. For others, their use of the ED may be a consequence of poor access to primary or specialty care. Regardless, the key point with these patients is to ensure that indeed their condition is chronic and that there are no high risk features associated with their acute presentation. The latter includes an absence of underlying or worsening renal function, and a lack of worrisome clinical consideration (i.e., minimal peripheral edema, no chest pain, and no dyspnea at rest). Once these considerations have been assessed, and an individually appropriate, achievable transitional care plan has been developed (i.e., one that will not

Acute Heart Failure Disposition

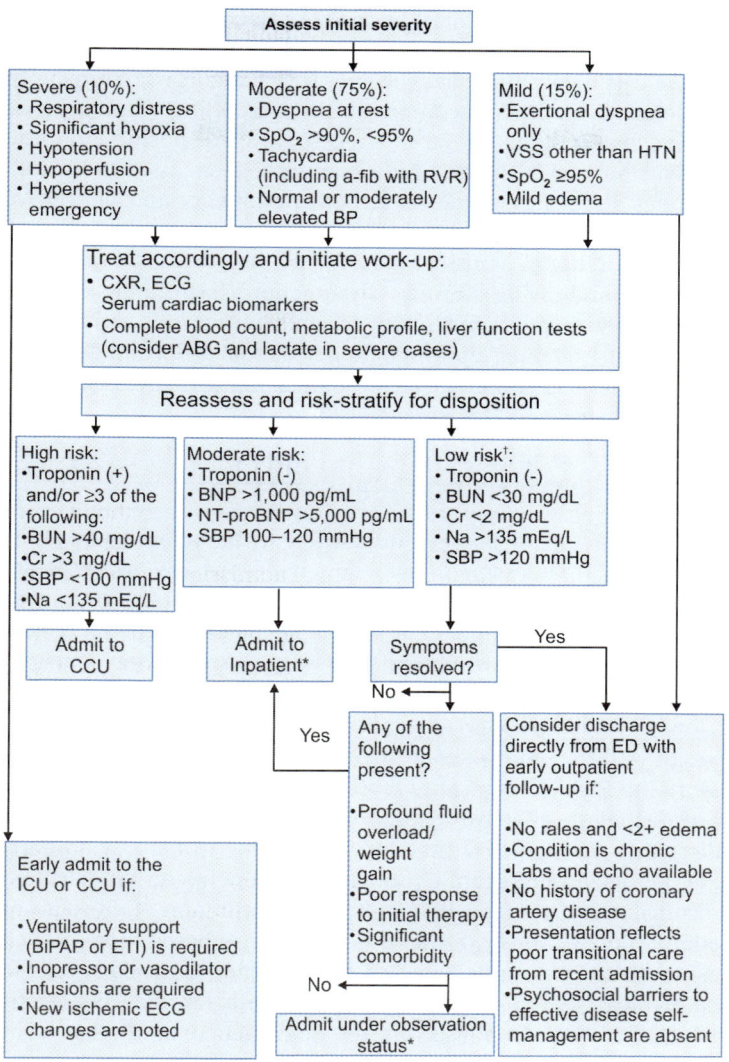

†Consider modified approach using EMHRG score.
*Telemetry criteria: arrhythmia, ICD firing, syncope, active chest pain, potassium ≤2.5 or ≥6.0, magnesium ≤1 mEq/L.

SpO$_2$, saturation of peripheral oxygen; a-fib, atrial fibrillation; RVR, rapid ventricular rate; BP, blood pressure; VSS, venous sinus stenting; HTN, hypertension; SBP, systolic blood pressure; CXR, chest X-ray; ECG, echocardiogram; ABG, arterial blood gas; CCU, coronary care unit; ICU, intensive care unit; BiPAP, bilevel positive airway pressure; ETI, endotracheal intubation, ED, emergency department; BUN, blood urea nitrogen; BNP, brain natriuretic peptide; NT-proBNP, N-terminal of the prohormone brain natrinretic peptide.

ALGORITHM 1: Evidence-based algorithm for acute heart failure patient disposition from the emergency department

be hindered by psychosocial barriers), discharge home is a viable option.

The true disposition challenge lies with patients who have more moderate symptoms accompanied by borderline respiratory or hemodynamic status. By far the largest group, disposition of these patients should be guided by a comprehensive assessment that includes an initial evaluation of both pulmonary and peripheral congestion along with a search for evidence of cardiac or renal injury. Additional considerations, such as heart failure (HF) etiology, underlying cardiac dysfunction (especially ejection fraction), suspected precipitant (i.e., hypertension, arrhythmia, myocardial ischemia, and worsening renal function), and degree of volume overload should be factored in, along with the therapeutic response to initial ED treatment.

STEP 2: PATIENT REASSESSMENT

Patient profiles can change dramatically within a few hours of ED arrival and reassessment involving both physical examination after initial therapy has been initiated and a review of laboratory or radiographic results encompasses the next step. For patients with chronic heart failure who experience symptom resolution or at least a return to baseline, meet the SCPC low risk criteria (Table 1) or have a low or very low (rate of 7-day mortality for patients discharged from the ED = 0.25% and 0.21%, respectively) Emergency Heart Failure Mortality Risk Grade score (Table 2), and do not have any other preclusions to effective disease self-management (Algorithm 1), discharge from the ED may be considered. To help avoid early ED revisits, arrangement of outpatient follow-up, and medication reconciliation, perhaps with short-term uptitration of diuretics or addition of previously unprescribed, evidence based therapy such as an aldosterone antagonist or a dual action β-blockers should be included as part of the discharge process. Further HF-specific education with emphasis on the importance of disease self-management may also be needed.

How do you know if your patient has experienced sufficient symptom resolution? While an improvement in fluid overload can be identified on physical examination by specific findings including a reduction in jugular venous pressure, resolution of pulmonary rales, a decrease in peripheral edema, diminished body weight, and an increase in urine output, there is no validated measure to assess dyspnea. Clinicians often assess dyspnea by simply asking the patient if they feel better, but responses are highly subjective

TABLE 2: Emergency Heart Failure Mortality Risk Grade model

Variable*	Unit or measure	Mathematical adjustment†
Age	Continuous in years	Multiply by 2
Transported by EMS	Categorical	Add 60, if yes
Systolic blood pressure	Continuous in mmHg (max = 160 mmHg)	Multiply by 1
Heart rate	Continuous in beats per minute (min = 80, max = 120 beats/min)	Multiply by 1
Oxygen saturation	Continuous as % (max = 92%)	Multiply by 2
Creatinine	Continuous as mg/dL (divide by 88.4 if reported as µmol/L)	Multiply by 20
Potassium	Categorical: • 4.0 to 4.5 mmol/L • ≥4.6 mmol/L • ≤3.9 mmol/L	If yes: • Add 0 • Add 30 • Add 5
Troponin	Categorical	Add 60, if above upper limit of normal
Active cancer	Categorical	Add 45, if yes
Metolazone at home	Categorical	Add 60, if yes
Adjustment factor	–	Add 12

*Based on initial or triage measurement
†Score derived from sum of all variables, including the adjustment factor: very low risk = ≤−15.9; low risk = −15.8–17.9; intermediate risk = 18.0–56.5; high risk = 56.6–89.3; very high risk = ≥89.4.
EMS, emergency medical services; min, minimum; max, maximum.

and such an approach is far from ideal. More objective measures such as 5 or 7 point Likert scales and 100 mm Visual Analogue Scales, correlate with dyspnea improvement when used in clinical trials but their uptake in real world practice has been limited. Typically, used in patients with chronic pulmonary disease, peak expiratory flow rate has also been evaluated as a way to standardize dyspnea measurement in AHF patients with data suggesting that it may be complimentary to Likert scales, especially within the first 24 hours of treatment. Provocative dyspnea assessment, a recently developed approach where patients self-report dyspnea in the upright and, after a brief equilibration period, supine positions, may be an additional useful adjunct enabling identification of "hidden" symptoms of persistent congestion that are gravity dependent.

Despite improvements at rest, dyspnea may still be present on exertion and assessing this provides an important measure of the potential need for further decongestion. For those who feel better and have objective evidence of reduced symptoms, simply having the patient ambulate in the ED without symptoms (e.g., dyspnea, dizziness, and chest pain) can be quite useful. Precisely how far and how long they should be able to ambulate prior to discharge has not been established, but in stable angina patients, the 6-minute walk test (6MWT), where the maximal ambulatory distance is measured over 6 minutes and compared to age-adjusted population norms, is considered a valid metric of cardiovascular risk. While the 6MWT has not been formally tested as a metric of "dischargeability", a modified version involving 3 minutes of ambulation with concurrent monitoring of heart rate, respiratory rate, pulse oximetry, and subjective dyspnea may be useful, helping to distinguish ED patients with AHF at risk for worse outcome in a small, single center feasibility study (n = 40).

Whatever the approach to reassessment, patients who have residual dyspnea at rest or cannot tolerate exertion after initial treatment in the ED clearly require more extensive, hospital-based treatment.

STEP 3: DETERMINING ADMISSION LOCATION

Once it has been decided that a patient requires admission, the specific location within the hospital must be determined. Whether a given patient should be directed to the observation unit, an inpatient ward, or the cardiac care unit can be guided by the anticipated duration of therapeutic intervention and the level of risk for inhospital adverse events. While duration of therapy can be difficult to predict, the presence of significant peripheral edema will likely require repeated doses of intravenous diuretic making the observation unit for such patients a poor choice. On the other hand, risk assessment models based on routinely collected variables, such as blood pressure, electrocardiography, and laboratory measures, including serum electrolytes, renal function (i.e., blood urea nitrogen and serum creatinine), and biomarkers of cardiac stress and injury (i.e., troponin and natriuretic peptides) are well-established. Consequently, patients can be easily classified into distinct risk subgroups (low, medium, and high) and disposition can be aligned with the location most appropriate for their level of risk.

Of note, while telemetry is often used for those admitted with AHF and is certainly indicated for high risk patients destined for a cardiac or intensive care unit setting, there is little evidence to support this as a routine practice for moderate or low risk patients. Limited telemetry bed availability is not uncommon and prolonged stays in the ED may be an unintended consequence of such resource utilization. Moreover, telemetry does provide the ability to monitor cardiac rate and rhythm, it does not equate with a higher level of nursing care per se and should not be used as a substitute for more intensive care when needed. As such, our algorithm includes criteria for use of telemetry based upon factors that increase the likelihood of developing potential cardiac rate or rhythm disturbances.

CONCLUSION

A stepwise, evidence based approach to the disposition of AHF patients can help improve the delivery of care, while avoiding potentially unnecessary utilization of valuable hospital resources. As outlined in our algorithm (Algorithm 1), such an approach must incorporate multiple facets of the patient encounter while remaining cognizant of the complex, dynamic nature of the disease process itself.

KEY POINTS

- Disposition of patients with acute heart failure can be challenging
- While many experience clinical improvement after initial treatment in the ED, admission to the hospital remains the default pathway with only one out of every six patients being discharged home
- The ideal approach to disposition should balance the potential risk for adverse events in the outpatient setting with the expected benefits of further, hospital based care
- To assist with this, we provide real-world insight into the process of ED disposition and propose a simplified approach to decision-making built on a foundation of multilevel, evidence based risk stratification.

SUGGESTED READINGS

1. Beatty AL, Schiller NB, Whooley MA. Six-minute walk test as a prognostic tool in stable coronary heart disease: data from the heart and soul study. Arch Intern Med. 2012;172:1096-102.
2. Collins SP, Lindsell CJ, Storrow AB, Fermann GJ, Levy PD, Pang PS, et al. Early changes in clinical characteristics after emergency department therapy for acute heart failure

syndromes: identifying patients who do not respond to standard therapy. Heart Fail Rev. 2012;17:387-94.
3. Collins SP, Pang PS, Fonarow GC, Yancy CW, Bonow RO, Gheorghiade M. Is hospital admission for heart failure really necessary?: the role of the emergency department and observation unit in preventing hospitalization and rehospitalization. J Am Coll Cardiol. 2013;61:121-6.
4. Collins SP, Storrow AB. Moving toward comprehensive acute heart failure risk assessment in the emergency department: the importance of self-care and shared decision making. JACC Heart Fail. 2013;1:273-80.
5. Ezekowitz JA, Hernandez AF, O'Connor CM, Starling RC, Proulx G, Weiss MH, et al. Assessment of dyspnea in acute decompensated heart failure: insights from ASCEND-HF (acute study of clinical effectiveness of nesiritide in decompensated heart failure) on the contributions of peak expiratory flow. J Am Coll Cardiol. 2012;59:1441-8.
6. Heart Failure Society of America, Lindenfeld J, Albert NM, Boehmer JP, Collins SP, Ezekowitz JA, et al. HFSA 2010 Comprehensive Heart Failure Practice Guideline. J Card Fail. 2010;16:e1-194.
7. Hogg KJ, McMurray JJ. Evaluating dyspnoea in acute heart failure: progress at last! Eur Heart J. 2010;31:771-2.
8. Lee DS, Stitt A, Austin PC, Stukel TA, Schull MJ, Chong A, et al. Prediction of heart failure mortality in emergent care: a cohort study. Ann Intern Med. 2012;156(11):767-75, W-261, W-262.
9. McCausland JB, Machi MS, Yealy DM. Emergency physicians' risk attitudes in acute decompensated heart failure patients. Acad Emerg Med. 2010;17:108-10.
10. Mebazaa A, Pang PS, Tavares M, Collins SP, Storrow AB, Laribi S, et al. The impact of early standard therapy on dyspnoea in patients with acute heart failure: the URGENT-dyspnoea study. Eur Heart J. 2010;31:832-41.
11. Pan AM, Stiell IG, Clement CM, Acheson J, Aaron SD. Feasibility of a structured 3-minute walk test as a clinical decision tool for patients presenting to the emergency department with acute dyspnoea. Emerg Med J. 2009;26:278-82.
12. Pang PS, Collins SP, Sauser K, Andrei AC, Storrow AB, Hollander JE, et al. Assessment of dyspnea early in acute heart failure: patient characteristics and response differences between likert and visual analog scales. Acad Emerg Med. 2014;21:659-66.
13. Peacock WF, Fonarow GC, Ander DS, Collins SP, Gheorghiade M, Kirk JD, et al. Society of Chest Pain Centers recommendations for the evaluation and management of the observation stay acute heart failure patient-parts 1-6. Acute Card Care. 2009;11:3-42.
14. Storrow AB, Jenkins CA, Self WH, Alexander PT, Barrett TW, Han JH, et al. The burden of acute heart failure on U.S. emergency departments. JACC Heart Fail. 2014;2:269-77.
15. Weintraub NL, Collins SP, Pang PS, Levy PD, Anderson AS, Arslanian-Engoren C, et al. Acute heart failure syndromes: emergency department presentation, treatment, and disposition: current approaches and future aims: a scientific statement from the American Heart Association. Circulation. 2010;122:1975-96.

CHAPTER 3

Using Natriuretic Peptides in the Emergency Department

Yang Xue, Elizabeth Lee, Jeffrey Chan, Sonal Sarkariya, Erik A Green, Alan S Maisel

INTRODUCTION

Acute heart failure is a complex syndrome. Despite major advances in heart failure (HF) therapy, challenges still remain in the timely diagnosis of acute heart failure (AHF). This is due to the blurred lines between pulmonary and cardiac causes of acute dyspnea, which can lead to delayed or erroneous diagnosis for AHF, longer hospital stay, greater healthcare costs, higher morbidity, and mortality. For these reasons, biomarkers are used for rapid and accurate diagnoses of patients with acute dyspnea.

Today, natriuretic peptides are the most validated biomarkers in AHF diagnosis. Relevant biomarkers in the natriuretic peptide family are B-type natriuretic peptide (BNP), N-terminal pro-B-type natriuretic peptide (NT-proBNP), atrial natriuretic peptide (ANP), and mid-region pro-atrial natriuretic peptide (MR-proANP). In this group, ANP is made in the atria and cardiac ventricles, while BNP is made predominantly in the cardiac ventricles. Atrial natriuretic peptide and BNP counteract the physiological abnormalities of AHF by increasing glomerular filtration rate, increasing sodium and water excretion, relaxing arterioles and venules, increasing diastolic relaxation, decreasing myocardial fibrosis, inhibiting cardiac hypertrophy, as well as inhibiting renin and aldosterone secretion. Of the four natriuretic peptides, BNP, and NT-proBNP are the most widely used in today's clinical practice (Table 1).

Since ANP and BNP are mostly produced by the left cardiac ventricle, elevations of natriuretic peptide concentrations correlate well with elevated pulmonary capillary wedge pressure (PCWP)

Algorithms in Heart Failure

TABLE 1: Characteristics of B-type natriuretic peptide and N-terminal prohormone B-type natriuretic peptide

	BNP	NT-proBNP
Components	BNP molecule	NT fragments (1–76) NT-proBNP (1–108)
Molecular weight	4 kD	8.5 kD
Genesis	Cleavage from NT-proBNP	Release from ventricular myocytes
Half-life	20 min	120 min
Clearance mechanism	Neutral endopeptidase clearance receptors	Renal clearance
Increase with normal aging	+	++++
Correlation with estimated glomerular filtration rate	−0.20	−0.60
Approved cutoff(s) for CHF diagnosis	100 pg/mL	Age <75: 125 pg/mL Age >75: 450 pg/mL
Studies completed	1,370	39
Entry on US market	November, 2000	December, 2002

B-type natriuretic peptide; NT-proBNP, N-terminal of the prohormone brain natriuretic peptide; CHF, congestive heart failure.

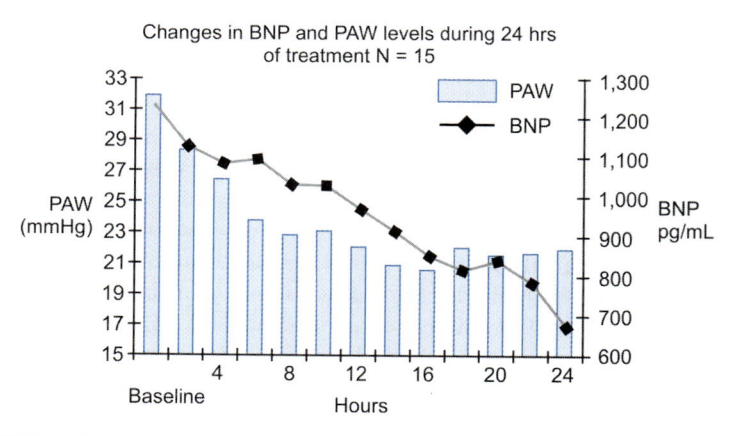

FIG. 1: Correlation between B-type natriuretic peptide and pulmonary artery wedge pressure

and increased left ventricular wall stress. This is seen in patients with severe aortic stenosis pre- and postaortic valve replacement, and in HF patients (Fig. 1). Increased ventricular wall stress leads to increased production of ANP and BNP by ventricular myocytes, typically in patients with hypertrophic cardiomyopathy. This correlation is the premise for using natriuretic peptide to diagnose for AHF in patients.

B-TYPE NATRIURETIC PEPTIDE: THE EVIDENCE

In 2002, the multicenter Breathing Not Properly trial demonstrated the effectiveness of BNP in the diagnosis of patients presenting to the emergency department (ED) with acute dyspnea. Patients with AHF had BNP levels of 675 ± 450 pg/mL, while patients without AHF had BNP levels of 110 ± 225 pg/mL. B-type natriuretic peptide was the single best predictor of AHF with an area under the receiver operating characteristic curve (AUC) of 0.91 (95% confidence interval: 0.90–0.93, $p < 0.001$). A BNP cutoff of 100 pg/mL had a sensitivity of 90%, specificity of 75%, and diagnostic accuracy of 83%. B-type natriuretic peptide levels <50 pg/mL were associated with a negative predictive value (NPV) of 96%. In multiple logistic regression analysis, BNP >100 pg/mL was the strongest independent predictor of AHF with an odds ratio of 29.6.

N-TERMINAL PRO-B-TYPE NATRIURETIC PEPTIDE: THE EVIDENCE

The proBNP Investigation of Dyspnea in the Emergency Department (PRIDE) study, similar to the BNP trial, was intended to evaluate the diagnostic power of NT-proBNP. The average NT-proBNP level in AHF patients was 4,054 pg/mL (AUC 0.94, $p < 0.0001$), while the average NT-proBNP level in patients without AHF was 131 pg/mL. Patients less than 50 years of age had an NT-proBNP cutoff of 450 pg/mL (sensitivity of 93%, specificity of 95%, diagnostic accuracy 95% for AHF). Patients more than 50 years of age, had an NT-proBNP cutoff of 900 pg/mL (sensitivity 91%, specificity 80%, diagnostic accuracy of 85% for AHF). In general, a concentration less than 300 pg/mL had a sensitivity of 99% and NPV of 99%. By multivariate analysis, NT-proBNP was the strongest predictor of AHF with an odds ratio of 44.0 ($p < 0.0001$) and was better than clinician estimated likelihood for the diagnosis of AHF (AUC = 0.94 vs. AUC = 0.90). Adding NT-proBNP to clinician estimated likelihood of AHF improved the AUC from 0.90 to 0.96. Different optimal cutpoints of NT-proBNP were analyzed among patients with the physician estimated AHF likelihood of 0–25% (sensitivity

96%, specificity 88% for AHF), 25–75% (sensitivity 93%, specificity 85% for AHF), more than 75% (sensitivity 93%, specificity 84% for AHF). Overall, NT-proBNP is a significant predictor of AHF.

ATRIAL NATRIURETIC PEPTIDE AND MID-REGION PRO-ATRIAL NATRIURETIC PEPTIDE: THE EVIDENCE

Although elevations of both BNP and ANP have been associated with AHF, ANP is inferior to BNP. Cowie et al. illustrated this difference between BNP [AUC 0.96, sensitivity 97%, specificity 84%, positive predictive value (PPV) 70%] and ANP (AUC 0.93, sensitivity 97%, specificity 72%, PPV 55%). The suboptimal result for ANP was due in part to its rapid clearance, thus limiting ANP's clinical application.

In comparison to ANP, mid-region (MR)-proANP is a much more stable and degradation resistant molecule. The diagnostic utility of MR-proANP in AHF was demonstrated in the Biomarker in Acute Heart Failure (BACH) trial. Midregional-proANP at cut point of 120 pmol/L (sensitivity 97%, specificity 59.9%, diagnostic accuracy 72.7%, PPV 56%, NPV 97.4) was superior to BNP at 100 pg/mL (sensitivity 95.6%, specificity 61.9%, diagnostic accuracy 73.6%, PPV 57%, NPV 96.4%) (Table 2). Furthermore, elevated MR-proANP added significantly to elevated BNP, increasing the C-statistic from 0.787 to 0.816 (p <0.001). When both MR-proANP and BNP were elevated, the overall diagnostic accuracy increased from 73.6% for BNP alone to 76.6%. In patients with intermediate BNP levels and obesity, MR-proANP added incremental predictive value to BNP for the prediction of AHF. In patients with intermediate NT-proBNP levels, renal insufficiency (creatinine >1.6 mg/dL), obesity, age more than 70, and edema, MR-proANP also added incremental predictive

TABLE 2: Mid-region pro-atrial natriuretic peptide (MR-proANP) versus B-type natriuretic peptide for diagnosis of acute heart failure in the Biomarkers in Acute Heart Failure trial

Measure	Sensitivity	Specificity	Accuracy
MR-proANP 120 pmol/L	95.56	59.85	72.64
BNP 100 pg/mL	96.98	61.90	73.50
Difference	1.42	2.05	0.86
Upper 95% limit	2.82	3.84	2.10
Noninferiority p	<0.0001	<0.0001	<0.0001

MR-proANP, mid-region pro-atrial natriuretic peptide; BNP, B-type natriuretic peptide.

Using Natriuretic Peptides in the Emergency Department

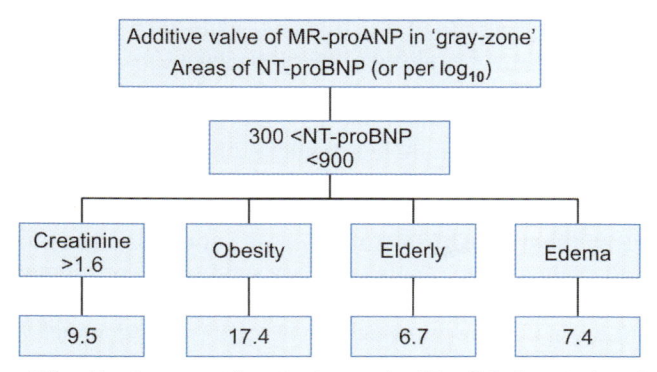

```
┌─────────────────────────────────────────┐
│ Additive value of MR-proANP in 'gray-zone' │
│ Areas of NT-proBNP (or per log₁₀)       │
└─────────────────────────────────────────┘
              │
    ┌─────────────────┐
    │ 300 <NT-proBNP  │
    │     <900        │
    └─────────────────┘
     │       │       │       │
 ┌───────┐ ┌──────┐ ┌──────┐ ┌──────┐
 │Creat. │ │Obesi-│ │Elder-│ │Edema │
 │>1.6   │ │ty    │ │ly    │ │      │
 └───────┘ └──────┘ └──────┘ └──────┘
     │       │       │       │
   ┌───┐   ┌────┐  ┌───┐   ┌───┐
   │9.5│   │17.4│  │6.7│   │7.4│
   └───┘   └────┘  └───┘   └───┘
```

MR-proANP, mid-region pro-atrial natriuretic peptide; NT-proBNP, N-terminal pro-B-type natriuretic peptide.

ALGORITHM 1: Incremental predictive value of adding mid-region pro-atrial natriuretic peptide to gray zone N-terminal pro-B-type natriuretic peptide for the diagnosis of acute heart failure

value to NT-proBNP for the prediction of AHF (Algorithm 1). In the subgroup of patients where the ED physicians were uncertain of the diagnosis, defined as 20–80% probability of AHF on a visual analog scale, the addition of MR-proANP reduced indecision by 29%.

USING NATRIURETIC PEPTIDES IN THE EMERGENCY DEPARTMENT

We propose the following algorithm in conjunction with history and physical examination for diagnostic evaluation. Patients with BNP levels less than 100 pg/mL or NT-proBNP less than 300 pg/mL would less likely have AHF (<2% likelihood). These patients should then be further evaluated for an alternative etiology for their acute dyspnea. In patients with acute dyspnea and BNP levels more than 500 pg/mL or NT-proBNP levels above an age dependent cutoff (>450 pg/mL in patients <50 years old or >900 pg/mL in patients 50–75 years of age, or >1,800 pg/mL in patients >75 years of age), AHF is very likely (>95% likelihood).

Acute heart failure therapy should be initiated immediately with diuretics to reduce the intravascular volume and left ventricular preload. If the patient has no cardiogenic shock, vasodilators can be added when hypertensive. Inotropes can also be considered in these patients if they need aid in diuresis. In patients with cardiogenic shock, both inotrope and vasodilators may be necessary to improve cardiac output by increasing contractility and decreasing afterload. For patients with natriuretic peptide levels in the gray zone (all ages: BNP 100–500 pg/mL; age >50: NT-proBNP 300–450 pg/mL; ages 50–75: NT-proBNP 300–900 pg/mL; age >75: NT-proBNP 300–1,800 pg/mL), history of HF, and left ventricular dysfunction, AHF is highly probable (90% likelihood). Consequently, these patients should receive empiric treatment for AHF with diuretics and vasodilators as needed and observed closely. If there is no history of HF or left ventricular dysfunction, then an evaluation for acute coronary syndrome, cor pulmonale, or acute pulmonary embolism should be considered and treated accordingly. If there is evidence of other cardiac issues, then the gray zone natriuretic peptide levels are unlikely to represent AHF (<25% likelihood), as these patients usually have higher natriuretic peptide levels during AHF. These patients should be closely observed and evaluated for an alternative diagnosis. In inconclusive patients, gray zone natriuretic peptide levels may still represent AHF (>75% likelihood) and therapy should be initiated (Algorithm 2).

Although not widely available, MR-proANP can also be used for the diagnostic evaluation of patients with acute dyspnea. Patients with MR-proANP levels less than 120 pg/mL are unlikely to have AHF. Patients with MR-proANP levels more than 600 pg/mL are very highly to have AHF. The gray zone for MR-proANP is 120–600 pg/mL. When available, MR-proANP levels should be measured in patients with BNP or NT-proBNP levels in the diagnostic gray zone to increase the diagnostic accuracy of natriuretic peptides in patients with obesity (intermediate BNP levels), renal insufficiency (intermediate NT-proBNP levels), and advanced age (intermediate NT-proBNP levels) (Algorithm 1).

In patients with chronic HF, diagnosing AHF using natriuretic peptides can be intricate. Patients with preexisting HF can have significantly elevated natriuretic peptide levels at baseline owing to chronically elevated PCWP from severe underlying HF and renal dysfunction. Thus, it is not unusual to see BNP levels more than 500 pg/mL and NT-proBNP levels more than 1,800 pg/mL in patients with existing HF who do not have AHF. In these patients, it would be very helpful to know their optivolemic or "dry" natriuretic peptide levels when they are clinically euvolemic. If their presenting natriuretic peptide levels are elevated more than 50% from baseline, then AHF is likely. Empiric therapy for AHF should be implemented as soon as possible. However, if their presenting natriuretic peptides levels are not elevated more than 50% from baseline, then AHF is unlikely. These patients should be observed (Algorithm 3).

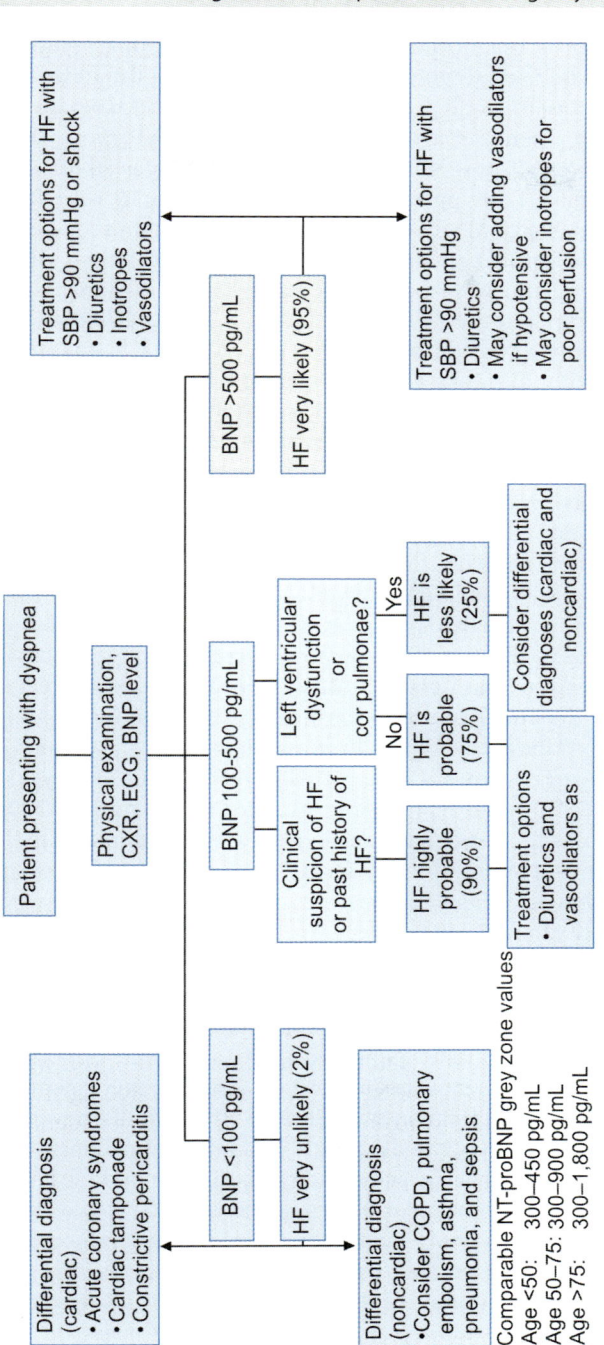

Using Natriuretic Peptides in the Emergency Department

Patient presenting with dyspnea
↓
Physical examination, CXR, ECG, BNP level

BNP <100 pg/mL → **HF very unlikely (2%)**

Differential diagnosis (cardiac)
- Acute coronary syndromes
- Cardiac tamponade
- Constrictive pericarditis

Differential diagnosis (noncardiac)
- Consider COPD, pulmonary embolism, asthma, pneumonia, and sepsis

Comparable NT-proBNP grey zone values
Age <50:   300–450 pg/mL
Age 50–75: 300–900 pg/mL
Age >75:   300–1,800 pg/mL

BNP 100–500 pg/mL

- Clinical suspicion of HF or past history of HF?
  - HF highly probable (90%)
  - Treatment options
    - Diuretics and vasodilators as

- Left ventricular dysfunction or cor pulmonae?
  - No → HF is probable (75%)
  - Yes → HF is less likely (25%)
  - Consider differential diagnoses (cardiac and noncardiac)

BNP >500 pg/mL → **HF very likely (95%)**

Treatment options for HF with SBP >90 mmHg or shock
- Diuretics
- Inotropes
- Vasodilators

Treatment options for HF with SBP >90 mmHg
- Diuretics
- May consider adding vasodilators if hypotensive
- May consider inotropes for poor perfusion

CXR, chest X-ray; BNP, B-type natriuretic peptide; ECG, electrocardiogram; HF, heart failure;; COPD, chronic obstructive pulmonary disease; systolic blood pressure.

ALGORITHM 2: Algorithm on using B-type natriuretic peptide and N-terminal B-type natriuretic peptide (NT-proBNP) levels to rule in and rule out acute heart failure.

Once AHF is diagnosed, serial measurements of natriuretic peptide can be used to guide therapy. We propose the following algorithm for natriuretic peptide guided therapy in AHF patients in the ED. In patients age less than 50 with BNP more than 1,000 pg/mL or NT-proBNP less than 900 pg/mL, ages 50–75 with BNP more than 1,800 pg/mL, and age more than 75 with BNP more than 3,600 pg/mL, the AHF is likely severe and these patients would benefit from inpatient therapy. However, if the patient's BNP is 500–1,000 pg/mL or NT-proBNP between 300 pg/mL and an age dependent upper limit (>900 pg/mL for age <50, >1,800 pg/mL for ages 50–75, and >3,600 pg/mL for age >75), an intensive treatment approach with diuretics and vasodilators in the ED can be considered. Meanwhile, natriuretic peptide levels should be checked every 3 hours. If the patient experiences improvement and a reduction in natriuretic peptide levels, then they can be discharged with close outpatient follow-up. Conversely, if the patient does not experience any improvement and stable natriuretic peptide levels, then the patient should be admitted for further therapy. For patients with known HF presenting with acute dyspnea and natriuretic peptide levels 50% higher than baseline, inpatient therapy is often necessary, especially if their presenting BNP level is more than 1,000 pg/mL or NT-proBNP level is greater than an age-dependent cutoff (>900 for age <50, >1,800 for ages 50–75, and >3,600 for age >75). Finally, for patients with gray zone NP levels (BNP 100–500 pg/mL, age <50: NT-proBNP 300–450 pg/mL, ages 50–75: NT-proBNP 300–900 pg/mL, age >75: NT-proBNP 300–1,800 pg/mL) who do not have an alternative explanation for their acute dyspnea, empiric therapy for AHF should be attempted in the ED. If they experience improvement in their symptoms with empiric AHF therapy, then they can be discharged with close outpatient follow-up and further evaluation for HF. If they do not experience improvement in their symptoms, then they should be admitted for continued observation and evaluation (Algorithm 3).

When using natriuretic peptides, there are some important caveats that clinicians must keep in mind. First, natriuretic peptide elevations are not pathognomonic for AHF. They should never be used in isolation during the diagnostic evaluation of patients with acute dyspnea. As shown by prior studies, natriuretic peptide levels can increase due to variety of other reasons such as age, weight, gender, renal dysfunction, and other cardiac and noncardiac ailments. Another aspect of natriuretic peptide levels that the clinician must keep in mind is that although there is a correlation between PCWP and natriuretic peptide levels, NP levels do not

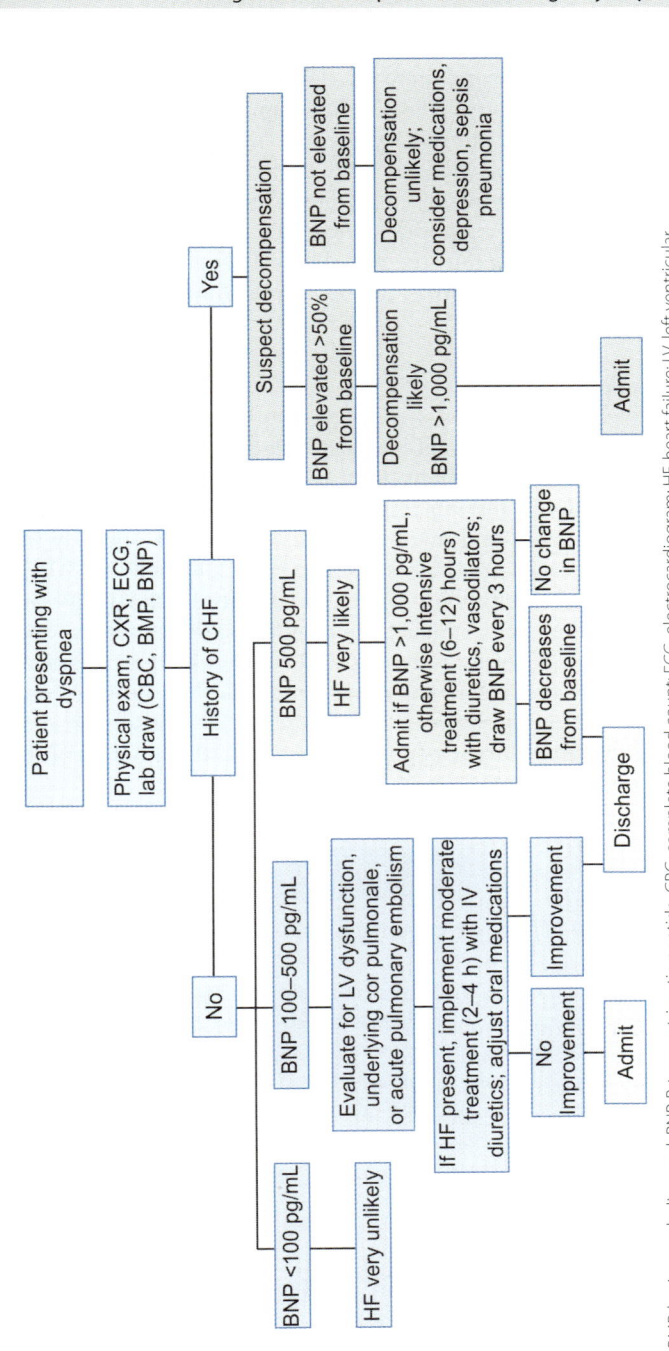

Using Natriuretic Peptides in the Emergency Department

```
Patient presenting with dyspnea
        │
Physical exam, CXR, ECG,
lab draw (CBC, BMP, BNP)
        │
   History of CHF
    ┌───┴───┐
   No      Yes
                │
         Suspect decompensation
         ┌──────────────┴──────────────┐
   BNP elevated >50%           BNP not elevated
   from baseline               from baseline
         │                           │
   Decompensation              Decompensation
   likely                      unlikely;
   BNP >1,000 pg/mL            consider medications,
         │                     depression, sepsis
       Admit                   pneumonia
```

No branch:
- BNP <100 pg/mL → HF very unlikely
- BNP 100–500 pg/mL → Evaluate for LV dysfunction, underlying cor pulmonale, or acute pulmonary embolism
  - If HF present, implement moderate treatment (2–4 h) with IV diuretics; adjust oral medications
    - No Improvement → Admit
    - Improvement → Discharge
- BNP 500 pg/mL → HF very likely
  - Admit if BNP >1,000 pg/mL, otherwise Intensive treatment (6–12 hours) with diuretics, vasodilators; draw BNP every 3 hours
    - BNP decreases from baseline → Discharge
    - No change in BNP

BMP, basic metabolic panel; BNP, B-type natriuretic peptide; CBC, complete blood count; ECG, electrocardiogram; HF, heart failure; LV, left ventricular.

ALGORITHM 3: Algorithm for the management of heart failure in an emergency department setting

change "instantaneously". In situations of acute increases in left ventricular filling pressure, there is a delay in the rise of NPs as the intracellular production of NPs is ramped up. Thus, in patients with clear evidence of flash pulmonary edema, a low natriuretic peptide level cannot be used to rule out AHF. Lastly, not all HF is caused by increases in left ventricular filling pressures. Conditions such as mitral stenosis and constrictive pericarditis can cause significant HF symptoms without causing elevations of left ventricular filling pressures. Thus, the natriuretic peptide levels may be low in these cases.

CONCLUSION

Natriuretic peptides with their low cost, objectivity, reproducibility, and accessibility are excellent adjuncts to physical examination, standard laboratory, and imaging studies in diagnosing both acute systolic heart failure and acute diastolic heart failure quickly in the ED. Besides having a high sensitivity and specificity for AHF, they have high discriminatory power in cases where the diagnosis is indeterminate. Additionally, natriuretic peptide assays are fast and reliable, thereby reducing ED evaluation time, hospital admission rates, hospital length of stay, and overall healthcare cost without increasing mortality or morbidity. Hence, we suggest the incorporation of natriuretic peptide to the standard evaluation of all patients presenting to the ED with acute dyspnea.

KEY POINTS

- Acute heart failure is a common diagnosis among hospitalized patients
- Although acute dyspnea is a common presenting symptom among patients with AHF, differentiating between patients with pulmonary diagnosis and AHF remains a challenge
- Natriuretic peptides are highly effective in assisting the diagnostic evaluation of patients with AHF in the emergency department
- Natriuretic peptide help not only in increasing the diagnostic accuracy of AHF and also decrease diagnostic uncertainty in the emergency department (ED)
- They can also decrease ED and hospital length of stay without increasing risk for adverse outcomes
- Furthermore, level of natriuretic peptides can be used to guide therapy for AHF patients in the ED.

SUGGESTED READINGS

1. Cowie MR, Struthers AD, Wood DA, Coats AJ, Thompson SG, Poole-Wilson PA, et al. Value of natriuretic peptides in assessment of patients with possible new heart failure in primary care. Lancet. 1997;350(9088):1349-53.
2. Haug C, Metzele A, Kochs M, V Hombach, Adolf Gruenert. Plasma brain natriuretic peptide concentrations correlate with left ventricular end-diastolic pressure. Clin. Cardiol. 1993;16(7):553-7.
3. Ikeda T, Matsuda K, Itoh H, Shirakami G, Miyamoto Y, Yoshimasa T, et al. Plasma levels of brain and atrial natriuretic peptides elevate in proportion to left ventricular end-systolic wall stress in patients with aortic stenosis. Am Heart J. 1997;133:307-14.
4. Januzzi JL, Camargo CA, Anwaruddin S, Baggish AL, Chen AA, Krauser DG, et al. The N-terminal Pro-BNP investigation of dyspnea in the emergency department (PRIDE) study. Am J Cardiol. 2005;95(8):948-54.
5. Kazanegra R, Cheng V, Garcia A, Krishnaswamy P, Gardetto N, Clopton P, et al. A rapid test for B-type natriuretic peptide correlates with falling wedge pressures in patients treated for decompensated heart failure: a pilot study. J Card Fail. 2001;7(1):21-9.
6. Lang CC, Choy AM, Turner K, Tobin R, Coutie W, Struthers AD. The effect of intravenous saline loading on plasma levels of brain natriuretic peptide in man. J Hypertens. 1993;11(7):737-41.
7. Maisel A, Mueller C, Nowak R, W. Frank Peacock, Judd W. Landsberg, Piotr Ponikowski, et al. Mid-region pro-hormone markers for diagnosis and prognosis in acute dyspnea: results from the BACH (Biomarkers in Acute Heart Failure) trial. J Am Coll Cardiol. 2010;55(19):2062-76.
8. Massie B, Ports T, Chatterjee K, Parmley W, Ostland J, O'Young J, et al. Long-term vasodilator therapy for heart failure: clinical response and its relationship to hemodynamic measurements, Circulation. 1981;63(2):269-78.
9. Yasue H, Yoshimura M, Sumida H, Kikuta K, Kugiyama K, Jougasaki M, et al. Localization and mechanism of secretion of B-type natriuretic peptide in comparison with those of A-type natriuretic peptide in normal subjects and patients with heart failure. Circulation. 1994;90(1):195-203.
10. Yoshimura M, Yasue H, Okumura K, Ogawa H, Jougasaki M, Mukoyama M, et al. Different secretion patterns of atrial natriuretic peptide and brain natriuretic peptide in patients with congestive heart failure. Circulation. 1993;87(2):464-9.

4
CHAPTER

Role of Ultrasound in the Management of Acute Heart Failure

Luna Gargani

INTRODUCTION

Ultrasound is the imaging technique of choice in emergencies, since it is readily and widely available at the bedside, providing noninvasively crucial information for the management of patients. Transthoracic echocardiography is the most commonly used sonographic examination in patients with acute heart failure (AHF), offering immediate and comprehensive assessment of cardiovascular morphology, function, and hemodynamics, with minimal discomfort or risk for the patient, without using contrast material or ionizing radiation.

Echocardiography in AHF can be useful at all stages of patient's in hospital management: immediately at admission, for in hospital follow-up, and at discharge.

AT ADMISSION

The main aim of echocardiography in patients admitted for AHF is to identify the cause of decompensation. The main parameters that should be assessed are shown in algorithm 1.

Left Ventricular Systolic Function

Main questions:
- Is left ventricular systolic function normal or reduced?
- What is the severity of left ventricular systolic dysfunction?
- Has the left ventricular systolic function changed from a previous exam?

Role of Ultrasound in the Management of Acute Heart Failure

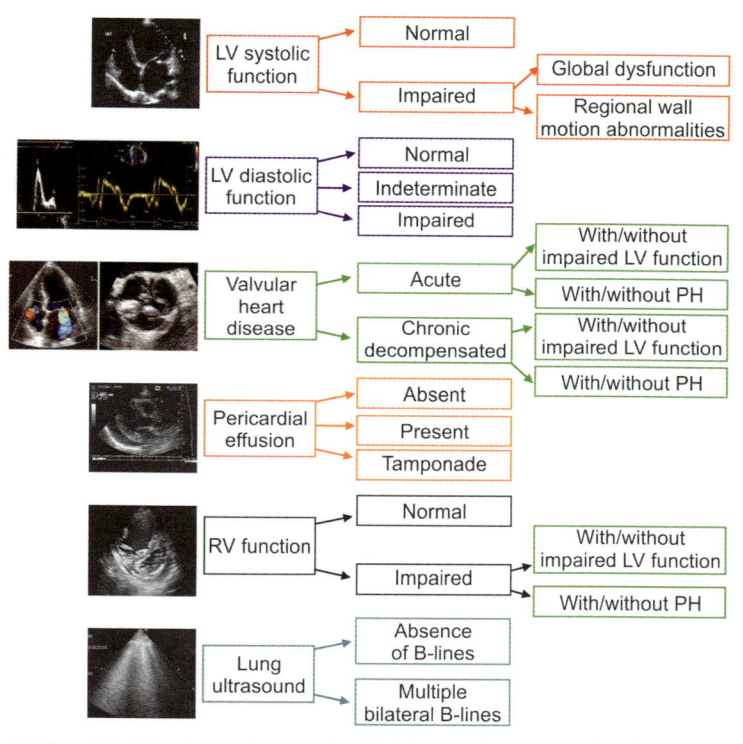

Algorithm flowchart:

- LV systolic function → Normal / Impaired → Global dysfunction / Regional wall motion abnormalities
- LV diastolic function → Normal / Indeterminate / Impaired
- Valvular heart disease → Acute (With/without impaired LV function; With/without PH) / Chronic decompensated (With/without impaired LV function; With/without PH)
- Pericardial effusion → Absent / Present / Tamponade
- RV function → Normal / Impaired (With/without impaired LV function; With/without PH)
- Lung ultrasound → Absence of B-lines / Multiple bilateral B-lines

LV, left ventricle; PH, pulmonary hypertension; RV, right ventricle; AHF, acute heart failure.

ALGORITHM: Schematic overview of the main echocardiographic parameters to evaluate in acute heart failure patients at admission

- Is it a global left ventricular systolic dysfunction or a localized wall motion abnormality (suggesting an acute coronary syndrome underlying AHF)?

Echocardiographic features of systolic heart failure include:
- A reduced LV ejection fraction (EF <45-50%)
- Dilatation of the left ventricular
- Diffuse or regional wall motion abnormalities
- Functional mitral and/or tricuspid regurgitation
- Low cardiac output.

Left Ventricular Diastolic Function

Noninvasive assessment of left ventricular diastolic function at admission is relevant especially for patients with severe symptoms and inconclusive clinical, radiographic, and biochemical data, with preserved LV ejection fraction and without a clear evident cause of decompensation. In these patients, heart failure with preserved ejection fraction (HFpEF) may be the diagnosis.

- In patients with depressed left ventricular systolic function, the mitral inflow pattern by itself can be used to estimate filling pressures with reasonable accuracy
- In patients with normal EF, as in HFpEF, E/e' ratio obtained by tissue Doppler imaging (TDI) should be calculated (mean value between septal and lateral e'). An average ratio less than or equal to 8 identifies patients with normal left ventricular filling pressures, whereas a ratio more than or equal to 13 indicates increased left ventricular filling pressures. When the ratio is between 9 and 13, other parameters are necessary, such as left atrial indexed volume less than or equal to 34 mL/m^2, Ar-A duration ≥30 ms, pulmonary artery systolic pressure more than 35 mmHg (in the absence of pulmonary disease).

Limitations

- E/e' allows only a semiquantitative assessment of left ventricular filling pressures
- E/e' is not accurate as an index of left ventricular filling pressures in patients with heavy annular calcification, surgical rings, mitral valve disease, basal left ventricular wall motion abnormalities related to left bundle branch block, paced-rhythm, myocardial infarction, cardiopulmonary bypass, and constrictive pericarditis.
- Absence of signs of diastolic disfunction on echocardiography dose not rule out the diagnosis of HFpEF.

Hemodynamics

A noninvasive hemodynamic assessment may be valuable in those AHF patients in whom the physical examination is discordant with symptoms, and can be used to monitor the patients after institution of appropriate therapy.

Useful noninvasive hemodynamic variables are:

- Stroke volume (SV) and cardiac output (CO) by pulsed-wave (PW) Doppler of the left ventricular outflow tract (LVOT)

$$SV = 0.785 \times Diameter_{(LVOT)}^2 \times VTI_{(LVOT)}$$

When serial measurements of SV and CO are performed, the baseline annulus measurement can be used for the repeated studies.

- Pulmonary capillary wedge pressure (PCWP) by the following regression equation:

$$PCWP = [1.24 \times (E/e')] + 1.9$$

- Right ventricular systolic pressure (RVSP), right atrial pressure (RAP) and pulmonary artery systolic pressures (PASP) from tricuspid valve velocity and inferior vena cava dimension and collapsibility

$$RVSP = 4 \times \text{maximum tricuspidal velocity}^2 \text{ (m/s)}$$

Right atrial pressure can be estimated from the end-expiratory diameter and respiratory changes of the inferior vena cava (IVC)

$$PASP = RVSP + RAP$$

Pericardial Effusion

Pericardial effusion can be visible as an echo-free space. When the effusion is big, the echo-free space extends circumferentially around the heart, and its size depends on the amount of fluid in the pericardial sac.

Echocardiography is crucial to:
- Differentiate between pericardial effusion and pericardial fat
- Differentiate between pericardial and pleural effusion
- Assess hemodynamic variations in clinical suspicion of cardiac tamponade
- Guide pericardiocentesis.

Valvular Dysfunction

Valvular dysfunction can be a cause and a consequence of AHF.
- Acute valvular heart disease can be the cause of AHF in a previously healthy patient (e.g., chordal rupture)
- Chronic valvular heart disease can be the cause of AHF in case of decompensation
- Valvular heart disease can be the consequence of AHF, when functional mitral or tricuspidal regurgitation occur in the setting of dilated cardiomyopathy or ischemic cardiac disease.

Acute Mitral Regurgitation

Main questions:
- Is mitral regurgitation (MR) severe?
- Is MR organic or functional?
- Is it acute MR or chronic decompensated MR?
- What is the cause of MR?
- Is MR amenable to surgical intervention?

- How urgent is surgical repair or replacement?

Most frequent causes of acute MR are:
- Ischemic MR due to rupture of a papillary muscle
- Ischemic MR due to regional left ventricular dysfunction with abnormal contraction of papillary muscle or underlying ventricular wall
- Spontaneous chordal rupture
- Infective endocarditis
- Blunt chest trauma
- Prosthetic valve dysfunction.

Color flow imaging: although not highly accurate (since the color flow display depends on many technical and hemodynamic factors), it is the most common technique to assess MR severity.

When feasible, the measurement of the *vena contracta*—the narrowest region of the regurgitant jet—is recommended to quantify MR.

The flow convergence method by evaluation of the proximal isovelocity surface area is up-to-date the most accurate sonographic approach to evaluate the severity of MR. Although it will not always be feasible in emergencies, it is recommended especially in those patients where MR is not clearly severe.

Transesophageal echocardiography should be performed, if mitral valve morphology and regurgitant severity are still in question after transthoracic echocardiography. It can also be helpful in demonstrating the anatomic cause of acute severe MR and directing successful surgical repair.

Acute Aortic Regurgitation

Similar to MR, when assessing aortic regurgitation (AR) in a patient with AHF, it is crucial to provide answers to the following key questions:
- Is AR severe?
- Is AR organic or consequent to aortic root dilation?
- Is it acute AR or chronic decompensated AR?
- What is the cause of AR?
- Is AR amenable to surgical intervention?
- How urgent is surgical intervention?

Most frequent causes of acute AR are:
- Infective endocarditis
- Blunt chest trauma
- Aortic root dissection, which is a surgical emergency
- Prosthetic valve dysfunction.

Color flow doppler provides a qualitative approach to evaluate AR severity. The color jet area is weakly correlated with the degree of AR, because it is affected by the aortic to left ventricular diastolic pressure gradient and left ventricular compliance.

The *vena contracta*—the smallest flow diameter at the level of the aortic valve in the LVOT —provides a semi-quantitative estimation of the size of the effective regurgitant orifice area (EROA).

Diastolic flow reversal in the descending aorta is a qualitative approach to diagnose severe AR. Significant holodiastolic reversal in the abdominal aorta is also a sensitive sign of severe AR.

The flow convergence method has been less extensively performed in AR than in MR. An EROA greater than or equal to 30 mm^2 or a regurgitant volume greater than or equal to 60 mL indicates severe AR.

The rate of deceleration of the diastolic AR jet and the derived pressure-half time (PHT) is related to the pressure difference between the aorta and the left ventricle during diastole. As the degree of AR increases, the aortic diastolic pressure decreases and the left ventricular end-diastolic pressure increases. A PHT less than 200 ms is consistent with severe AR.

Decompensated Chronic Valvular Heart Disease

Patients with chronic valvular heart disease may survive in a compensated phase for a long time, until a concomitant alteration of the cardiopulmonary homeostasis leads to rapid decompensation, such as in hypertensive crisis, sodium or volume overload, decreased compliance with medical therapy, anemia, exacerbation of chronic obstructive pulmonary disease, inflammation, or infection.

In decompensated chronic MR, the forward SV decreases and the LA pressure increases significantly. The presence of TR permits the estimation of PASP, which is generally high.

Decompensated chronic aortic stenosis (AS) is a frequent cause of AHF in the elderly population.

When left ventricular systolic dysfunction coexists with severe AS, the AS velocity and transaortic gradient may be low, despite a small valve area, a condition termed "low-flow low-gradient AS". In these patients, calculation of the stenotic orifice area or aortic valve area (AVA) is helpful because it is flow-independent. Aortic valve area can be calculated based on the continuity-equation, according to the following formula:

$$AVA = \frac{0.785 \times (\text{Diameter}_{LVOT})^2 \times VTI_{LVOT}}{VTI_{AV}}$$

A simplified approach to reducing error related to LVOT diameter measurements is the dimensionless ratio, that can be performed both by using VTI or jet maximum velocities.

$$\text{VTI ratio} = \frac{\text{VTI}_{\text{LVOT}}}{\text{VTI}_{\text{AV}}}$$

or

$$\text{Velocity ratio} = \frac{\text{Vel. max}_{\text{LVOT}}}{\text{Vel. max}_{\text{AV}}}$$

In the absence of valve stenosis, the ratio approaches 1, with smaller numbers indicating more severe stenosis. Severe stenosis is present when the ratio is 0.25 or less, corresponding to a valve area 25% of normal.

The Right Ventricle

When performing an echocardiogram to an AHF patient at admission, the right heart should always be addressed.
The questions to be answered are:
- Is the RV dilated and is RV systolic function normal?
- Is there a specific right heart abnormality?
- Is there pulmonary hypertension?

Functional tricuspid regurgitation is very frequent in patients with left ventricular dysfunction, and PASP values can be useful for hemodynamic monitoring of therapy. In case of abnormal RV function without evidence of left ventricular dysfunction or valvular heart disease in a patient admitted with shortness of breath, the suspicion of pulmonary embolism should be raised. In a patient with chest pain and suspected acute coronary syndrome, a dysfunctional RV can be concomitant to inferior ischemia/infarction. Arrhythmogenic right ventricular dysplasia is a rare cause of isolated RV dysfunction.

Techniques that can be employed at the bedside to evaluate right ventricular dysfunction include:
- Tricuspid annular plane systolic excursion
- Tricuspid systolic annular TDI velocity
- Right ventricular fractional area change (FAC) = (end-diastolic area – end-systolic area/end-diastolic area)

Pulmonary Congestion

In the last few years, lung ultrasound has been proposed for the evaluation of pulmonary congestion in patients with heart failure, through the assessment of B-lines, which are the sonographic sign of extravascular lung water. B-lines are useful for the differential diagnosis of cardiogenic versus noncardiogenic dyspnea. They could be a plausible alternative in acute settings when clinical findings are inconclusive, and natriuretic peptide analysis is not readily available or levels are in the "gray zone". Their negative predictive value to exclude the presence of pulmonary edema is particularly high. B-lines assessment can be performed with any type of echographic platform, including pocket size device. Convex or microconvex probes are more appropriate, but also cardiac and linear probes can be successfully employed.

In heart failure patients, lung ultrasonography may also enable the detection of pleural effusion. The effusion should firstly be sought in dependent zones. In presence of a radiopacity on chest X-ray, lung ultrasonography is able to better differentiate pleural effusion from atelectasis, consolidations, masses, or an elevated hemidiaphragm, and can be repeated serially at the bedside to detect the effusion, evaluate its extension, and indicate the appropriate area for an eventual thoracentesis.

CONCLUSION

Being readily available at the bedside, echocardiography is the imaging technique of choice in patients with AHF. The critical information about left and right ventricular morphology and function, valvular function, pericardium, noninvasive hemodynamics, and pulmonary interstitial edema or pleural effusion by lung ultrasound can be crucial to establish the correct etiology of the acute decompensation, to start appropriate treatment, to follow-up patients and to establish prognosis.

KEY POINTS

- Echocardiography is the single most useful diagnostic test in the evaluation of patients with heart failure, providing useful information at all stages of patient's management: immediately at admission, for in hospital follow-up and at discharge
- The main aim of echocardiography in patients admitted for AHF is to identify the cause of decompensation, establish its severity, and guide management
- Main parameters to be considered are systolic and diastolic function, valvular function, right ventricular function, noninvasive hemodynamics, pericardial and pleural effusion, and pulmonary congestion by lung ultrasound.

SUGGESTED READINGS

1. Baumgartner H, Hung J, Bermejo J, Chambers JB, Evangelista A, Griffin BP. EAE/ASE. Echocardiographic assessment of valve stenosis: EAE/ASE recommendations for clinical practice. J Am Soc Echocardiogr. 2009;22(1):1-23.
2. Bonow RO, Carabello BA, Chatterjee K, de Leon AC, Faxon DP, Freed MD. 2008 focused update incorporated into the ACC/AHA 2006 guidelines for the management of patients with valvular heart disease: a report of the American College of Cardiology/American Heart Association Task Force on Practice Guidelines (Writing Committee to revise the 1998 guidelines for the management of patients with valvular heart disease). Endorsed by the Society of Cardiovascular Anesthesiologists, Society for Cardiovascular Angiography and Interventions, and Society of Thoracic Surgeons. J Am Coll Cardiol. 2008;52(13):e1-142.
3. Galiuto L, Badano L, Fox K, Sicari R, Zamorano JL. The EAE Textbook of Echocardiography, 1st edition. Oxford University Press; 2011.
4. Gargani L, Volpicelli G. How I do it: lung ultrasound. Cardiovasc Ultrasound. 2014;12:25.
5. Jessup M, Abraham WT, Casey DE, Feldman AM, Francis GS, Ganiats TG, et al. 2009 focused update: ACCF/AHA Guidelines for the Diagnosis and Management of Heart Failure in Adults: a report of the American College of Cardiology Foundation/American Heart Association Task Force on Practice Guidelines: developed in collaboration with the International Society for Heart and Lung Transplantation. Circulation. 2009;119(14):1977-2016.
6. Lancellotti P, Moura L, Pierard LA, Agricola E, Popescu BA, Tribouilloy C, et al. European Association of Echocardiography recommendations for the assessment of valvular regurgitation. Part 2: mitral and tricuspid regurgitation (native valve disease). Eur J Echocardiogr. 2010;11(4):307-32
7. Lancellotti P, Tribouilloy C, Hagendorff A, Moura L, Popescu BA, Agricola E, et al. European Association of Echocardiography. European Association of Echocardiography recommendations for the assessment of valvular regurgitation. Part 1: aortic and pulmonary regurgitation (native valve disease). Eur J Echocardiogr. 2010;11(3):223-44.
8. Lang RM, Bierig M, Devereux RB, Flachskampf FA, Foster E, Pellikka PA, et al. Recommendations for chamber quantification: a report from the American Society of Echocardiography's Guidelines and Standards Committee and the Chamber Quantification Writing Group, developed in conjunction with the European Association of Echocardiography. J Am Soc Echocardiogr. 2005;18(12):1440-63.
9. Nagueh SF, Appleton CP, Gillebert TC, Marino PN, Oh JK, Smiseth OA, et al. Recommendations for the evaluation of left ventricular diastolic function by echocardiography. Eur J Echocardiogr. 2009;10(2):165-93.
10. Neskovic AN, Hagendorff A, Lancellotti P, Guarracino F, Varga A, Cosyns B, et al. Emergency echocardiography: the European Association of Cardiovascular Imaging. Emergency echocardiography. Eur Heart J Cardiovasc Imaging. 2013;14(1):1-11.
11. Rudski LG, Lai WW, Afilalo J, Hua L, Handschumacher MD, Chandrasekaran K, et al. Guidelines for the echocardiographic assessment of the right heart in adults: a report from the American Society of Echocardiography endorsed by the European Association of Echocardiography and the Canadian Society of Echocardiography. J Am Soc Echocardiogr. 2010;23(7):685-713.
12. Volpicelli G, Elbarbary M, Blaivas M, Lichtenstein DA, Mathis G, Kirkpatrick AW, et al. International evidence-based recommendations for point-of-care lung ultrasound. Intensive Care Med. 2012;38(4):577-91.

CHAPTER 5

Use of Bioelectrical Impedance Vector Analysis in the Dyspneic Patient

Salvatore Di Somma, Silvia Navarin

INTRODUCTION

The bioelectrical impedance vector analysis (BIVA) method measures in 30 seconds the opposition of body tissues to the flow of an alternating current of 300 µA, called bioelectrical impedance, administered by four surface electrodes at an operating frequency of 50 kHz. This bioelectrical impedance (Z) consists of two components—resistance (Rz) and reactance (Xc). While Rz is inversely related with the amount of total body water, the Xc is considered proportional to body mass. Fluids are good conductors so the length of Z vector, which represents body's impedance, is inversely related to fluid volume.

BIOELECTRICAL IMPEDANCE VECTOR ANALYSIS DEVICE

Bioelectrical impedance vector analysis device is handy and portable (Fig. 1).

Thus, it can be easily applied in every critical setting, because it does not require to be plugged, it can be carried at the patient's bedside, and its measurement results are immediately displayed on the monitor in two ways—as a vector or as a single number expressed in percentage, called hydration index (HI). The first method represents the bivariate vector with its two components (Rz and Xc), adjusted by the patient's height, in a monogram that is different for men and women. In the same coordinate system, three tolerance ellipses are plotted and they correspond to the 50th,

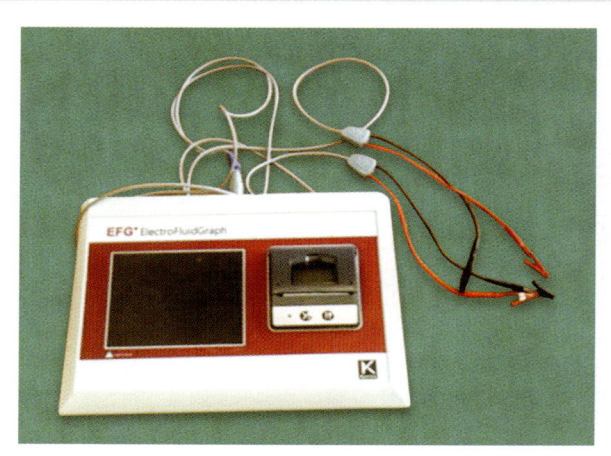

FIG. 1: Bioelectrical impedance vector analysis device

75th and 95th vector percentile of the healthy reference population. The major axis of this tolerance ellipses represents hydration status while the minor axis reflects tissue mass. In the second method, the 50th percentile corresponds to the values included in the range between 72.7 and 74.3%. Bioelectrical impedance vector analysis results are very accurate and easy, and rapid to be interpreted (Fig. 2).

Several studies have agreed on the delineation of the 75% tolerance ellipse as the boundary of normal tissue hydration. Consequently, vectors outside the upper pole of the 75% ellipse indicate dehydration, whereas vectors outside the lower pole of 75% confidence ellipse represent overhydration and shorter is the vector, more severe is the condition of fluid overload. Bioelectrical impedance vector analysis also allows to stratify the severity of both overhydration and dehydration subdividing these two classes into mild, moderate, or severe volume abnormalities (Fig. 2).

Due to its characteristics of manageability, cheapness, accuracy and velocity, and its ability to detect the change of the amount of body fluid in different kind of patients, the use of BIVA for assessing hydration status is spreading outside from its original application in the nephrology to all departments, and especially to the emergency settings, as intensive care unit and emergency department (ED), where total body fluid balance is essential (Algorithm 1). Bioelectrical impedance vector analysis showed to be able to easily monitor fluid loss, not only after hemodialysis or peritoneal dialysis but also after diuretic therapy, and fluid gain, due to renal impairment or heart failure. The lengthening of the

Use of Bioelectrical Impedance Vector Analysis in the Dyspneic Patient

Step 1: Patient

The human body is approximated as a sum of five interconnected cylinders that act as conductors in parallel. The subject must be supine and avoid skin contacts with the trunk or with the stretcher. Free fluid in thorax and abdomen, as pleural effusion, ascites and urine does not influence BIVA assessment

A bivariate vector (Rz and Xc), adjusted by the patient's height, in a nomogram that is different for men and women. The major axis of the tolerance ellipses represents hydration status while the minor axis reflects tissue mass

Step 2: Electrodes

Four cutaneous electrodes, two on the wrist and two on the ipsilateral ankle, are applied with an inter-electrodes distance of at least 5 cm to prevent electrodes interaction

Step 3: Results

A single number expressed in percentage in a scale, called hydrograph (or hydrogram). The 50th percentile corresponds to the values included in the range between 72.7% and 74.3%

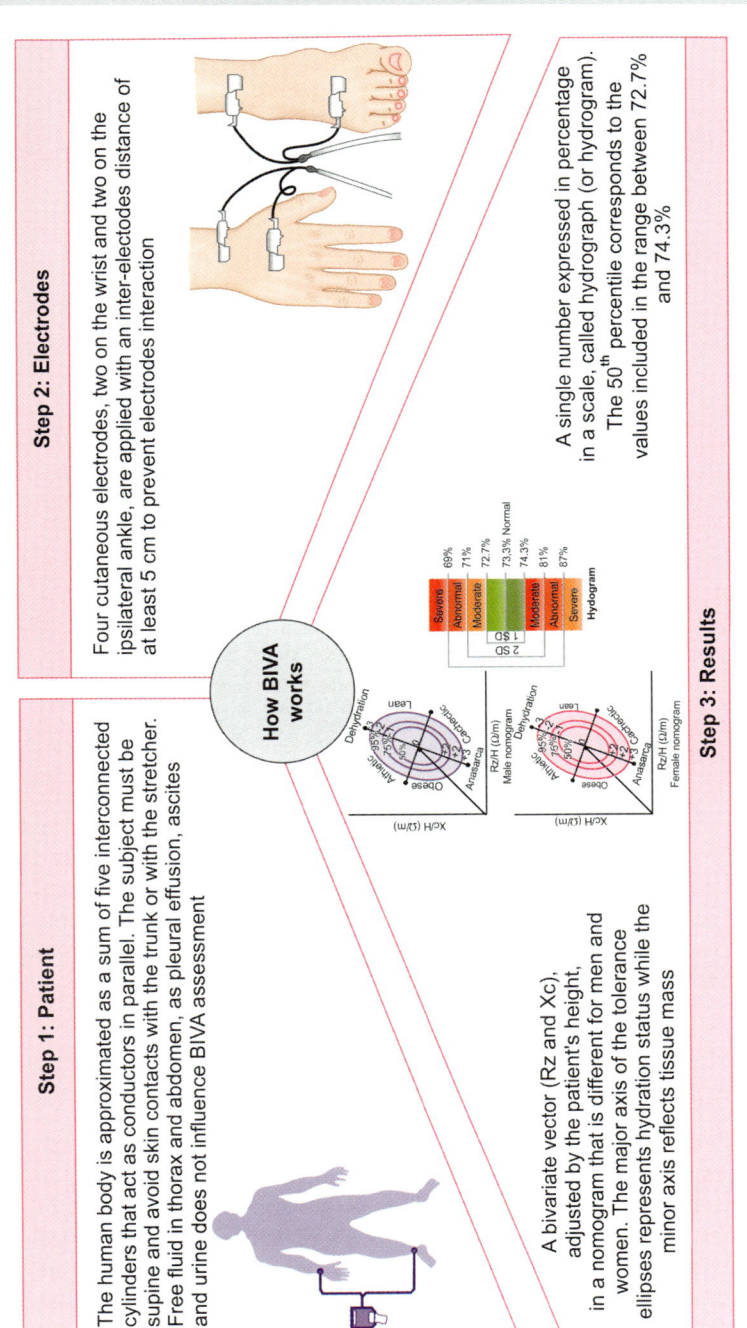

FIG. 2: Bioelectrical impedance vector analysis measurement and results

Algorithms in Heart Failure

Nephrology
BIVA technique proved to be able to detect the change of the amount of body fluid by the lengthening of the vector after hemodialysis and after peritoneal dialysis in chronic renal failure patients (p <0.001)

Intensive care unit	Emergency department
BIVA measurements were related to the CPV • CVP >12 mmHg → shorter BIVA vectors in 93% of patients, reflection overhydration • CVP >12 mmHg → longer vectors in 10% of patients, indicating dehydration • The progressive increase of CVP values was associated with shorter and down-sloping impedance vectors on the monogram	BIVA proved its diagnostic and predictive value in AHF • AHF patients had a significantly higher value of hydration status (77% ± 4) as compared with controls (73→ ± 2) • HI >80%→ events (death or rehospitalization) at 3 months after admission • BIVA confirmed its predictive value, independently from other variables • BIVA proved to be able to guide emergency physician's decisions about diuretic therapy, thus reducing renal complications

BIVA, bioelectrical impedance vector analysis; CVP, central venous pressure; AHF, acute heart failure; HI, hydration index.

ALGORITHM 1: Bioelectrical impedance vector analysis widespread application

vector reflects fluid loss, while its shortening reflects fluid gain. Furthermore, BIVA seems to have not only a diagnostic role but also a predictive value in dyspneic patients. For example, it was found a significant correlation of hydration values higher than 80% with events (death or rehospitalization) at 3 months after admission. Other trials confirmed BIVA predictive value, independently from other variables.

USE OF BIOELECTRICAL IMPEDANCE VECTOR ANALYSIS IN THE DYSPNEIC PATIENTS

All over the world dyspnea is one of the most frequent symptoms of admission in the ED and it is well known that dyspnea can hide severe, life-threatening, or fatal diseases and that the treatment must be started as soon as possible. By now, physicians classified dyspnea in cardiogenic or noncardiogenic on the basis of the "classical methods", such as physical examination and chest X-ray. Despite the growing, innovative, and advantageous introduction in the last years in the clinical practice of thoracic ultrasound (TUS) and of natriuretic peptides, dyspnea still represents a challenge for physicians in several conditions, especially because the population aging has led to an increase of comorbidities. Thoracic ultrasound identifies interstitial and/or alveolar edema by sonographic artifact, called B-lines or comet tails. These artifacts reflect a condition of congestion, typically caused by acute heart failure (AHF) and they thus allow to distinguish cardiogenic from noncardiogenic dyspnea. Natriuretic peptides, especially the 32 amino acids active hormone, called brain natriuretic peptide (BNP) and the 76 amino acids inactive form, named N-terminal proBNP (NT-proBNP), have already confirmed themselves as useful aids not only for dyspnea differential diagnosis but also for stratifying the risk in the ED, predicting death and rehospitalization, and guiding therapy. A cutoff value for BNP less than 100 pg/mL (and <400 pg/mL for NT-proBNP) is traditionally used to rule out cardiogenic dyspnea, whereas a cutoff value of BNP more than 400 pg/mL (NT-proBNP >2,000 pg/mL) to rule in. Values of BNP between 100 pg/mL and 400 pg/mL (or between 400 pg/mL and 2,000 pg/mL for NT-proBNP) represent the "gray zone", thus requiring further analysis. However, natriuretic peptides show their measurement limitations in certain conditions, including renal dysfunction, obesity, and atrial fibrillation. Moreover, it has been recently proposed an interesting differentiation of BNP levels in AHF patients into two components: a baseline value, called BNP dry, which reflect heart failure, and a BNP wet value that increases in acute decompensation and is related to volume or pressure overload.

Therefore, despite the unquestionable importance of clinical judgment and other classical methods, several international trials demonstrated their limitations. Typical signs of cardiogenic dyspnea, such as elevated jugular venous pressure, third heart sound, rales, and peripheral edema, are present in just few patients and chest X-ray is often nondiagnostic. In this complex scenario, it seems to be fundamental to resort to other innovative tools, as TUS, natriuretic peptides and BIVA. Their combined use, coupled with an accurate and essential physical examination, proved to overcome the limitations of each single method. For example, it was demonstrated that BIVA plays an important role in detecting BNP dichotomy between wet and dry and it was recently proved the additive diagnostic and prognostic role of HI obtained by BIVA measurements for AHF patients with BNP values in the gray zone. One more time, BIVA assessments, coupled with TUS, proved to improve the effectiveness in discriminating between

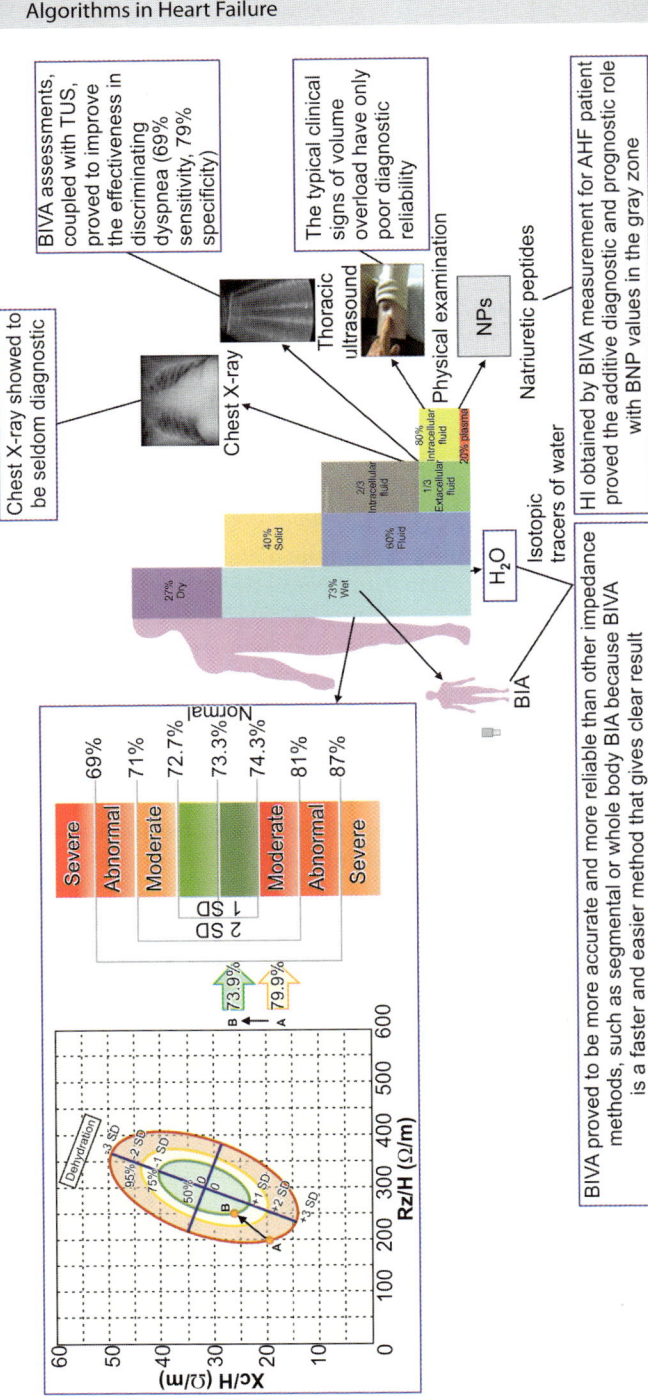

Algorithms in Heart Failure

FIG. 3: The additive value of bioelectrical impedance vector analysis, compared to other methods

BIVA, bioelectrical impedance vector analysis; BIA, bioimpedance analysis; TUS, thoracic ultrasound; AHF, acute heart failure; HI, hydration index; NP, natriuretic peptide; BNP, brain-type natriuretic peptide.

Use of Bioelectrical Impedance Vector Analysis in the Dyspneic Patient

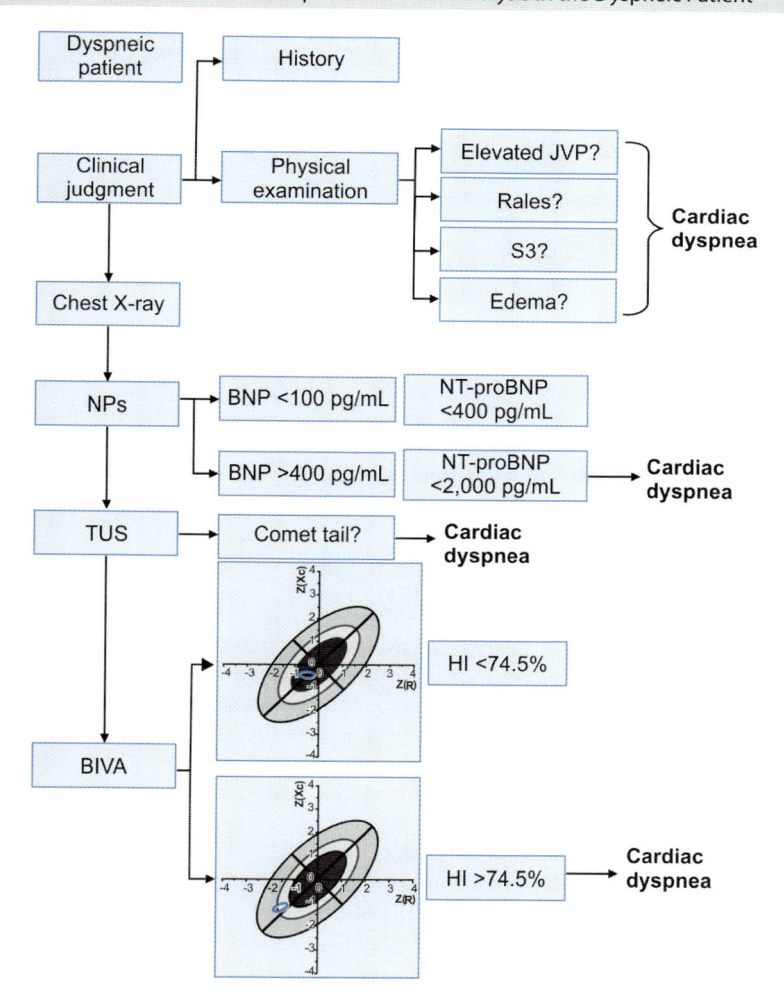

BIVA, bioelectrical impedance vector analysis; BNP, brain natriuretic peptide; HI, hydration index; JVP, jugular venous pressure; NPs, natriuretic peptides; TUS, thoracic ultrasound.

ALGORITHM 2: Diagnostic algorithm proposal for dyspneic patients

cardiogenic dyspnea and noncardiogenic dyspnea. Compared to other impedance methods, such as segmental or whole body bioimpedance analysis, BIVA showed to be more useful and reliable because it represents a faster, easier, and handier method that gives clear results (Algorithm 3).

Further trials and additional publications about BIVA measurements in patients with shortness of breath are required to standardize its diagnostic and prognostic role in the management of dyspneic patients. The combined use of classical and new methods, such as BIVA, natriuretic peptides, and TUS, could improve the management of patients with dyspnea in ED because their matched application could allow to assess different but complementary aspects of cardiogenic dyspnea (Algorithm 2).

CONCLUSION

Due to its characteristics, BIVA proved to be a promising device in different medical fields. It is handy, portable, easy-to-use, and accurate. BIVA alone is not the definitive answer to the challenge of dyspneic patients but it showed its unquestionable adding value in the early evaluation of patients with dyspnea.

KEY POINTS

- Bioelectrical impedance vector analysis (BIVA) technique has proved to be a promising method for the management of dyspneic patients, obviously in addition to the classical methods, such as clinical judgment and chest X-ray, and to the emerging tools, as natriuretic peptides and thoracic ultrasound
- Bioelectrical impedance vector analysis widespread availability is due to its favorable characteristics of accuracy, noninvasiveness, cheapness, velocity and manageability
- In patients with cardiogenic dyspnea BIVA vector is shorter and it is placed outside the lower pole of the 75% tolerance ellipse and the hydration index value is higher than 74.3%
- Bioelectrical impedance vector analysis demonstrated to be able to stratify the risk of dyspneic patients, to guide a proper therapy, and to avoid death or rehospitalization.

SUGGESTED READINGS

1. Di Somma S, De Berardinis B, Bongiovanni C, Marino R, Ferri E, Alfei B. Use of BNP and bioimpedance to drive therapy in heart failure patients. Congestive Heart Failure. 2010;Suppl 1:S56-S61.
2. Di Somma S, Lalle I, Magrini L, Russo V, Navarin S, Castello L, et al. Additive diagnostic and prognostic value of bioelectrical impedance vector analysis (BIVA) to brain natriuretic peptide 'grey-zone' in patients with acute heart failure in the emergency department. Eur Heart J Acute Cardiovasc Care. 2014;l3(2):167-75

3. Di Somma S, Navarin S, Giordano S, Spadini F, Lippi G, Cervellin G,et al. The emerging role of biomarkers and bio-impedance in evaluating hydration status in patients with acute heart failure. Clin Chem Lab Med. 2012;0(0):1-13.
4. Liteplo AS, Marill KA, Villen T, Miller RM, Murray AF, Croft PE, et al. Emergency thoracic ultrasound in the differentiation of the etiology of shortness of Breath (ETUDES): sonographic B-lines and N-terminal Pro-brain-type natriuretic peptide in diagnosing congestive heart failure. Acad Emerg Med. 2009;16:201-10.
5. Lukasky HC, Johnson PE, Bolonchuk WW. Assesment of fat-free mass using bioelectrical impedance measurements of human body. Am J Clin Nutr. 1985;41:810-7.
6. Maisel A, Mueller C, Adams K, Anker SD, Aspromonte N, Cleland JG, et al. State of the art: using natriuretic peptide levels in clinical practice. Eur J Heart Fail. 2008;10:824-9.
7. Maisel AS, Nakao K, Ponikowski P, Peacock WF, Yoshimura M, Suzuki T, et al. Japanese-Western consensus meeting on Biomarkers. Int Heart J. 2011;53:253-65.
8. Piccoli A, Pittoni G, Facco E. Relationship between central venous pressure and bioimpedance vector analysis in critically ill patients. Crit Care Med. 2000;28:132-7.
9. Piccoli A. Bioeletric impedance vector distribution in peritoneal dialysis patient with different hydration status. Kidney Int. 2004;65:1050-63.
10. Piccoli A. Identification of operational clues to dry weight prescription in hemodialysis using bioimpedance vector analysis. Kidney Int. 1998;53:1036-2043.
11. Talluri T, Lietdke RJ, Evangelisti A, Talluri J, Maggia G. Fat-free mass qualitative assessment with bioelectrical impedance analysis (BIA). Ann N Y Acad Sci. 1999;20:873-94.
12. Valle R, Aspromonte N, Milani L, Peacock FW, Maisel AS, Santini M, et al. Optimizing fluid management in patient with acute decompensated heart failure (ADHF): the emerging role of combined measurement of body hydration status and brain natriuretic peptide(BNP) levels. Heart Fail Rev. 2011;16:519-29.

6
CHAPTER

Mechanical Ventilation in Acute Heart Failure: The Role of Noninvasive Ventilation

Josep Masip, Kenneth Planas

INTRODUCTION

Clinical use of mechanical ventilation (MV) depends on the health care facility. In general intensive care units (ICUs), invasive mechanical ventilation (IMV) is mostly used to treat patients with acute respiratory failure (ARF),, followed by patients with coma or exacerbations of chronic diseases (Box 1). Conversely,

> **Box 1: Main diseases treated with mechanical ventilation according to the type of critical care unit**
>
> **Intensive care unit**
> - Acute respiratory failure (65%)
>   - Pneumonia
>   - Sepsis
>   - Trauma
>   - Surgical complications
>   - Heart failure
>   - Acute respiratory distress syndrome
> - Coma
> - Chronic obstructive pulmonary disease
> - Neuromuscular disorders
> - Postoperative high risk interventions
>
> **Cardiovascular intensive care unit**
> - Cardiogenic shock (acute coronary syndromes or myocarditis)
> - Acute pulmonary edema
> - Cardiorespiratory arrest
> - Postoperative cardiac surgery

in cardiovascular intensive care units (CICUs), the diseases that require IMV are essentially cardiogenic shock, acute pulmonary edema (APE), cardiopulmonary arrest, and postoperative cardiac surgery. Noninvasive ventilation (NIV) is used in multiple scenarios to treat acute and chronic respiratory disorders, but exacerbation of chronic obstructive pulmonary disease (COPD) and APE are the main indications. In the CICU, NIV is used almost exclusively in patients with APE and in selected cases as a support therapy in the postoperative of cardiac surgery or in the ventilator weaning.

Overall, the aim of MV is to decrease the work of breathing and to reverse acute hypoxemia and progressive acidosis. The reduction in the work of breathing, which in severe acute situations, may involve 20–50% of the total body oxygen consumption, allows the recovery of respiratory muscles.

INVASIVE MECHANICAL VENTILATION IN PATIENTS WITH HEART FAILURE

Patients with heart failure (HF) and reduced left ventricular systolic function may have significant hemodynamic instability resulting in abnormal responses to MV (Box 2). First, endotracheal intubation (EI) is poorly tolerated since the loss of adrenergic stimuli and the vasodilation produced by sedative agents lead to a more pronounced hypotension, which often requires the administration of vasoactive drugs. Second, during IMV, patients with HF have frequent oscillations in blood pressure and higher incidence of rhythm disturbances, especially atrial fibrillation, complicating ventilation. Hemodynamic instability induced by IMV is greater if it is associated with myocardial ischemia. Third, some patients, especially those with preserved left ventricular systolic function may experience an increase in cardiac output when applying MV due to the decrease in left ventricle preload and afterload, which are

> **Box 2: Possible adverse effects of invasive mechanical ventilation**
> - Hypotension secondary to vasodilation (loss of adrenergic stimuli, effect of sedative drugs, and decrease in venous return)
> - Blood pressure oscillations, need for vasoactive drugs
> - Rhythm disturbances, especially atrial fibrillation
> - Heart failure decompensation when positive intrathoracic pressure is withdrawn during weaning (loss of the hemodynamic protective effect)
> - Right ventricular failure in predisposed patients due to an increase in pulmonary vascular resistances and right ventricular afterload

usually elevated in patients with HF. Positive intrathoracic pressure acts in most cases as a protection for HF and when removed, acute decompensation may occur. This is common in weaning. It has been reported that 30–40% of weaning failures are due to HF. Adequate compensation with previous negative cumulative fluid balance the administration of vasodilators and diuretics, avoiding tachycardia and hypertension, and using NIV in some cases, are measures that may prevent this complication. It should be emphasized that the prognosis of patients with APE treated with IMV does not depend on the severity of ARF, but on myocardial injury and the consequent degree of myocardial dysfunction. Finally, IMV has occasionally to be used in patients with right ventricular failure associated to acute (severe pulmonary embolism or right ventricular infarction) or chronic pulmonary hypertension. The increase in right ventricular afterload imposed by the positive intrathoracic pressure, impairs right ventricular function resulting extremely difficult management of these patients.

Noninvasive Ventilation

Noninvasive ventilation can be defined as the application of positive intrathoracic pressure without EI. There are three components: (i) a source of oxygen or air (generally a ventilator); (ii) transmission tubes; and (iii) the interface, which is the key element of the technique. There are multiple interfaces such as masks, helmets, oral clamps, or nasal pillows (Fig. 1). The most commonly used are masks, which can be nasal, oronasal, partial full-face or total face. Noninvasive ventilation has its advantages and complications over IMV (Box 3).

When using a ventilator, synchronization between the ventilator and the patient's inspiratory effort is fundamental. The majority of current ventilators have mechanisms that facilitate ventilation, including leakage compensation, modulation of pressure ramp, trigger and inspiration and cycling-off times.

With few exceptions, when using NIV, respiratory rate (RR) is not programmed, because it is the patient who activates the system with his inspiratory effort. This requires a sufficient level of awareness and collaboration, one of the primary advantages of NIV. Avoiding sedation and EI, NIV permits interruptions, communication, and oral feeding.

There is a therapeutic window in which NIV is indicated that is located in the boundaries between good response to conventional oxygen therapy and extremely severe situations requiring

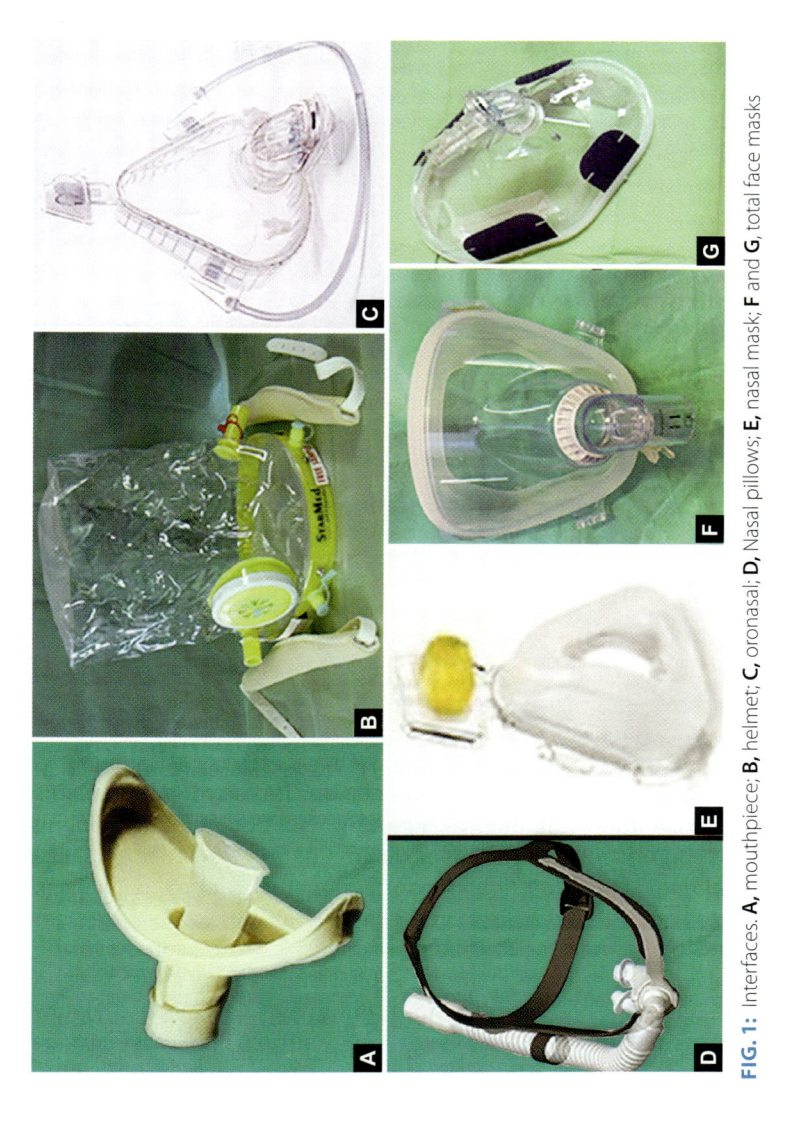

FIG. 1: Interfaces. **A,** mouthpiece; **B,** helmet; **C,** oronasal; **D,** Nasal pillows; **E,** nasal mask; **F** and **G,** total face masks

> **Box 3: Advantages and complications of noninvasive ventilation**
>
> - Inconvenients related to the interface
>   - Discomfort
>   - Facial erythema
>   - Claustrophobia
>   - Skin ulcers
>   - Noise, ear irritation (Helmet)
> - Inconvenients related to the flow or pressure
>   - Nasal congestion
>   - Sinus or ear pain
>   - Dryness (nasal/oral)
>   - Ocular irritation
>   - Gastric distension
>   - Hypotension
> - Possible advantages
>   - Reduction in the need for EI
>   - Decrease the length of stay in CICU
>   - Decrease mortality in some cases
>   - Reduction of infections, especially VAP
> - Complications
>   - Bronchoaspiration
>   - Pneumothorax
>
> EI, endotracheal intubation; CICU, cardiovascular intensive care units; VAP, ventilator associated pneumonia.

immediate EI (Fig. 2). It is important to identify early patients unresponsive to NIV. Continuous monitoring of physiological variables and evaluation of patient status minutes is crucial, at minimum every 1–2 hours, to avoid undue delay in EI for poor responders as such a delay may worsen the prognosis in some cases.

Modalities of Noninvasive Ventilation

Continuous positive airway pressure (CPAP) can be applied without the aid of a ventilator, only requiring a source of air or oxygen to renew the air and a hermetical mask equipped with a positive end-expiratory pressure (PEEP) valve or with a Boussignac system, which generates PEEP through a transversal high flow that creates a barrier effect. Continuous positive airway pressure is, therefore, the simplest technique (Fig. 3).

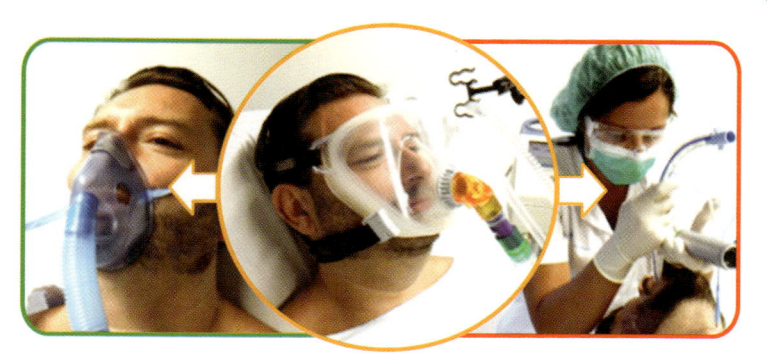

FIG. 2: Therapeutic window for noninvasive ventilation

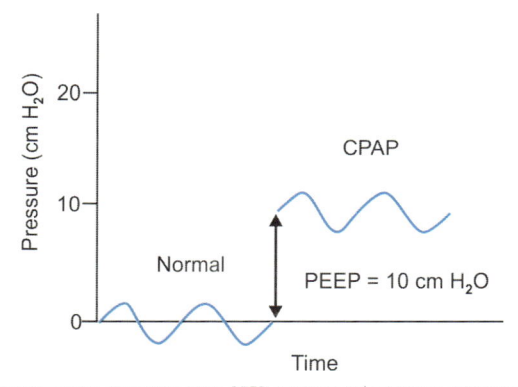

CPAP, continuous positive airway pressure; PEEP, positive end expiratory pressure

FIG. 3: Continuous positive airway pressure. Pressure-time curve of a patient with continuous positive airway pressure

Pressure support ventilation (PSV) with positive end expiratory pressure (PEEP), also called biphasic, bilevel or two-level pressure [inspiratory positive airway pressure (IPAP) and expiratory positive airway pressure (EPAP)] (Fig. 4). When the patient starts the inspiratory effort, the ventilator delivers pressure support using a decelerated flow, which keeps the prefixed IPAP constant. When the patient finishes the inspiratory effort or the flow has decreased below a preset percentage of its maximum value (usually 25%), the ventilator assistance ceases and the pressure drops down to the predetermined EPAP. Tidal volumes (Vt) change with each breath according to the patient's effort. This method requires some experience for setting the ventilator to the changing needs of the patient. Adequate synchrony is essential.

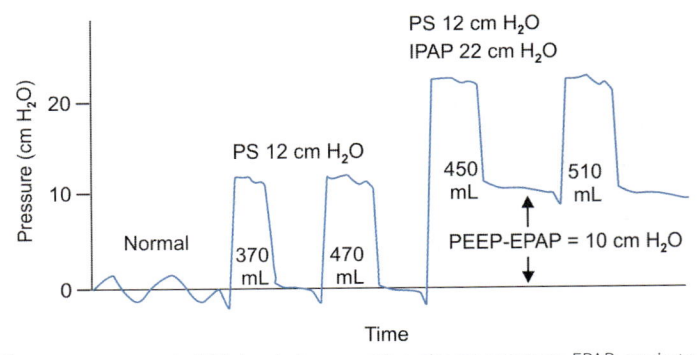

PS, pressure support; IPAP, inspiratory positive airway pressure; EPAP, expiratory positive airway pressure; PEEP, positive end expiratory pressure

FIG. 4: Pressure support ventilation. Pressure-time curves of a patient breathing normally, with pressure support (PS) and after the application of PEEP (bilevel)

Other Modalities

Proportional assist ventilation: the inspiratory support is regulated by integrating the elastance and resistance of the patient's lung, delivering assisted ventilation proportional to the patient's effort. Although it seems to be more comfortable to the patients, it is not commonly used in clinical practice.

- Adaptive-pressure-control: the ventilator adjusts the inspiratory pressure to the patient's inspiratory effort to maintain a target tidal volume. It has been used in patients with hypercapnic encephalopathy (Glasgow Coma Score <10).
- Adaptative servo ventilation: it used in patients with HF and mixed sleep disturbances, combining central and obstructive apneas. A multicenter randomized trial has been prematurely interrupted recently after showing some negative effects
- High flow nasal cannula: the delivery of intranasal heating and humidification high flow (up to 35 L), produces a low CPAP effect, reducing upper airflow resistance and renewing upper airway dead space. It is used in subacute and prolonged respiratory support and recently it has been demonstrated to be superior to NIV in hypoxemic ARF.

Current Indications for Noninvasive Ventilation

Although home NIV is used extensively in chronic patients with obstructive sleep apnea and pulmonary or neuromuscular diseases, the technique is used primarily in patients with ARF (Box 4).

> **Box 4: Acute diseases with some evidence of benefit with the use of noninvasive ventilation**
>
> - Chronic obstructive pulmonary disease (COPD) exacerbation
> - Acute pulmonary edema
> - Pneumonia (especially in COPD and hypercapnic patients)
> - Acute respiratory distres syndrome at initial phases
> - Weaning:
>   - Direct method in difficult weaning
>   - To prevent postextubation acute respiratory failure
> - Acute respiratory failure in immunocompromised patients
> - Postoperative patients
> - Do not intubate patients
> - Severe asthma

Noninvasive ventilation has been shown to be superior to conventional oxygen therapy in terms of reduced mortality in COPD exacerbations, APE, hypercapnic COPD patients with pneumonia, immunocompromised patients (hematologic or post solid organ transplantation), and weaning. In regard to weaning, the results have been favorable as a preventive measure of postextubation ARF in individuals at risk and as a direct method of weaning in patients who have failed several spontaneous breathing trials. It has not proven to be useful in treating postextubation ARF once established.

Noninvasive Ventilation in Acute Heart Failure

Noninvasive ventilation is restricted to APE or in initial low cardiac output states. Most patients with APE present with a mixed acidosis. It has been reported that hypercapnia and improvement after the first hour of NIV are predictors of a good response to the technique in these patients. Acute pulmonary edema is the second most frequent indication for NIV, primarily in the emergency room. For APE patients, use of nasal masks is not recommended due to severity of dyspnea driving patients to breathe orally, making airway pressurization impossible. However, there is experience with both modalities of NIV.

Continuous positive airway pressure: the CPAP level used in APE patients varies between 5 and 15 cm H_2O, although the most common pressure used in clinical practice is 10 cm H_2O. Fraction of inspired oxygen (FiO_2) is usually recommended to be high

(50–100%) and should be titrated according to clinical status and evaluation. The early use of CPAP in the prehospital setting improves oxygenation and may reduce the rate of EI with respect to conventional oxygen therapy.

Pressure support-positive end-expiratory pressure: Commonly used inspiratory pressure support is 10–20 cm H_2O and PEEP of 4–7 cm H_2O with high FiO_2 (50–100%). It is convenient to start with lower pressures and increase PSV progressively as patient's adaptation improves, to ensure Vt is more than or equal to 350–500 mL. In ventilators with a single tube, EPAP or PEEP more than or equal to 4 cm H_2O should be used to prevent rebreathing. Different types of masks should be available to check optimal adjustment to patients' faces. Modern ventilators are equipped with leakage compensation and display screens, with a wide set of alarms and curves. It is essential to achieve and maintain good synchronicity between patient and ventilator. Every effort must be followed by an inspiratory cycle. In tachypneic patients, it may be useful to reduce the IPAP, with the shortest ramp and inspiratory time possible. In many cases, while giving instructions to the patient, manual support of the mask to the face is recommended at the onset to reduce excessive leakage (>30 L/m). In those who are very anxious or show excessive tachypnea, supplemental doses of morphine or remifentanil may be useful to decrease RR and achieve better synchrony. In any case, the application of NIV should not delay the concomitant administration of vasodilators and diuretics.

In the last European Society of Cardiology (ESC) guidelines from 2012, NIV was considered class IIa, level of evidence B for APE. A recent consensus paper of the ESC and Emergency Societies recommended the use of NIV in prehospital and early treatment of patients with APE.

Controversies

In 2008, the Three Interventions in Cardiogenic Pulmonary Oedema (3CPO) trial, the largest study ever done on NIV was published. This study included more than 1,000 patients with APE and pH less than 7.35, divided into three groups: (i) CPAP, (ii) PS-PEEP, and (iii) conventional therapy. Patients in both groups of NIV showed faster improvement in ARF, but no difference in mortality at 30 days, which was the primary end-point. The very low rate of EI in this study (2.9%), the absence of hypoxemia at study entry (average PaO_2 was 100 mmHg in the three groups), the high rate of crossovers (the conventional group was significantly higher due to respiratory distress), the high rate of intolerance to NIV (up to 25%) equating low experience with technique, determined these results. Despite the discrepancy with previous meta-analyses, some new meta-analyses including the 3CPO have shown that both methods reduce the rate of EI and that CPAP also reduces mortality by about 30%.

No differences have been demonstrated in the outcomes in trials comparing CPAP and PS-PEEP. However, since a more significant improvement of some respiratory parameters has been described with the use of PS-PEEP compared to CPAP in some randomized studies, and PS-PEEP has been usefully applied as rescue therapy when CPAP has failed in others, PS-PEEP may be preferable in patients with fatigue or significant hypercapnia. No study has shown that NIV can precipitate a higher rate of myocardial infarction and conversely, NIV has been successfully used in these patients.

Early NIV treatment (CPAP preferably in the ambulance) is recommended in appropriate patients with APE who show respiratory distress (increased work of breathing, SpO_2 <90% and RR >25), particularly those already treated with conventional oxygen therapy (Algorithm 1). In patients with persistent respiratory

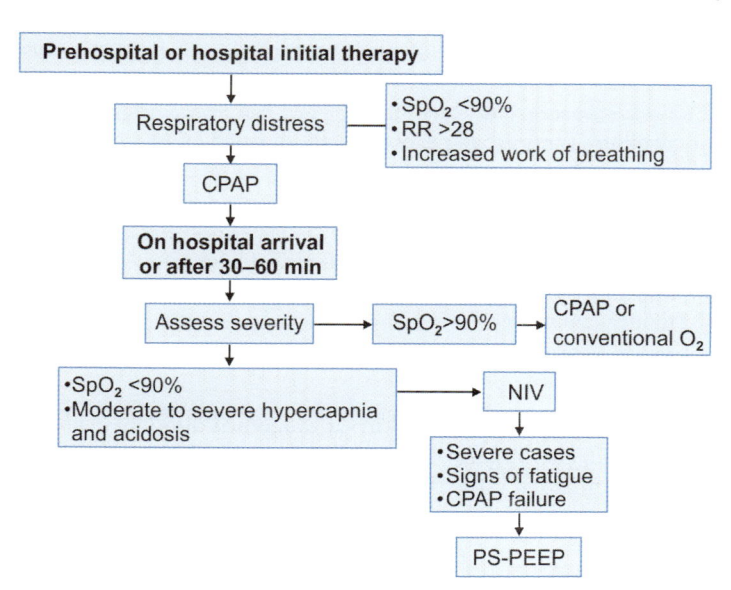

NIV, noninvasive ventilation; CPAP, continuous positive airway pressure; RR, respiratory rate; PS-PEEP, pressure-support positive end-expiratory pressure.

ALGORITHM 1: Algorithm for oxygen therapy and noninvasive ventilation in patients with acute pulmonary edema

distress after 30–60 minutes and particularly in those with acidosis and hypercapnia, NIV (either CPAP or PS-PEEP) must be continued or initiated, if it had not been started yet. As previously mentioned, PSV may be preferable in severe cases with significant hypercapnia or in patients with signs of fatigue or CPAP failure.

CONCLUSION

For the treatment of APE, currently available evidence supports the benefit of NIV compared to conventional treatment in terms of improvement from ARF, reduction in the rate of endotracheal intubation and even death in some cases. Invasive mechanical ventilation should be considered in NIV-failure, after cardiorespiratory arrest or established cardiogenic shock.

KEY POINTS

- A substantial proportion of patients with acute heart failure develop severe acute respiratory failure (ARF) requiring ventilatory support
- In the last decade, noninvasive ventilation via an interface (mask, pillow, cannula, helmet, etc.) has been progressively used in this setting
- Two main modalities—continuous positive airway pressure and pressure support ventilation—with a positive end-expiratory pressure (bilevel) are utilized
- Both techniques and some others recently introduced technological innovations have extensively demonstrated a faster improvement of ARF, facilitating the release of conventional mechanical ventilation, frequently avoiding endotracheal intubation, and in some cases, reducing mortality
- Acute heart failure is currently the second indication of this technique
- Noninvasive ventilation is also used in a wide range of acute settings such as critical care unit, emergency department, and in prehospital care. The appropriate selection of patients and the adaptation to the technique are the keys to success.

SUGGESTED READINGS

1. Ducros L, Logeart D, Vicaut E, Henry P, Plaisance P, Collet JP, et al. CPAP for acute cardiogenic pulmonary oedema from out-of-hospital to cardiac intensive care unit: a randomised multicentre study. Intensive Care Med. 2011;37:1501-9.

2. Esteban A, Anzueto A, Frutos F, Alía I, Brochard L, Stewart TE, et al. Characteristics and outcomes in adult patients receiving mechanical ventilation: a 28-day international study. JAMA. 2002;287:345-55.
3. Esteban A, Frutos-Vivar F, Ferguson ND, Arabi Y, Apezteguía C, González M, Epstein SK, et al. Noninvasive positive-pressure ventilation for respiratory failure after extubation. N Engl J Med. 2004;350:2452-60.
4. Fedullo AJ, Swinburne AJ, Wahl GW, Bixby K. Acute cardiogenic pulmonary edema treated with mechanical ventilation. Factors determining in-hospital mortality. Chest. 1991;99:1220-6.
5. Frat JP, Thille AW, Mercat A, Girault C, Ragot S, Perbet S, et al. High-flow oxygen through nasal cannula in acute hypoxemic respiratory failure. N Engl J Med. 2015;372:2185-96.
6. Gray A, Goodacre S, Newby DE, Masson M, Sampson F, Nicholl J. Noninvasive ventilation in acute cardiogenic pulmonary edema. N Engl J Med. 2008;359:142-51.
7. Liesching T, Kwok H, Hill NS. Acute applications of noninvasive positive pressure ventilation. Chest. 2003;124:669-713.
8. Masip J. The patient who needs mechanical ventilation. In the session : The difficult patient in the CICU. European Congress of Cardiology. Paris, 2011
9. McMurray JJ, Adamopoulos S, Anker SD, Auricchio A, Böhm M, Dickstein K, et al. ESC guidelines for the diagnosis and treatment of acute and chronic heart failure 2012: The Task Force for the Diagnosis and Treatment of Acute and Chronic Heart Failure 2012 of the European Society of Cardiology. Developed in collaboration with the Heart Failure Association (HFA) of the ESC. Eur Heart J. 2012;33(14):1787-847.
10. Mebazaa A, Yilmaz MB, Levy P, Ponikowski P, Peacock WF, Laribi S, et al. Recommendations on pre-hospital & early hospital management of acute heart failure: a consensus paper from the Heart Failure Association of the European Society of Cardiology, the European Society of Emergency Medicine and the Society of Academic Emergency Medicine. Eur Heart J. 2015;17(6):544-58.
11. Pinsky MR, Summer WR, Wise RA, Permutt S, Bromberger-Barnea B. Augmentation of cardiac function by elevation of intrathoracic pressure. J Appl Physiol. 1983;54:950-5.
12. Rodriguez L, Carrillo A, Melgarejo A, Renedo Villarroya A, Párraga Ramírez M, Jara Pérez P, et al. Predictive factors related to success of noninvasive ventilation and mortality in the treatment of acute cardiogenic pulmonary edema. Med Clin (Barc). 2005;124:126-31.
13. Tobin, MJ. Mechanical ventilation. New Engl J Med. 1994;330:1056-61.
14. Weng CL, Zhao YT, Liu QH, Fu CJ, Sun F, Ma YL, et al. Meta-analysis: Noninvasive ventilation in acute cardiogenic pulmonary edema. Ann Intern Med. 2010;152:590-600.

7
CHAPTER

When to Employ Cardiac Magnetic Resonance Imaging and Cardiac Computed Tomography in the Evaluation of Heart Failure?

Kimberly C Atianzar, Joel R Wilson

INTRODUCTION

Advanced cardiovascular imaging using computed tomography (CT) and magnetic resonance imaging (MRI) are valuable tools in the initial diagnosis, risk stratification, and management of patients with heart failure. Cardiac MRI is considered to be a gold standard for quantification of biventricular volumes and systolic function, with standard errors of around 5%. Cardiac MRI is unencumbered by sonographic windows, allowing for complete visualization of the blood pool and myocardium. Myocardial fibrosis, myocardial edema/inflammation and iron deposition can be readily identified with MRI. The presence and pattern of findings helps differentiate between ischemic and nonischemic etiologies, and further distinguishes between subtypes of nonischemic cardiomyopathy. Additionally, the presence of myocardial fibrosis has prognostic implications in nearly every form of heart failure. If ischemic cardiomyopathy is known or suspected, stress testing with cardiac MRI can be performed either with myocardial perfusion imaging using gadolinium contrast agent during vasodilator administration, or with functional imaging by assessing contractile response to graded rates of dobutamine infusion. Cardiac MRI can quantify blood-flow velocities, allowing for evaluation of cardiac output and shunt severity in patients with anatomic defects. Although Cardiac CT has less of a role than cardiac MRI in the management of patients with heart failure, it is well suited for the evaluation of coronary arteries and for delineating morphologic abnormalities. It can also accurately quantify biventricular volumes and function in patients with contraindications to cardiac MRI.

The specific test to order, cardiac MRI versus cardiac CT, will not only depend upon the diagnostic question but also on what technologies and expertise are available. The 2013 Appropriate Utilization of Cardiovascular Imaging in Heart Failure document outlines time points during the care of heart-failure patients, when imaging techniques are typical. This document covers appropriate utilization of echocardiography, radionucleotide ventriculography, single photon emission computed tomography (SPECT), positron emission tomography (PET), and invasive angiography in addition to cardiac MRI and cardiac CT. Advanced cardiovascular imaging is usually indicated when the etiology of heart failure is not well-established on the basis of initial tests; for example, when echocardiography is suboptimal or did not fully address the specific question, or when results will affect management. Cardiac MRI is also uniquely able to assess for myocardial involvement of systemic conditions.

PATIENT PREPARATION AND SCREENING

Refer to table 1 for a list of preprocedure patient selection questions.

Metallic Implants

Most nonelectronic implanted metallic medical devices are compatible with the MRI environment, but some devices are potentially dangerous. Devices compatible with MRI at 1.5 Tesla include all prosthetic heart valves, coronary and peripheral stents, aortic stent grafts, sternal wires, epicardial pacing wires, septal occluder devices and coils, artificial joint replacements and Harrington rods. Some inferior vena cava filters are weakly ferromagnetic, and MRI should be deferred for 6 weeks after implantation of such devices. Cerebral aneurysm clips may be a contraindication to MRI, depending upon the specific type of clip used. Devices that are contraindications for MRI include, retained endovascular pacing wires, intra-aortic balloon pumps, most neurostimulators, and thermodilution Swan-Ganz catheters. Magnetic resonance imaging compatible pacemakers and implantable cardioverter defibrillator (ICDs) are available. The safety of performing cardiac MRI studies in patients with pacemakers and ICDs is currently being debated. The American Heart Association

TABLE 1: Checklist of questions to ask in preparation for cardiac MRI or CT

Questions to ask before cardiac MRI	If yes
Does the patient have an implanted pacemaker, cardiac defibrillator or retained transvenous leads?	Cardiac MRI is contraindicated
Does patient require a thermodilution Swan-Ganz catheter?	Study must be deferred until catheter can be removed or exchanged for an MRI compatible device
Is the patient's ability to hold their breath and/or lay supine compromised, for example, by volume overload?	Consider deferring cardiac MRI until heart failure is compensated
Does the patient have severe claustrophobia?	Consider premedication with a benzodiazepine
Is atrial fibrillation present?	Consider deferring until after cardioversion, if planned. If not, proceed with study
Does the patient has acute renal failure, or stable chronic renal failure with eGFR <30 mL/min?	Either defer cardiac MRI until renal function stabilizes, or proceed with noncontract study
Does the patient has a history of an allergic-type reaction to gadolinium-based contrast agents?	Consider premedication, e.g. prednisone 50 mg PO Q6H for three doses (preferred) or hydrocortisone 200 mg IV Q6H for three doses (second-line) ending 1 hour prior to procedure; plus diphenhydramine 50 mg PO or IV once with final dose of steroid

Continued

Continued

Questions to ask before cardiac CT	If yes
Is atrial fibrillation present?	Consider deferring until after cardioversion, if planned. If not, consult the advanced imaging practitioner regarding feasibility
Is resting heart rate >60 bpm?	Most patients should be premedicated with beta blockade, e.g. 50–100 mg of metoprolol, for optimal image quality unless contraindicated
Are beta-blockers contraindicated?	Consider premedication with diltiazem to suppress heart rate to <60, unless contractile function is tenuous
Does the patient has a history of a moderate to severe allergic-type reaction to iodinated contrast?	Consider premedication, e.g. prednisone 50 mg PO Q6H for three doses (preferred) or hydrocortisone 200 mg IV Q6H for three doses (second-line) ending 1 hour prior to procedure; plus diphenhydramine 50 mg PO or IV for one dose with final dose of steroid
Does patient take metformin?	Metformin should be held for 48 hours or more starting at the time of CT scan in most patients with heart failure to prevent lactic acidosis
Is acute renal insufficiency or moderate to severe chronic renal insufficiency (CRI) present?	Risks of contrast-induced nephropathy must be weighed against information to be gained. Some experts recommend a threshold for creatinine of 2 mg/dL in patients with sable CRI. Anuric patients on hemodialysis can undergo contrast study

IV, intravenous; PO, orally; bpm, beats per minute; eGFR, estimated glomerular filtration rate; Q6H, every 6 hourly; CT, computed tomography.

has issued a scientific statement on safety of cardiovascular devices during MRI, and an extensive list of implanted medical devices and their MRI compatibility is maintained at www.mrisafety.com. Medical devices can create artifacts in both CT and MRI images, but generally these are not of major concern.

Contrast Agents

Renal Function

Although gadolinium contrast agents used in MRI do not appreciably alter renal function, patients with chronic renal failure and a glomerular filtration rate of less than 30 mL/minute or acute renal failure cannot undergo gadolinium-enhanced cardiac MRI due to the rare and life-threatening complication of nephrogenic systemic sclerosis.

Iodinated contrast is required for most cardiac CT assessments. The risk of worsening renal dysfunction with contrast exposure must be balanced against the value of the information to be gained. Baseline renal insufficiency is the most consistently identified risk factor for developing contrast induced nephropathy (CIN). A threshold of 2.0 mg/dL has been recommended by some authorities as safe in most patients with chronic stable renal dysfunction.

Hypersensitivity Reactions

Immediate hypersensitivity reactions to gadolinium contrast agents are rare and tend to be mild. Severe reactions occur at a rate of less than 0.01%. Immediate hypersensitivity reactions to low osmolar iodinated CT contrast agents occur between 0.18% and 0.7% of administrations, with serious reactions at a rate of 0.04%. Patients with a history of allergic-type reaction to a contrast agent should be premedicated prior to the study, although premedication does not prevent all recurrences. Typical premedication regimens include prednisone 50 mg by mouth every 6 hours for three doses ending 1 hour prior to procedure (start 13 hours in advance), plus diphenhydramine 50 mg orally or intravenously (IV) once with the final dose of steroid. Oral prednisone is preferable to intravenous steroid, but 200 mg hydrocortisone IV may be substituted for prednisone if required. Patients with history of hypersensitivity to iodinated contrast agents generally do not require premedication prior to gadolinium-contrast exposure, and vice versa, as there does not appear to be significant cross-reactivity.

Claustrophobia

Mild claustrophobia is relatively common. It is severe enough to prevent completion of the MRI study in less than 1% of cases, but approximately 2% of patients will require sedation with benzodiazepines to complete the study. Claustrophobia generally does not limit CT scanning.

IMAGE ACQUISITION

Cine cardiac MRI sequences offer high intrinsic contrast between blood pool and myocardium; thus no contrast is needed for analysis of myocardial function. Gadolinium contrast is required to assess myocardial perfusion for imaging fibrosis or damaged myocardium. Iodinated contrast is required for CT assessment of coronary arteries and functional analysis, but not for assessing coronary artery calcification alone.

For both cardiac MRI and cardiac CT, images are generally acquired with the patient holding the breath and timed to the cardiac cycle (cardiac gated). This means that image quality and/or acquisition parameters are affected by presence of arrhythmia and conditions leading to dyspnea; MRI, more so.

For evaluation of coronary arteries, most patients without a contraindication to beta blockade receive a dose of oral beta-blocker about an hour prior to the procedure. If needed, the heart rate is further lowered with the patient on the CT table using IV beta blockade to achieve goal heart rate less than 60 beats per minute. Patients who are undergoing evaluation of coronary arteries are then given 0.4 mg nitroglycerin sublingually, a few minutes before coronary assessment.

GENERAL UTILITY OF ADVANCED IMAGING

Cardiac MRI has a demonstrable impact on management the majority of the time it is used, and only about 15% of patients require subsequent imaging. Cardiac MRI has several advantages over other modalities. It does not use ionizing radiation, and has the flexibility to characterize tissues, quantify blood flow and myocardial perfusion, strain, and infarct size. As a stress modality, it has higher special resolution than SPECT and is not limited by attenuation artifact. Both cardiac MRI and CT have the advantage over echocardiography of having no limitations to tomographic planes. Both also have the ability to quantify cardiovascular performance measures like ventricular volumes and mass and to accurately represent anatomy, including coronary artery course and origins. Cardiac CT has the additional advantage of being helpful in evaluating for coronary atherosclerosis.

WHEN TO USE ADVANCED CARDIOVASCULAR IMAGING

Advanced cardiovascular imaging can be useful when questions about etiology, severity or prognosis of cardiac condition remain after the initial evaluation. Advanced cardiovascular imaging techniques are rarely the first tests employed in the evaluation of patients with heart failure. Approximately two-thirds of patients referred for cardiac MRI have undergone transthoracic echocardiography and a quarter have had prior invasive angiography. When employed, results of cardiac MRI suggest an entirely new diagnosis about 16% of the time in a large registry series, and result in a change in medications over 23% of the time.

Some form of cardiovascular imaging is invariably indicated during the initial evaluation of patients with a possible cardiac condition. Appropriate use criteria documents exist to guide when to employ echocardiography, invasive coronary angiography, and stress testing. An extensive discussion of these modalities is beyond the scope of this chapter. Most patients will undergo echocardiogram as a baseline test in evaluation of heart failure (Algorithm 1, step 1). However, patients with acute myocardial infarction or cardiogenic shock will often proceed directly to invasive catheterization and/or positioning of mechanical support (Algorithm 1, step 2). Echocardiography (Algorithm 1, step 3) or cardiac MRI (Algorithm 1, step 4) for functional analysis and/or viability testing is typically performed during triage or after initial stabilization. The specific indications for obtaining cardiac MRI will be covered in greater detail below.

Most patients with heart failure with reduced ejection fraction (HFrEF) will undergo evaluation for presence of coronary artery disease. How best to accomplish this, depends in part upon the pretest probability for coronary artery disease. In patients with HFrEF who are at high pretest probability for coronary artery disease, early referral to invasive coronary angiography (Algorithm 1, step 2 or step 3) is the most appropriate option. If the pretest probability for coronary artery disease is low to intermediate, cardiac CT (Algorithm 1, step 6) or stress testing (Algorithm 1, step 7) are both reasonable options. Stress testing with cardiac

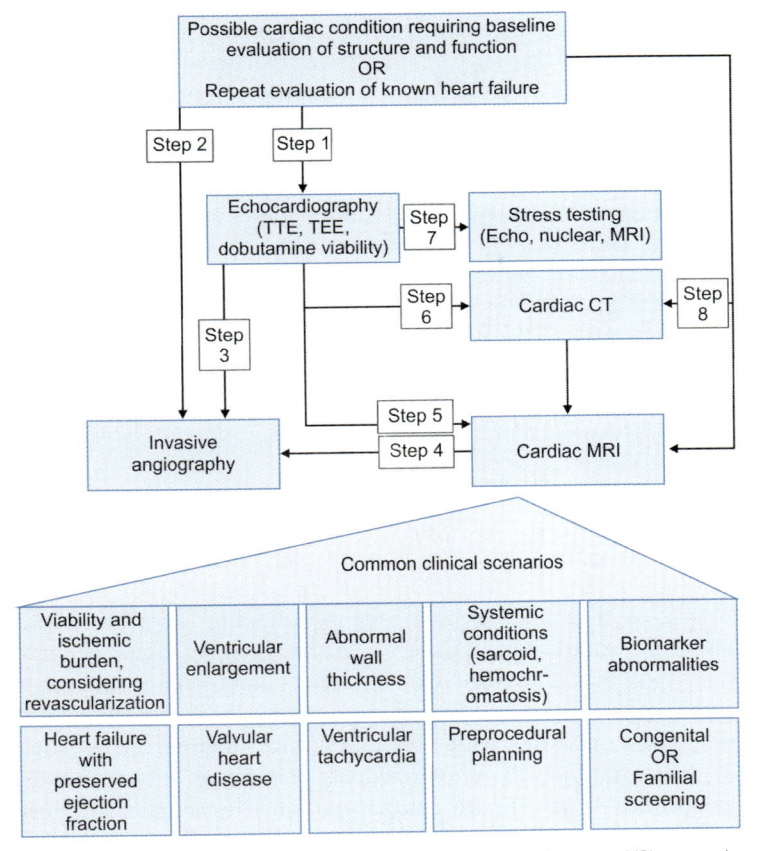

```
                    ┌─────────────────────────────────┐
                    │ Possible cardiac condition      │
                    │ requiring baseline evaluation   │
                    │ of structure and function       │
                    │            OR                   │
                    │ Repeat evaluation of known      │
                    │ heart failure                   │
                    └─────────────────────────────────┘
```

Flow chart with steps:
- Step 1 → Echocardiography (TTE, TEE, dobutamine viability)
- Step 2 → (from top box)
- Step 3 → Invasive angiography
- Step 4 → Cardiac MRI → Invasive angiography
- Step 5 → Cardiac MRI
- Step 6 → Cardiac CT
- Step 7 → Stress testing (Echo, nuclear, MRI)
- Step 8 → Cardiac CT

Common clinical scenarios:

Viability and ischemic burden, considering revascularization	Ventricular enlargement	Abnormal wall thickness	Systemic conditions (sarcoid, hemochromatosis)	Biomarker abnormalities
Heart failure with preserved ejection fraction	Valvular heart disease	Ventricular tachycardia	Preprocedural planning	Congenital OR Familial screening

TTE, transthoracic echocardiogram; TEE, transesophageal echocardiograms; MRI, magnetic resonance imaging; CT, computed tomography;

ALGORITHM 1: Algorithm for ordering advanced cardiac imaging studies. Numbers in white boxes correspond to numbered steps outlined in text. The clinical scenarios at the bottom of the algorithm are the most common indications for cardiac MRI. Cardiac CT may be to MRI in some of these scenarios, as in preprocedural planning studies, or in patients with contraindications to MRI (implantable cardioverter defibrillator/pacemakers)

MRI is not widely available, but can either be performed with noncontrast dobutamine study or with vasodilator stress during first pass myocardial perfusion with gadolinium contrast. Cardiac MRI stress testing offers a "one stop shop" for assessing for ischemic and nonischemic etiologies for heart failure, since viability and functional assessment are typically performed in the same setting.

In patients with extensive wall motion abnormalities and known coronary artery disease, viability testing can assist in determining which territories are likely to improve function following revascularization. Viability testing can be performed using one of several modalities: nuclear imaging with PET or SPECT (not shown in algorithm), echocardiography or cardiac MRI with low-dose dobutamine infusion to assess contractile reserve (Algorithm 1, step 3 or #4) or cardiac MRI (Algorithm 1, step 4) with gadolinium contrast to assess extent of fibrosis. The method for imaging fibrosis using cardiac MRI is called late gadolinium enhancement. In patients with ischemic cardiomyopathy, the transmural extent of fibrosis correlates inversely with likelihood of functional recovery after revascularization. Myocardial infarction can be identified by MRI in nearly all patients whose systolic dysfunction is primarily due to coronary artery disease.

In addition to providing information about viability in the setting of ischemic cardiomyopathy, the presence and pattern of late gadolinium enhancement in patients with nonischemic cardiomyopathy provides prognostic and diagnostic information. Indicators may be present on echocardiogram or other initial tests that would suggest need for further imaging. These include the presence of ventricular chamber enlargement or other structural disorder; abnormal myocardial thickness; presence of systemic diseases with potential cardiac manifestations such as hemochromatosis or sarcoidosis; biomarker abnormalities in absence of obstructive coronary atherosclerosis; heart failure with preserved systolic function, especially when attempting to differentiate between restrictive and constrictive etiologies; congenital heart disease or screening for structural heart disease in familial syndromes; valvular disorders; cardiac masses, evaluation for etiology of ventricular tachycardia especially when considering ablation or ICD implantation; and increasingly as preoperative planning in patients requiring surgeries or procedures.

Ventricular Enlargement or Structural Heart Disease

Cardiac MRI is the gold standard for evaluating biventricular size and function. In patients with suboptimal sonographic windows or in whom accurate assessment of cardiac function is especially critical, it is reasonable to obtain cardiac MRI (Algorithm 1, step 5 or Algorithm 1, step 8). Commonly, this would include evaluation of systolic function in patients undergoing potentially cardiotoxic chemotherapy, or for evaluating ejection fraction (EF) in patients who are candidates for ICDs, but whose EF assessment by echocardiography is borderline. In patients with contraindications to MRI, cardiac CT with retrospective gating also provides accurate volumetric assessment.

The differential for isolated right ventricular enlargement includes pulmonary hypertension, severe prolonged tricuspid regurgitation, right ventricular dysfunction in association with left heart failure, arrhythmogenic right ventricular cardiomyopathy and shunt. If an anatomic shunt is identified, such as an atrial septal defect, the volume and direction of flow through the shunt can be directly measured with cardiac MRI. Additionally, flow through the pulmonary artery and aorta can be directly measured to estimate Qp: Qs. Cardiac CT is also well-suited for the evaluation of many anatomic lesions such as pulmonary venous drainage anomalies, and can assist in understanding septal defects in three dimensions, which can be helpful in determining suitability for percutaneous closure. In patients with risk factors for ARVC, cardiac MRI can identify regions of right ventricular akinesia/dyskinesia and is the gold standard for right ventricular EF assessment. Fibrous or fatty infiltration of right or left ventricular myocardium can also sometimes be seen by cardiac MRI, but this is not currently a diagnostic criteria for ARVC. Cardiac CT can provide right ventricular volumes and regional function assessment in patients who are unable to undergo cardiac MRI.

Increased Left Ventricular Wall Thickness

Cardiac MRI can accurately describe distribution of hypertrophy and quantify maximal wall thickness and myocardial mass. The distribution of hypertrophy along with the pattern of late gadolinium enhancement can help distinguish hypertensive heart disease from infiltrative disorders, like cardiac amyloidosis and cardiac sarcoidosis, or from genetic disorders such as hypertrophic cardiomyopathy and the lysosomal storage disorder—Fabry disease. Cardiac MRI is playing an increasing role in the diagnosis and management of hypertrophic cardiomyopathy. Approximately 60% of patients with hypertrophic cardiomyopathy will have evidence of fibrosis on cardiac MRI. The presence of myocardial fibrosis in patients with hypertrophic cardiomyopathy has been associated with adverse outcomes including cardiac death. Fibrosis assessment is useful for risk stratification when the clinical risk profile does not clearly indicate whether implanted cardiodefibrillator is advisable. Although most patients with hypertrophic cardiomyopathy undergo echocardiogram, presence of a characteristic murmur and clinical findings would be reasonable grounds to refer directly for cardiac MRI (Algorithm 1, step 8).

Predisposing Conditions

Amyloidosis, sarcoidosis, and iron-overload states are systemic conditions with potential cardiac manifestations. When myocardium is involved in one of these conditions, there may be characteristic findings on cardiac MRI before symptoms or echocardiographic findings are present. Of patients with extracardiac sarcoidosis, for example, approximately 5% of patients have cardiac signs or symptoms, yet evidence of cardiac involvement is present in approximately one-quarter of patients by MRI. The presence of myocardial fibrosis in patients with systemic sarcoidosis is associated with death, aborted sudden cardiac death, and appropriate ICD discharge. In patients with iron-overload cardiomyopathy, the risk of arrhythmia is present at lower myocardial iron concentrations than when systolic dysfunction typically develops. Therefore, echocardiography is not an effective screening tool for arrhythmic risk in this setting. In some cases of cardiac amyloidosis, abnormalities in late gadolinium enhancement can precede left ventricular hypertrophy. In all three of these conditions, characteristic findings on MRI may obviate the need for myocardial biopsy. The presence of one of these systemic conditions is reasonable justification to refer directly for cardiac MRI without prior echocardiography (Algorithm 1, step 8).

Evaluating Patients with Biomarker Abnormalities and Nonobstructive Coronary Artery Disease

The differential for systolic dysfunction in patients with abnormalities in cardiac biomarkers including troponin in patients with nonobstructive coronary artery disease most commonly includes myocarditis, stress-induced (takotsubo) cardiomyopathy, embolic myocardial infarction, drug-induced cardiac dysfunction (commonly methamphetamine or cocaine), and rarely prolonged vasospasm, although conditions such as pulmonary embolism should also be considered. The pretest probability for one entity versus another is influenced by clinical factors such as gender, age of presentation, predisposing factors such as preceding viral illness or extreme emotional stressor, toxicology results and electrocardiogram abnormalities. Most commonly coronary arteries will be evaluated with invasive angiography, but in patients with low pretest probability for coronary artery disease, cardiac CT angiography is an appropriate alternative. Distinguishing between these entities can have important treatment considerations and prognostic implications. For example, presence of late gadolinium enhancement in patterns indicative of myocarditis is associated with long-term cardiac death compared to patients with myocarditis who lack fibrosis; or a myocardial infarction by MRI in a patient with nonobstructive coronary artery disease might trigger an evaluation for thrombophilia or cause initiation of antithrombotic therapy.

Heart Failure with Preserved Ejection Fraction—Differentiating Restrictive Cardiomyopathy from Constrictive Pericarditis

In patients with heart failure signs and symptoms out of proportion to the degree of systolic dysfunction, cardiac MRI can be very helpful in distinguishing restrictive cardiomyopathy from constrictive pericarditis. Restrictive cardiomyopathy, when due to cardiac amyloidosis, can usually be identified by a characteristic pattern of late gadolinium enhancement. In cases, where late gadolinium enhancement is either absent or when restrictive and constrictive physiology may be overlapping, cardiac MRI can identify anatomic and physiologic effects of pericardial disease, including abnormal pericardial thickening, pericardial enhancement, presence of pericardial effusion, distortions in ventricular shape, pericardial tethering to myocardium, and exaggerated ventricular interdependence during free-breathing cine images. Cardiac CT is superior to other modalities for evaluating the presence of pericardial calcification, and is also probably more accurate than cardiac MRI in gauging pericardial thickness due to its superior spatial resolution.

Valvular Heart Disease

Echocardiography is generally the preferred modality for assessing valvular disease, however recent studies have expanded the role for cardiac MRI in assessment of valvular heart disease. Magnetic resonance imaging has the capability of directly quantifying blood flow and regurgitant fractions, especially of the semilunar valves. Additionally, patients with bicuspid valves benefit from assessing the size of the ascending thoracic aorta using either CT or MRI at least once to correlate with echocardiographic measurements.

Ventricular Tachycardia

After evaluation for coronary artery disease by either stress testing or CT or invasive angiography, cardiac MRI is reasonable to assess for myocardial fibrosis.

Preprocedural Planning

As procedures become less invasive, preprocedural imaging has assumed a larger role in helping to plan for the procedure. Computed tomography has become the primary modality for this. Procedures with relevance to heart-failure patients which typically require three dimensional preprocedural imaging include transcatheter aortic valve implantation, mitral-clip procedure, percutaneous left atrial appendage closure devices, and minimally-invasive or robotically-assisted cardiac and aortic surgeries.

Congenital Heart Disease

Many complex congenital heart diseases require serial monitoring with imaging, often including MRI. A complete appraisal of the utility of advanced imaging in complex congenital heart disease is outside the scope of this chapter.

Evaluation of Left Ventricular Masses and Thrombus

Tissue characterization techniques take advantage of the differences in MRI signal between tissues of varying composition which can help identify thrombus and characterize extent and invasion of myocardial masses.

CONCLUSION

Advanced cardiac imaging with cardiac MRI and CT play an important role in the diagnosis and management of heart failure. Both provide more accurate volumetric assessments of biventricular function than echocardiography. Cardiac CT is usually employed for coronary artery assessment, but is also effective in evaluating structural heart disease. Cardiac MRI is most often employed when questions about heart failure etiology remain after initial diagnostic tests are performed. Cardiac MRI in particular offers significant prognostic information beyond echocardiography.

KEY POINTS

- When to order an advanced cardiovascular imaging study and what type of exam to order are directed by pretest probability, prior imaging findings, and local availability of technologies and expertise
- Cardiac magnetic resonance imaging (MRI) is a gold standard for assessing biventricular volumes and function. Direct and indirect measurements of flows, including Qp: Qs and regurgitant fractions, are possible
- Magnetic resonance imaging can readily identify fibrosis, the presence of which is an adverse prognostic indicator in most cardiac conditions. The pattern of fibrosis also provides diagnostic information
- Most metallic medical implants are compatible with cardiac MRI; the most significant exceptions are pacemakers and implantable cardioverter defibrillators
- Cardiac computed tomography (CT) is most helpful in assessing for coronary atherosclerosis in patients with low pretest probability, but is also extensively used for preprocedural planning
- Cardiac CT can provide accurate biventricular volumes and function in patients with contraindications to cardiac MRI and suboptimal echocardiographic images.

SUGGESTED READINGS

1. ACR Manual on Contrast Media: American College of Radiology. Version 9 (2013). Available from www.acr.org/Quality-Safety/Resources/Contrast-Manual [Accessed Jan, 2016].
2. Assomull RG, Prasad SK, Lyne J, Smith G, Burman ED, Khan M, et al. Cardiovascular magnetic resonance, fibrosis, and prognosis in dilated cardiomyopathy. J Am Coll Cardiol. 2006;48(10):1977-85.
3. Bruder O, Schneider S, Nothnagel D, Dill T, Hombach V, Schulz-Menger J, et al. EuroCMR (European cardiovascular magnetic resonance) registry: results of the German pilot phase. J Am Coll Cardiol. 2009;54(15):1457-66.
4. Chan RH, Maron BJ, Olivotto I, Pencina MJ, Assenza GE, Haas T, Lesser, et al. Prognostic value of quantitative contrast-enhanced cardiovascular magnetic resonance for the

evaluation of sudden death risk in patients with hypertrophic cardiomyopathy. Circulation. 2014;130(6):484-95.
5. Flett AS, Westwood MA, Davies LC, Mathur A, Moon JC. The prognostic implications of cardiovascular magnetic resonance. Circ Cardiovasc Imaging. 2009;2(3):243-50.
6. Gersh BJ, Maron BJ, Bonow RO, Dearani JA, Fifer MA, Link MS, et al. 2011 ACCF/AHA guideline for the diagnosis and treatment of hypertrophic cardiomyopathy: a report of the American College of Cardiology Foundation/American Heart Association Task Force on Practice Guidelines. Developed in collaboration with the American Association for Thoracic Surgery, American Society of Echocardiography, American Society of Nuclear Cardiology, Heart Failure Society of America, Heart Rhythm Society, Society for Cardiovascular Angiography and Interventions, and Society of Thoracic Surgeons. J Am Coll Cardiol. 2011;58(25):e212-60.
7. Greulich S, Deluigi CC, Gloekler S, Wahl A, Zurn C, Kramer U, et al. CMR imaging predicts death and other adverse events in suspected cardiac sarcoidosis. JACC Cardiovasc Imaging. 2013;6(4):501-11.
8. Grun S, Schumm J, Greulich S, Wagner A, Schneider S, Bruder O, et al. Long-term follow-up of biopsy-proven viral myocarditis: predictors of mortality and incomplete recovery. J Am Coll Cardiol. 2012;59(18):1604-15.
9. Hundley WG, Bluemke DA, Finn JP, Flamm SD, Fogel MA, Friedrich MG, et al. ACCF/ACR/AHA/NASCI/SCMR 2010 expert consensus document on cardiovascular magnetic resonance: a report of the American College of Cardiology Foundation Task Force on Expert Consensus Documents. J Am Coll Cardiol. 2010;55(23):2614-62.
10. Kwon DH, Hachamovitch R, Popovic ZB, Starling RC, Desai MY, Flamm SD, et al. Survival in patients with severe ischemic cardiomyopathy undergoing revascularization versus medical therapy: association with end-systolic volume and viability. Circulation. 2012;126(11 Suppl 1):S3-8.
11. Levine GN, Gomes AS, Arai AE, Bluemke DA, Flamm SD, Kanal E, et al. Safety of magnetic resonance imaging in patients with cardiovascular devices: an American Heart Association scientific statement from the Committee on Diagnostic and Interventional Cardiac Catheterization, Council on Clinical Cardiology, and the Council on Cardiovascular Radiology and Intervention: endorsed by the American College of Cardiology Foundation, the North American Society for Cardiac Imaging, and the Society for Cardiovascular Magnetic Resonance. Circulation. 2007;116(24):2878-91.
12. Mahrholdt H, Wagner A, Judd RM, Sechtem U, Kim RJ. Delayed enhancement cardiovascular magnetic resonance assessment of non-ischaemic cardiomyopathies. Eur Heart J. 2005;26(15):1461-74.
13. McCrohon JA, Moon JC, Prasad SK, McKenna WJ, Lorenz CH, Coats AJ, et al. Differentiation of heart failure related to dilated cardiomyopathy and coronary artery disease using gadolinium-enhanced cardiovascular magnetic resonance. Circulation. 2003;108(1):54-9.
14. McMurray JJ, Adamopoulos S, Anker SD, Auricchio A, Bohm M, Dickstein K, et al. ESC guidelines for the diagnosis and treatment of acute and chronic heart failure 2012: The task force for the diagnosis and treatment of acute and chronic heart failure 2012 of the European Society of Cardiology. Developed in collaboration with the Heart Failure Association (HFA) of the ESC. Eur J Heart Fail. 2012;14(8):803-69.
15. Patel MR, White RD, Abbara S, Bluemke DA, Herfkens RJ, Picard M, et al. 2013 ACCF/ACR/ASE/ASNC/SCCT/SCMR appropriate utilization of cardiovascular imaging in heart failure: a joint report of the American College of Radiology Appropriateness Criteria Committee and the American College of Cardiology Foundation Appropriate Use Criteria Task Force. J Am Coll Cardiol. 2013;61(21):2207-31.

16. Pennell DJ, Udelson JE, Arai AE, Bozkurt B, Cohen AR, Galanello R, et al. Cardiovascular function and treatment in beta-thalassemia major: a consensus statement from the American Heart Association. Circulation. 2013;128(3):281-308.
17. Soriano CJ, Ridocci F, Estornell J, Jimenez J, Martinez V, De Velasco JA. Noninvasive diagnosis of coronary artery disease in patients with heart failure and systolic dysfunction of uncertain etiology, using late gadolinium-enhanced cardiovascular magnetic resonance. J Am Coll Cardiol. 2005;45(5):743-8.
18. Syed IS, Glockner JF, Feng D, Araoz PA, Martinez MW, Edwards WD, et al. Role of cardiac magnetic resonance imaging in the detection of cardiac amyloidosis. JACC Cardiovasc Imaging. 2010;3(2):155-64.
19. Taylor AJ, Cerqueira M, Hodgson JM, Mark D, Min J, O'Gara P, et al. ACCF/SCCT/ACR/AHA/ASE/ASNC/NASCI/SCAI/SCMR 2010 appropriate use criteria for cardiac computed tomography. A report of the American College of Cardiology Foundation appropriate use criteria task force, the society of cardiovascular computed tomography, the American College of Radiology, the American Heart Association, the American Society of Echocardiography, the American Society of Nuclear Cardiology, the North American Society for Cardiovascular Imaging, the Society for Cardiovascular Angiography and Interventions, and the Society for Cardiovascular Magnetic Resonance. J Am Coll Cardiol. 2010;56(22):1864-94.
20. Warnes CA, Williams RG, Bashore TM, Child JS, Connolly HM, Dearani JA, et al. ACC/AHA 2008 guidelines for the management of adults with congenital heart disease: a report of the American College of Cardiology/American Heart Association Task Force on Practice Guidelines (writing committee to develop guidelines on the management of adults with congenital heart disease). Developed in Collaboration With the American Society of Echocardiography, Heart Rhythm Society, International Society for Adult Congenital Heart Disease, Society for Cardiovascular Angiography and Interventions, and Society of Thoracic Surgeons. J Am Coll Cardiol. 2008;52(23):e143-263.
21. Wu KC, Weiss RG, Thiemann DR, Kitagawa K, Schmidt A, Dalal D, et al. Late gadolinium enhancement by cardiovascular magnetic resonance heralds an adverse prognosis in nonischemic cardiomyopathy. J Am Coll Cardiol. 2008;51(25):2414-21.
22. Yancy CW, Jessup M, Bozkurt B, Masoudi FA, Butler J, McBride PE, et al. 2013 ACCF/AHA guideline for the management of heart failure: A report of the American College of Cardiology Foundation/American Heart Association Task Force on practice guidelines. J Am Coll Cardiol. 2013;62(16):1495-539.
23. Zikria JF, Machnicki S, Rhim E, Bhatti T, Graham RE. MRI of patients with cardiac pacemakers: a review of the medical literature. AJR Am J Roentgenol. 2011;196(2):390-401.

8
CHAPTER

When to Discharge the Heart Failure Patient?

Benjamin A Kipper

INTRODUCTION

Heart failure (HF) is one of the leading causes of hospital admission, morbidity, and mortality in the United States. Acute exacerbations of HF often lead to hospitalizations and adverse outcomes of morbidity and mortality. Once admitted and stabilized, the next question in managing these patients is determining when they can be discharged. One in four patients hospitalized with HF is readmitted within the first 30 days and many of these hospitalizations can be prevented if care is optimized prior to the patient leaving the hospital. This problem is further complicated by the fact that the frequency of hospitalizations is directly correlated with risk of death. Decreasing hospital readmission rates will aid in the better management of these HF patients and help reduce the morbid course of their disease. Reducing readmission rates also decreases the financial burden faced by patients and the health care. This chapter aims at discussing a particular algorithm that helps identify ideal conditions for discharge (Algorithm 1).

INITIAL PATIENT EVALUATION

Precipitating Event

Upon initial presentation of the HF patient, it is vital to determine the underlying cause of the acute exacerbation. Regardless of symptoms, it is vital that underlying disease etiology be identified

When to Discharge the Heart Failure Patient?

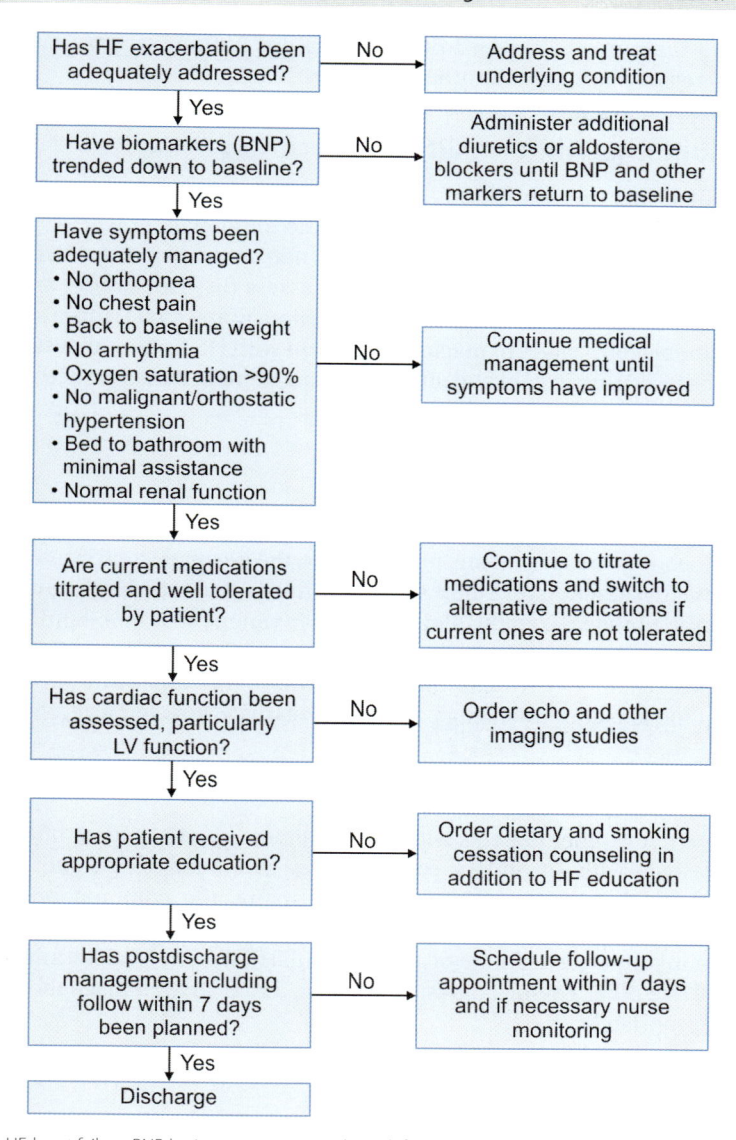

```
Has HF exacerbation been adequately addressed?
  │ No → Address and treat underlying condition
  │ Yes
  ▼
Have biomarkers (BNP) trended down to baseline?
  │ No → Administer additional diuretics or aldosterone blockers until BNP and other markers return to baseline
  │ Yes
  ▼
Have symptoms been adequately managed?
  • No orthopnea
  • No chest pain
  • Back to baseline weight
  • No arrhythmia
  • Oxygen saturation >90%
  • No malignant/orthostatic hypertension
  • Bed to bathroom with minimal assistance
  • Normal renal function
  │ No → Continue medical management until symptoms have improved
  │ Yes
  ▼
Are current medications titrated and well tolerated by patient?
  │ No → Continue to titrate medications and switch to alternative medications if current ones are not tolerated
  │ Yes
  ▼
Has cardiac function been assessed, particularly LV function?
  │ No → Order echo and other imaging studies
  │ Yes
  ▼
Has patient received appropriate education?
  │ No → Order dietary and smoking cessation counseling in addition to HF education
  │ Yes
  ▼
Has postdischarge management including follow within 7 days been planned?
  │ No → Schedule follow-up appointment within 7 days and if necessary nurse monitoring
  │ Yes
  ▼
Discharge
```

HF, heart failure; BNP, brain natriuretic peptide; LV, left ventricular.

ALGORITHM 1: When to discharge heart failure patient-algorithm

so as to correct, and not just mask the underlying problem. If the underlying cause of the exacerbation is not managed properly, and the acute event is only managed symptomatically, the patient will undoubtedly return to the hospital for future exacerbations, increasing both morbidity and mortality.

Biomarker Abnormalities

Initial labs drawn upon admission to the hospital provide valuable prognostic and diagnostic value to the patient with a HF exacerbation. Markers such as brain natriuretic peptide (BNP), troponins, and others can be used to assess disease severity and shift from patient baseline values (if previously assessed). These are valuable tools when managing the patient with HF, as they allow for lab-based assessment and efficacy of management in this particular cohort of people.

Weight Gain or Fluid Retention

Due to the frequency of hemodynamic instability often seen in the HF patient, many patients presenting to the hospital show signs of renal dysfunction and fluid retention. This is evidenced frequently in the physical exam by elevated jugular venous pressure, fluid in the lungs, lower extremity edema, ascites, and most frequently rapid weight gain. When determining ideal discharge time, physicians should aim at normalizing patient fluid status to euvolemic levels.

Secondary Comorbidities

Like many other patients with chronic illness, the HF patient often presents with secondary comorbidities that often contribute to disease progression. While there are many, the common ones include diabetes, renal dysfunction, and respiratory infections. Upon primary evaluation of a patient with HF, it is vital to determine if these other comorbidities are present, and if so to manage them appropriately.

Cognitive Assessment

Cognitive impairment is frequently seen in the HF patient as the heart can fail to provide adequate blood supply to the brain causing delirium. Because this can present similar to dementia and drug use, it is increasingly important to identify cognitive impairments, which can then be compared to baseline. A cognitive assessment allows physicians to assess if cognitive decline is caused by the exacerbation or another underlying condition.

WHEN TO DISCHARGE

Trending Biomarkers: Brain Natriuretic Peptide

The traditional biomarker for HF and volume overload is BNP, elevations of which have been shown to correlate with HF exacerbations. In a patient without significant HF, BNP levels are usually below 100 pg/mL; however, during an exacerbation, levels often rises to greater than 400 pg/mL. These cutoff values are considered ideal, unfortunately, many patients presenting with HF may have baseline BNP value well above 100 pg/mL due to the chornic nature of their disease. This makes it increasingly important to determine a baseline or "dry" value of BNP that allows physicians to determine significant deviations that may indicate excess fluid retention. A BNP level that is significantly deviated from baseline indicates fluid retention and an ongoing HF exacerbation. This is commonly known as a "wet" BNP because BNP is a strong predictor of adverse events, it is vital that high values be driven down prior to discharge. By lowering the BNP values back to baseline (or as close as possible), future and immediate exacerbations can be prevented. If BNP values remain elevated at discharge (>400 pg/mL), this may indicate an elevated "dry" BNP value or a need for further volume depletion. If the BNP value remains high despite aggressive treatment another approach is to use aldosterone blockers along with home monitoring and a return visit within one week to reduce readmission rates.

Because of the high prognostic and diagnostic value of BNP, it can be used as a guide for appropriate treatment and may help identify ideal physiologic conditions for discharge (once it has returned to near baseline).

Other Biomarkers to be Considered

Recent evidence has identified additional biomarkers useful in the management of patients with HF. These include markers such as: ST-2, neutrophil gelatinase-associated lipocalin (NGAL), galectin-3, and mid-regional-proadrenomedullin. High levels of these markers have all been shown to correlate with high mortality rates, some even outperforming the HF standard BNP. While these markers are not yet standards of care in patients with HF, they are available and can be ordered if traditional tools and assessments are inadequate in the assessment of a particular HF patient.

Symptom Management

One of the keys to determine if a patient with HF is ready for discharge is symptom management and control. Symptoms that should be adequately managed are listed below:

- Orthopnea: patients should be able to lie flat (or at least near their baseline), comfortably, before being discharged from the hospital
- Chest pain: while chest pain is not a common symptom of HF, it may indicate coronary artery disease which indicates a need for further evaluation. Prior to discharge, patients should be experiencing no chest pain
- Hypertension: patients with orthostatic or malignant hypertension should have these issues addressed prior to discharge to prevent future adverse events caused by these conditions
- Arrhythmia: patients should receive medications to control problematic dysrhythmias and to prevent emboli formation, if indicated
- Oxygen saturation: a baseline oxygen saturation of 90% with or without additional oxygen should be achieved prior to discharge, depending on if they were previously using supplemental oxygen (again, knowledge of baseline value is helpful)
- Ambulatory capacity: many patients with HF are confined to a wheelchair or have difficulty walking, but, if possible, patients should be able to move from bed to toilet with minimal assistance, particularly, if they will be taking a diuretic
- Weight gain: before discharge, patients should be returned to baseline weight and euvolemic status. This is often achieved through aggressive diuresis
- Treatment of secondary medical issues: as many patients with HF have other compounding illnesses and comorbidities that can contribute to readmission, it is vital that these be managed prior to discharge.
- Renal function assessment: one of the main comorbidities associated with HF is renal dysfunction. Because the kidneys are susceptible to irreversible damage it is vital to determine renal function prior to discharge. Biomarkers such as creatinine and blood urea nitrogen are traditionally used to assess renal dysfunction. Recently, other biomarkers, such as NGAL, show promise in identifying kidney injury and dysfunction much sooner than the traditional marekers.

Pharmacologic Management and Education

Medical management of the HF patient is vital for proper discharge conditions. Standard guidelines state patients with HF should be started on β-blockers and an angiotensin converting enzyme inhibitor, especially if there is reduced ejection fraction. Additionally, before discharge, patient should demonstrate tolerance to new medications and be transitioned from intravenous to oral medications. Due of the complicated drug regimens many of these patients face, education about medication should also be provided to ensure appropriate dosing and scheduling.

Complicated drug regimens that are used to treat HF and other comorbidities are very specific and sensitive to dosage timing. These complex schedules can be conducive to mistakes as well as nonadherence. Medication nonadherence is a growing concern and is a leading cause of negative patient outcomes, higher readmission rates, and higher healthcare costs. Frequently, it may be important for the patient to be educated by the treating staff about the medications they will be taking and about the health consequences of nonadherence. Postdischarge follow-up appointments should be scheduled before discharge which should include reminders of drug schedules and adherence reports. Additionally, much research is being conducted to develop effective predischarge and postdischarge systems to help patients take their medications correctly. Reducing medication nonadherence is a challenging task, but it does significantly improve patient outcomes and reduce hospital readmissions.

ASSESSMENT OF CARDIAC FUNCTION

Patients coming into the hospital for exacerbations of HF often have previously documented assessments of cardiac function. However, if undocumented, it is vitally important to determine baseline cardiac parameters, particularly, left ventricular ejection fraction. This type of useful information can often be achieved through echocardiography, ECG, biomarker levels, and magnetic resonance imaging. This allows physicians to determine if patients are presenting with new abnormalities and pathologies during future clinical visits and hospital readmissions.

Assessing Functional Status

Physical and cognitive functional status is an important consideration when planning to discharge a patient with HF.

Common among patients with HF are frailty, cognitive impairment, and limited social and financial support. Depression is also a common condition among patients with HF. Because of these factors, patients can find it difficult to comply with plans for new lifestyle changes they may need to make or with their new and often complicated medication regimens. In this situation, a multidisciplinary team is, especially, useful in addressing each difficulty in hopes of increasing motivation and overall compliance.

Management of Other Comorbidities

Especially in elderly patients, comorbidities can further complicate HF treatment. Improper management of these complications can ultimately contribute to readmission rates. Common comorbidities, such as respiratory disease, renal dysfunction, and diabetes mellitus, need to be monitored closely by the treating staff. Polypharmacy is often unavoidable when treating patients with HF and multiple comorbidities. Because of this, systems need to be in place which allows the treating staff to review a patient's medication list, ensure efficacy of the medications, and to identify and avoid adverse drug interactions. Properly recognizing and treating any and all comorbidities does significantly improve outcome for patients with HF.

PATIENT EDUCATION

Often, patients with HF are discharged with an inadequate understanding about their health, medications, and plan of action. Compliance with low salt diets, exercise regimens, smoking cessation, and medication schedules requires lifestyle changes, which can be very difficult. By engaging with the patient and their support group in two-way communication, trained staff can more effectively tailor education sessions to best fit the needs of the patient. Many studies have also shown that using a multidisciplinary approach to therapy can boost compliance. Ensuring proper education to the patient and their families can help drastically reduce hospital readmission rates.

POSTDISCHARGE MANAGEMENT

Postdischarge management of patients with HF is crucial in decreasing morbidity, mortality, and future hospital readmission in these patients. Discharge management should include: patient monitoring via telephone within 3 days of discharge, clinical evaluation within 1 week of discharge, daily weight assessments to identify shifts in volume status, and if indicated blood pressure recordings. Studies have demonstrated that only 37.5% of patients discharged from the hospital with HF receive a follow-up appointment within 7 days. This number is not ideal, as recent evidence has shown that hospitals that have low rates of early physician follow-up have higher rates of rehospitalization compared to those with higher rates of early physician follow-up. Adequate postdischarge management is vital and may help decrease frequency of future adverse events and hospitalizations.

CONCLUSION

The management of a patient with heart failure should be approached with the goal of returning the patient back to their normal baseline, or as close to that normal baseline as possible. When contemplating discharge for this group of patients it is vital to ensure: the patient is euvolemic, optimally managed on their medication, treated for associated comorbidities, functioning as close to their baseline as possible, and scheduled for appropriate follow up. This will help prevent hospital readmission and decrease the morbidity associated with heart failure and its acute exacerbations.

KEY POINTS

- Clinical evaluation to determine the underlying cause of a heart failure (HF) exacerbation is necessary for appropriate management and care of the HF patient
- Treatment should be aimed at treating the underlying cause of the exacerbation in addition to treating symptoms
- The use of biomarkers like brain natriuretic peptide, creatinine, blood urea nitrogen, neutrophil gelatinase-associated lipocalin, and others combined with physical examination can help physicians identify optimal volume status and patient baseline. These markers can also be used to follow disease progression and efficacy of treatment
- Optimal volume status should be attained and maintained prior to leaving the hospital
- Prior to discharge, all patients should be free of acute HF symptoms, be able to perform activities of daily living, and tolerate oral medications
- After being discharged, postdischarge care and follow-up is vital in preventing future hospital readmissions and HF exacerbations.

SUGGESTED READINGS

1. Aghel A, Shrestha K, Mullens W, Borowski A, Tang WH. Serum neutrophil gelatinase-associated lipocalin (NGAL) in predicting worsening renal function in acute decompensated heart failure. J Card Fail. 2010;16(1):49-54.
2. Damman K, Masson S, Hillege HL, Maggioni AP, Voors AA, Opasich C, et al. Clinical outcome of renal tubular damage in chronic heart failure. Eur Heart J. 2011;32(21):2705-12.
3. Hernandez AF, Greiner MA, Fonarow GC, Hammill BG, Heidenreich PA, Yancy CW, et al. Relationship between early physician follow-up and 30-day readmission among Medicare beneficiaries hospitalized for heart failure. JAMA. 2010;303(17):1716-22.
4. Ho PM, Bryson CL, Rumsfeld JS. Medication adherence: its importance in cardiovascular outcomes. Circulation. 2009;119(23):3028-35.
5. Jaarsma T. Inter-professional team approach to patients with heart failure. Heart. 2005;91(6):832-8.
6. Lang CC, Mancini DM. Non-cardiac comorbidities in chronic heart failure. Heart. 2007;93(6):665-71.
7. Logeart D, Thabut G, Jourdain P, Chavelas C, Beyne P, Beauvais F, et al. Predischarge B-type natriuretic peptide assay for identifying patients at high risk of re-admission after decompensated heart failure. J Am Coll Cardiol. 2004;43(4):635-41.
8. Macdonald S, Arendts G, Nagree Y, Xu XF. Neutrophil Gelatinase-Associated Lipocalin (NGAL) predicts renal injury in acute decompensated cardiac failure: a prospective observational study. BMC Cardiovasc Disord. 2012;12:8.
9. Maisel A, Mueller C, Nowak R, Peacock WF, Landsberg JW, Ponikowski P, et al. Mid-region pro-hormone markers for diagnosis and prognosis in acute dyspnea: results from the BACH (biomarkers in acute heart failure) trial. J Am Coll Cardiol. 2010;55(19):2062-76.
10. Maisel AS, Mueller C, Fitzgerald R, Brikhan R, Hiestand BC, Iqbal N, et al. Prognostic utility of plasma neutrophil gelatinase-associated lipocalin in patients with acute heart failure: The NGAL EvaLuation along with B-type NaTriuretic Peptide in acutely decompensated heart failure (GALLANT) trial. Eur J Heart Fail. 2011;13(8):846-51.
11. Paul S. Hospital discharge education for patients with heart failure: What really works and what is the evidence? Crit Care Nurse. 2008;28(2):66-82.
12. Phillips CO, Wright SM, Kern DE, Singa RM, Shepperd S, Rubin HR. Comprehensive discharge planning with postdischarge support for older patients with congestive heart failure: a meta-analysis. JAMA. 2004;291(11):1358-67.
13. Setoguchi S, Stevenson LW, Schneeweiss S. Repeated hospitalizations predict mortality in the community population with heart failure. Am Heart J. 2007;154(2):260-6.
14. van Kimmenade RR, Januzzi JL Jr, Ellinor PT, Sharma UC, Bakker JA, Low AF, et al. Utility of amino-terminal pro-brain natriuretic peptide, galectin-3, and apelin for the evaluation of patients with acute heart failure. J Am Coll Cardiol. 2006;48(6):1217-24.

વિભાગ 2

SECTION

Heart Failure in the Hospital

9
CHAPTER

Approach to Diuretics in the Hospital

Meghana G Halkar, Wai Hong W Tang

INTRODUCTION

Patients with heart failure often get admitted to the hospital when they have signs and symptoms of worsening congestion, fluid retention, dyspnea, exercise intolerance, or failure to thrive. As such, treatment to relieve congestion is still the mainstay. For the goal to remove salt and volume, diuretic drugs (particularly loop diuretics) are very effective. Currently available diuretics are divided into five main classes, with a brief outline of their pharmacologic features (Table 1) and key effects (Table 2). A glance at the mechanisms of action helps us better understand their effects—both therapeutic and adverse, as they shuttle electrolytes across channels at various levels of the renal tubule (Fig. 1).

EVIDENCE BASED MEDICINE FOR USING DIURETICS IN THE HOSPITAL

Two reassuring landmark studies help shed light on safety of aggressive diuretic use in the hospital for acute decompensated heart failure (ADHF) (Table 3).

GENERAL CONCEPTS

- The overarching goal should always be long-term maintenance of euvolemia than seeking short-term gratification without considering adverse consequences

TABLE 1: Pharmacokinetics and dosing of diuretics

Diuretics	Bioavailability	Onset of action		Time to peak		Elimination of half-life ($t_{1/2}$)			Duration of action		Oral dose	
	Oral	Oral	IV	Oral	IV	Normal subjects Oral	Patients with renal insufficiency Oral	Patients with congestive heart failure Oral	Oral	IV	Initial dose	Maximal dose
Loop diuretics												
Bumetanide	80–100%	30–60 min	2–3 min	1–2 h	15–30 min	1 hour	1.6 h	1.3 h	4–6 h	2–3 h	1 mg QD or BID	10 mg/day
Furosemide	60–64%	30–60 min	5 min	1–2 h	30 min	1.5–2 h	2.8 h	2.7 h	6–8 h	2 h	40 mg QD or BID	400 mg/day
Torsemide	80%	<60 min	<10 min	1–2 h	<1 hour	3–4 h	4–5 h	6 h	18–24 h	18–24 h	10 mg QD or BID	200 mg/day
Thiazide diuretics												
Chlorthiazide	30–50%	2 h	15 min	4 h	30 min	45–120 min	Prolonged	No change	6–12 h	6–12 h	500 mg	1,000 mg
Chlorthalidone	64%	2 h	NA	2–6 h	NA	40 h	Prolonged	ND	48–72 h	NA	50–100 mg/day	200 mg/day
Hydrochlorothiazide	65–75%	2 h	NA	4–6 h	NA	5–14 h	Prolonged	No change	6–12 h	NA	25 mg QD	200 mg/day
Indapamide	93%	1–3 h	NA	2 h	NA	Biphasic 14 and 25 h	ND	ND	36 h	NA	2.5 mg QD	5 mg/day

Continued

Approach to Diuretics in the Hospital

Continued

Diuretics	Bioavailability	Onset of action		Time to peak		Elimination of half-life ($t_{1/2}$)			Duration of action		Oral dose	
						Normal subjects	Patients with renal insufficiency	Patients with congestive heart failure				
	Oral	Oral	IV	Oral	IV	Oral	Oral	Oral	Oral	IV	Initial dose	Maximal dose
Metolazone	40–65%	1 hour	NA	2 h	NA	14 h	Prolonged	No change	12–24 h	NA	2.5–5 mg QD or BID	20 mg/day
Potassium-sparing diuretics												
Amiloride	15–25%	2–3 h	NA	6–10 h	NA	17–26 h	100 h	ND	24 h	NA	5 mg QD	15–20 mg/day
Eplerenone	69%	Unknown	NA	1.5 h	NA	4–6 h	No change	Oral	Unknown	NA	25 mg QD	50 mg/day
Spironolactone	65%	Unknown	NA	3–4 h	NA	1.4 h	No change	No change	2–3 days	NA	12.5–25 mg QD	25–50 mg/day
Triamterene	50%	2–4 h	NA	3 h	NA	2–5 h	Prolonged	ND	7–9 h	NA	100 mg BID	300 mg/day
Carbonic anhydrase inhibitors												
Acetazolamide		2 h	2 min	2–4 h	15 min	3–6 h	Prolonged	Unknown	8–12 h	4–5 h	250–375 mg QD	375 mg/day
Vasopressin antagonists												
Conivaptan	100%	NA	Unknown	NA	2–4 h	5–8 h	No change	Unknown	NA	12 h	NA	NA
Tolvaptan	ND	2–4 h	NA	4–8 h	NA	5–12 h	No change	No change	24 h	NA	15 mg QD	60 mg/day

IV, intravenous; NA, not applicable; ND, not determined; QD, once daily; BID, twice daily; min, minute; h, hour.

TABLE 2: Key features of different diuretic classes

Diuretic	Site of action	Effect	Role in acute decompensated heart failure
Loop diuretic	Loop of Henle: Medullary thick ascending limb	Natriuresis, diuresis, PG up-regulation	Most powerful and first line
Thiazide diuretic	Distal convoluted tubule	Natriuresis, hypokalemia: aldosterone and RAAS activation	Conjunction with loop to overcome resistance
Potassium sparing diuretic	Collecting duct	Natriuresis, diuresis	Conjunction with thiazide and loop for K$^+$ sparing effects
Vasopressin receptor antagonist	V1a and V2 receptors	Diuresis	To overcome euvolemic and hypervolemic hyponatremia
Carbonic anhydrase inhibitors	Proximal convoluted tubule	Inhibit bicarbonate absorption	Weak diuretics, very rarely used to overcome alkalosis

RAAS, renin-angiotensin-aldosterone system; PG, prostaglandin.

Approach to Diuretics in the Hospital

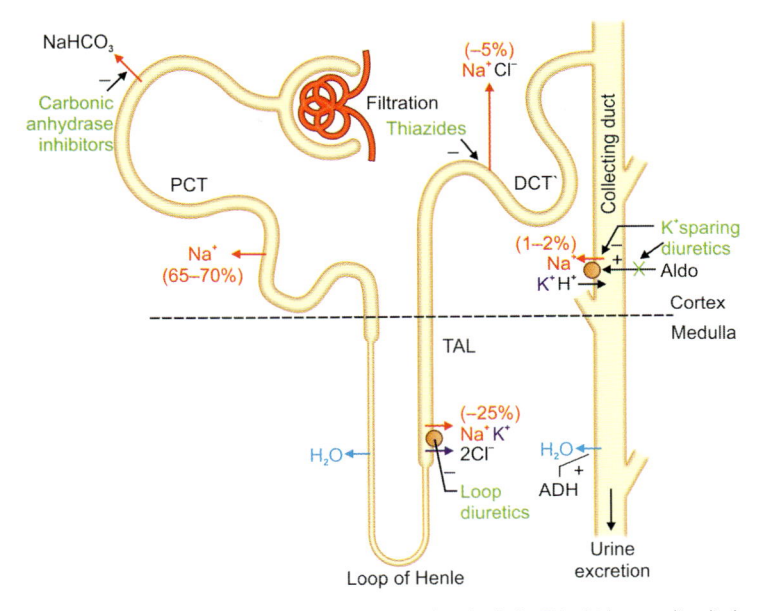

PCT, proximal convoluted tubule; DCT, distal convoluted tubule; TAL, thick ascending limb; ADH, antidiuretic hormone.

FIG. 1: Different types of diuretics and their sites of action in the nephron

- It is important to distinguish between intravascular and total body volume overload
- Diuretics can only be effective if there is excess salt and water in the body and if this excess is accessible and can be refilled through the vasculature
- It is paramount to assess and adequately estimate volume status regularly in order to monitor treatment progress, also bearing in mind that certain forms of restrictive and constrictive cardiomyopathies have far less reserve since their mobilizable volume is often reduced
- The pace of salt and water removal is a crucial determinant of balance between maintenance of perfusion and adequate decongestion
- Diuretic resistance can often be overcome by simply increasing the dosage of the drug in the short term
- Not all congestive signs and symptoms require immediate pharmacologic therapy with diuretics. A good example is dependent edema which is more chronic developing over weeks to months can often be treated by nonpharmacologic measures.

TABLE 3: Landmark randomized control trials on diuretic therapy in acute decompensated heart failure

Clinical trial	Design	Study Scheme	Outcomes assessed	Results
DOSE-AHF	Prospective double blind RCT	2 × 2 factorial design: high vs. low dose IV loop diuretics and continuous vs. bolus infusion	Global assessment of symptoms and mean change of creatinine at 72 h	No significant difference in continuous vs. bolus infusion. High dose better than low dose in terms of GAS and secondary endpoints
CARRESS-HF	Prospective RCT	1:1 randomization of patients with ADHF and worsening renal function to UF vs. stepped pharmacologic care	Change in serum creatinine and weight at day 4	Comparable effects in two groups. UF associated with worsening adverse events, with no advantage over stepped pharmacologic approach

DOSE-AHF, Diuretic Optimization Strategies Evaluation in Acute Heart Failure; CARRESS-HF, Cardiorenal Rescue Study in Acute Decompensated Heart Failure; RCT, randomized controlled trials; HF, heart failure; UF, ultrafiltration; ADHF, acute decompensated heart failure; GAS, global assessment scale.

APPROACH TO USING DIURETICS IN THE HOSPITAL

A general approach to using diuretic therapy in the hospital is summarized below (Algorithm 1).

Does the patient need intravenous diuretic therapy?
- Not all patients admitted with heart failure have congestion as the underlying cause
- Some forms of congestion are easily amenable to oral diuretics without causing adverse consequences [heart failure with a preserved ejection fraction (HFpEF)].

Does the patient have evidence of congestion?
- An objective assessment of the degree of congestion is vital, in order to distinguish volume redistribution from overload

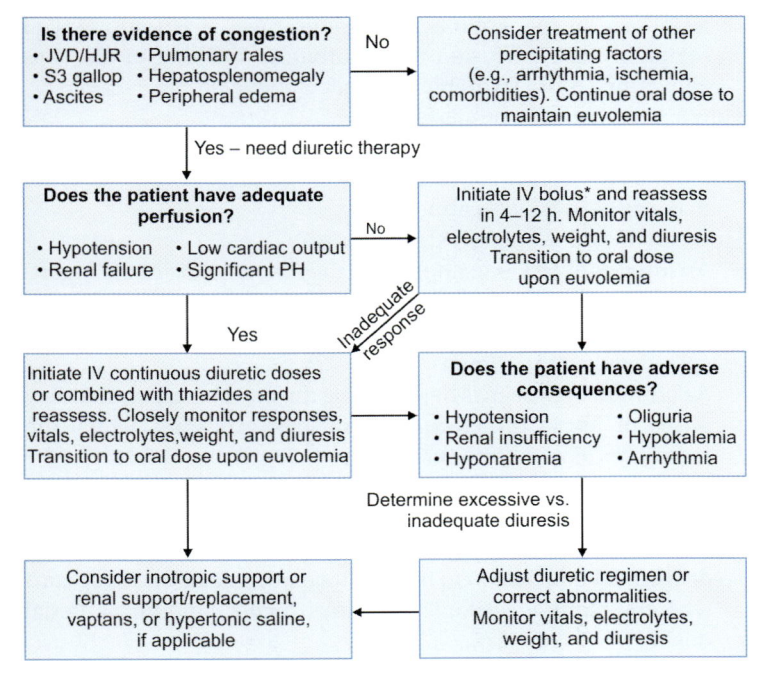

```
Is there evidence of congestion?
• JVD/HJR    • Pulmonary rales
• S3 gallop  • Hepatosplenomegaly
• Ascites    • Peripheral edema
       │                    No → Consider treatment of other precipitating factors
       │                         (e.g., arrhythmia, ischemia, comorbidities). Continue oral dose to maintain euvolemia
       ↓ Yes – need diuretic therapy

Does the patient have adequate perfusion?
• Hypotension    • Low cardiac output
• Renal failure  • Significant PH
       │                    No → Initiate IV bolus* and reassess in 4–12 h. Monitor vitals, electrolytes, weight, and diuresis. Transition to oral dose upon euvolemia
       ↓ Yes                      ↓ Inadequate response

Initiate IV continuous diuretic doses or combined with thiazides and reassess. Closely monitor responses, vitals, electrolytes, weight, and diuresis. Transition to oral dose upon euvolemia
                              →  Does the patient have adverse consequences?
                                 • Hypotension          • Oliguria
                                 • Renal insufficiency  • Hypokalemia
                                 • Hyponatremia         • Arrhythmia

                              Determine excessive vs. inadequate diuresis

Consider inotropic support or      ←   Adjust diuretic regimen or correct
renal support/replacement,             abnormalities. Monitor vitals,
vaptans, or hypertonic saline,         electrolytes, weight, and diuresis
if applicable
```

*Treatment dose: 1–2.5 × home oral daily in IV (DOSE-AHF); Goal: target 2–3 L/day urine output (CARRESS-HF).

JVD, jugular venous distention; HJR, hepatojugular reflux; IV, intravenous; PH, pulmonary hypertension; DOSE-AHF, Diuretic Optimization Strategies Evaluation in Acute Heart Failure study; CARRESS-HF, Cardiorenal Rescue Study in Acute Decompensated Heart Failure; S3, third heart sound.

ALGORITHM 1: General approach to using diuretic therapy in the hospital (in cases of flash pulmonary edema from ischemic mitral regurgitation, atrial fibrillation with rapid ventricular rate, or defibrillator shock, where vasodilator therapy or rate or rhythm control may be more appropriate, respectively). Home diuretics can be continued at the same doses in such cases.

Jugular venous distention (JVD), third heart sound (S3) and hepatojugular reflux (HJR) are far more indicative of the need for diuretics.

Is the congestion amenable to removal?
- This is an essential question, especially, in settings of marginal hemodynamics where it might be beneficial to initiate continuous infusion of loop diuretics in order to maintain renal perfusion while optimizing volume removal
- Although the Diuretic Optimization Strategies Evaluation in Acute Heart Failure (DOSE-AHF) study did not show any advantage of this approach for routine use, it is important to maintain renal perfusion and continuous infusion of diuretics allows for a more favorable pharmacokinetic profile.

How should diuretics be started?
- This involves a careful assessment of volume status and parameters that can be followed through the treatment in order to construct a good treatment plan.

How can the kidney handle the diuretics?
- An important task is to appreciate the functionality of the organs which diuretics are dependent on—the kidneys.
- There is limited consensus on this topic and no standard specified dosing regimen
- A common approach is determining the dose based on standing doses of home diuretics and previous exposures which are surrogates of renal responsiveness
- For most instances, intravenous loop diuretics (furosemide and bumetanide) are common choices of therapy
- In the case of furosemide with a bioavailability of 50% for oral drugs, a 1:1 conversion to bolus intravenous dosing is a safe start whereby many elect for 2–2.5 times higher amount as initial dosing
- The DOSE-AHF study demonstrated that there were no detrimental consequences and a trend toward more prompt symptomatic relief with higher dosing approach
- In many instances, bolus administration of diuretics several times a day may further achieve decongestive purposes.

How much volume does one aim to remove and over how long?

- In congestive states, patients can easily achieve 1–2 L of net negative fluid balance that corresponds to a 1–3 kg drop in body weight
- However, both tracking methods may be grossly inaccurate and, therefore, inquiring about subjective improvement of congestive symptoms and signs is often helpful
- The pace and duration of decongestive therapy will depend largely on determining how to optimally remove maximal amount of fluid without jeopardizing end-organ perfusion or electrolyte imbalance.

How does the patient respond?
- The first 4–12 hours are perhaps the most crucial in making interim decisions to tailor therapy to the individual condition and response
- In many instances, care transition from the emergency department to the floor may lead to interruptions in meticulous monitoring of drug responses and should be avoided
- Inadequate responses may sometimes be evident requiring increase in the drug doses or transition to continuous infusion strategies.

What to monitor during diuresis?
- Hours after administration: urine output, weight loss, and symptom relief
- Blood pressure monitoring: to avoid hypotensive response and adjustment of regime accordingly by slowing diuretic or concomitant drug dose lowering
- Electrolyte imbalances to be watched: hyponatremia, hypokalemia, and hypomagnesemia, with appropriate repletion to avoid arrhythmias
- Watch for contraction alkalosis and azotemia
- Nonsensitive and nonspecific measures sometimes indicative of diuresis include: hemoconcentration, reflected by rise in hemoglobin, total protein, or albumin.

How to handle excessive diuresis?
Handling of excessive diuresis is explained in algorithm 2.

How to handle inadequate diuresis?
- The concept of diuretic resistance has no formal definition other than a clinically recognized phenomenon of inability to achieve euvolemia despite high or increasing diuretic dosing
- Most cases are due to inadequate diuretic dosing and can be overcome by higher doses greater frequencies and more consistent administration (i.e., continuous infusion)

Algorithms in Heart Failure

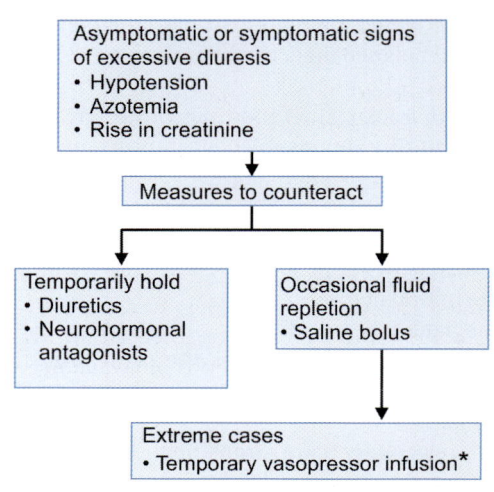

```
┌─────────────────────────────────┐
│ Asymptomatic or symptomatic     │
│ signs of excessive diuresis     │
│ • Hypotension                   │
│ • Azotemia                      │
│ • Rise in creatinine            │
└────────────────┬────────────────┘
                 ▼
      ┌──────────────────────┐
      │ Measures to counteract│
      └──────┬────────┬───────┘
             ▼        ▼
┌────────────────────┐  ┌────────────────────┐
│ Temporarily hold   │  │ Occasional fluid   │
│ • Diuretics        │  │ repletion          │
│ • Neurohormonal    │  │ • Saline bolus     │
│   antagonists      │  └─────────┬──────────┘
└────────────────────┘            ▼
                        ┌────────────────────────────────┐
                        │ Extreme cases                  │
                        │ • Temporary vasopressor infusion* │
                        └────────────────────────────────┘
```

*Supportive evidence for renovascular effects of dopamine is still lacking.

ALGORITHM 2: Handling of excessive diuresis

- In more serious cases, type 1 (acute) cardiorenal syndrome may preclude effective decongestive therapy:
    ○ The first task is to tackle "diuretic resistance" is to determine if inadequate renal perfusion in the cause leading to diminished delivery of the drug to the kidney. Increasing the diuretic dosing and frequent spacing of doses to avoid rebound sodium retention is important
    ○ Another phenomenon called "braking phenomenon" occurs whereby the distal renal tubular cells undergo hypertrophy during chronic diuretic use resulting in increased sodium and water absorption at this level. Here, pretreatment with thiazides in combination with loop diuretics helps overcome the problem
    ○ Activation of renin-angiotensin-aldosterone system (RAAS) and sympathetic response due to intravascular volume depletion from diuretic therapy may cause a vasoconstrictor response and further decrease in renal perfusion, thereby worsening resistance
- Other common methods to overcome diuretic resistance are addition of thiazide and carbonic anhydrase inhibitors to loop diuretics achieving sequential blockade of nephrons, with careful monitoring of electrolytes and acid-base balance.

What should be done when the creatinine rises?

Approach to Diuretics in the Hospital

- The most important step is to confirm if there is still volume overload
- This can be achieved by paying attention to clinical signs such as body weight above dry weight, markedly elevated natriuretic peptide levels above baseline, and reproducible symptoms on exertion, even if the JVD is flat
- A volume directed stepwise approach of diuretic administration, whereby the pace of diuretic therapy is decreased, is helpful in cases of persistent Congestion and Worsening Renal Function as Illustrated in the Cardiorenal Rescue study in Acute Decompensated Heart Failure (CARRESS-HF) study
- Sometimes, a long-acting and more bioavailable oral diuretic (torsemide) may help and at other times temporarily with holding the dose to allow "refill" subsequently starting a lower dose may help
- One of the biggest mistakes is to hold neurohormonal antagonists (especially at discharge) while maintaining perfusion with ongoing diuretics
- When the evidence of intravascular depletion is clear, selectively individualized options include:
  - Holding diuretic
  - Holding nephrotoxins
  - Holding RAAS antagonists
  - Bolus saline infusion
- The key is to cautiously monitor and determine how to re-establish guideline directed medical therapy and achieve euvolemia prior to discharge.

Box 1: Side effects during diuretic therapy

Hypokalemia
- Goal K^+ >4 mEq/L to avoid lethal arrhythmias
- Aim for adequate total body magnesium (which does not correlate with serum magnesium and is difficult to measure)

Hypernatremia
- Due to increase in proportion of water excretion compared to sodium

Hyperuricemia
- Due to reduced glomerular filtration rate and solute excretion as well as decreased uric acid secretion into the tubular lumen
- Potential for acute gout flare: diuretic therapy should be continued while treating underlying gout flare

Ototoxicity
- Dose-dependent phenomenon
- Common with rapid intravenous bolus compared with slow continous infusion

What side effects to watch for?

How and when should home dosing be transitioned?

- Most often after achieving euvolemia, oral diuretic regimen restarted in order to maintain adequate intravascular volume
- Although there is no clear conversion guideline many follow the reverse intravenous to oral equivalent dosing conversion
- Contributors to rebound congestion include: noncompliance with salt restriction, use of nonsteroidal anti-inflammatory drugs which cause prostaglandin inhibition (normally responsible for afferent renal vasodilation). More serious cases of recurrent congestion include advanced cardiorenal compromise possibly requiring renal replacement therapy versus palliative care.

What we do not know yet?

- How can diuretic response be adequately assessed?
  - We do not have reliable measures of *in vivo* natriuresis. Input and output measurements are often inaccurate and for now, weight is a surrogate measure, which too can often be highly variable
- Do different modalities of removing salt and water make any differences on long-term consequences?
  - The first few days of aggressive diuretic therapy may not translate into long-term maintenance of euvolemia.

CONCLUSION

Diuretics have been the core of acute heart failure therapy and their use has largely been guided by expert opinion. The Diuretic Optimization Strategies Evaluation in Acute Heart Failure (DOSE-AHF) trial has helped us in understanding the permissible use of high dose loop diuretics with a finite yet tolerable detrimental effect on renal function. This has so far served as an important tool in managing patients with ADHF, but optimal management strategies still remain a challenge due to lack of long randomized control trials evaluating specific diuretic protocols, especially with respect to cardiorenal syndrome. Cardiorenal syndrome continues to remain a challenge in diuretic therapy; the precise role of ultrafiltration besides salvage therapy still remains to be determined. Further studies are required to answer the question of minimizing worsening renal function and mortality while treating the volume overload effectively in this progressive syndrome. Until then, the best practice would be based on expert opinion and individualized to the clinical scenario.

Approach to Diuretics in the Hospital

KEY POINTS

- The long term goal of diuretic therapy in congestive heart failure is relief of acute congestion and maintenance of euvolemia
- Acute decompensated heart failure does not always mean overt volume overload; it is important to recognize that scenarios where only minimal use diuretics can achieve euvolemia with simultaneous treatment of precipitating factors
- Congestion must be approached keeping in mind the perfusion status with continuous infusion of loop diuretics being beneficial in hypotensive patients or those with underlying renal impairment
- In settings of normal perfusion initiating bolus dosing of intravenous loop diuretics at double the home dose and titrating the frequency and dosing per the initial 4–12 hour response is an effective method
- Transient worsening of renal function has no detrimental consequences as shown in the Diuretic Optimization Strategies Evaluation in Acute Heart Failure trial
- Rise in creatinine with diuretic therapy should be approached keeping in mind the volume status; excessive diuresis handled by temporarily holding diuretics and inadequate diuresis overcome by transition to continuous infusion of loop diuretics or ultrafiltration to slow down the pace of volume removal
- Diuretic resistance can be overcome by one of the followng methods: higher dosing, continuous infusion or addition of a different diuretic class for sequential nephron blockade
- Side effects including electrolyte imbalances should be treated during acute decongestive therapy with transition to oral diuretics once euvolemia is achieved.

SUGGESTED READINGS

1. Abraham WT, Hasan A. Diagnosis and management of heart failure. In: Fuster V, Walsh RA, Harrington RA, HurstrstA, (Eds). HMcGraw Hill Companies, Inc.; 2011.
2. Bart BA, Goldsmith SR, Lee KL, Givertz MM, O'Connor CM, Bull DA, et al. Ultrafiltration in decompensated heart failure with cardiorenal syndrome. N Engl J Med. 2012;367(24):2296-304.
3. Brater DC. Update in diuretic therapy: clinical pharmacology. Semin Nephrol. 2011;31(6):483-94.
4. Cavalcante JL, Khan S, Gheorghiade M. EVEREST study: Efficacy of Vasopressin Antagonism in Heart Failure Outcome Study with Tolvaptan. Expert Rev Cardiovasc Ther. 2008;6(10):1331-8.
5. Felker GM, Lee KL, Bull DA, Redfield MM, Stevenson LW, Goldsmith SR, et al. Diuretic strategies in patients with acute decompensated heart failure. N Engl J Med. 2011;364(9):797-805.

6. Heart Failure Society of America, Lindenfeld J, Albert NM, Boehmer JP, Collins SP, Ezekowitz JA, et al. HFSA 2010 Comprehensive Heart Failure Practice Guideline. J Card Fail. 2010;16(6):e1-194.
7. Jessup M, Abraham WT, Casey DE, Feldman AM, Francis GS, Ganiats TG, et al. 2009 focused update: ACCF/AHA Guidelines for the Diagnosis and Management of Heart Failure in Adults: a report of the American College of Cardiology Foundation/American Heart Association Task Force on Practice Guidelines: developed in collaboration with the International Society for Heart and Lung Transplantation. Circulation. 2009;119(14):1977-2016.
8. McMurray JJ, Adamopoulos S, Anker SD, Auricchio A, Böhm M, Dickstein K, et al. ESC Guidelines for the diagnosis and treatment of acute and chronic heart failure 2012: The Task Force for the Diagnosis and Treatment of Acute and Chronic Heart Failure 2012 of the European Society of Cardiology. Developed in collaboration with the Heart Failure Association (HFA) of the ESC. Eur Heart J. 2012;33(14):1787-847.
9. Volz EM, Felker GM. How to use diuretics in heart failure. Curr Treat Options Cardiovasc Med. 2009;11(6):426-32.

10
CHAPTER

Vasodilators in Acute Heart Failure

Shiro Ishihara, Alexandre Mebazaa

INTRODUCTION

According to large registries such as those of the GREAT network, many heart failure patients are hospitalized with normal or elevated blood pressure at presentation. Basically, vasoconstriction is the most important pathogenesis in patients with heart failure.

EFFECTS OF VASODILATORS IN ACUTELY DECOMPENSATED HEART FAILURE

Beneficial acute hemodynamic effects of vasodilators (VDs) are mostly related to the relief of vasoconstriction. Venodilation also leads to decrease in venous pressure and increase in organ's (kidney or liver) flow. Furthermore, a decrease in left ventricular afterload can lead to increase in cardiac output.

Accordingly, VDs can relief symptoms of dyspneic patients with acutely decompensated heart failure (ADHF) faster than diuretics do. Because of these favorable effects, the European Society of Cardiology guidelines and practical recommendations for the management of ADHF recommend VDs use with normal-to-high blood pressure (BP) at the time of admission.

CURRENTLY AVAILABLE VASODILATORS IN ACUTE DECOMPENSATED HEART FAILURE AND HOW TO USE IT (TABLE 1, ALGORITHM 1)

Spray, Sublingual, and Intravenous Nitroglycerin

Nitroglycerin mainly acts on venous side and also acts on arterial side. Nitroglycerin can unload the heart through lowering preload and afterload and increase cardiac output. Effects of nitroglycerin occur immediately after initiation and eliminate immediately after cessation. Intravenous nitroglycerin starts at 10 µg/min and should subsequently be titrated. Tachyphylaxis can be developed within 24 hours, and tolerance can be occurred on continuous use.

Nesiritide

Nesiritide, human brain natriuretic peptide, has variable effects, including on urinary output and sodium excretion. However, its main action is vasodilatory effect. Nesiritide can also reduce preload and afterload, and increase cardiac output. Nesiritide does not have tachyphylaxis.

Sodium Nitroprusside

Sodium nitroprusside acts on arterial side and venous side with balanced fashion. Nitroprusside can also reduce preload and afterload, and increase cardiac output. Invasive hemodynamic monitoring (arterial line) is needed to avoid hypotension. In general, nitroprusside starts at 0.3 µg/kg/min and titrates gradually. nitroprusside syringe must be covered because of its light sensitivity. Long-term use, in high doses, or renal dysfunction have been associated with the risk of isocyanate toxicity. To avoid rebound vasoconstriction, nitroprusside must be tapered gradually.

TABLE 1: Recommended dose of vasodilators

Drug	Full starting dose	Half dose
Nitroglycerin	Start with 10 µg/min, increase if needed	Start with 5 µg/min, increase if needed
Nesiritide	Bolus 2 µg/kg + infusion 0.01 µg/kg/min*	Bolus 1 µg/kg + infusion 0.005 µg/kg/min*
Nitroprusside	Start with 0.3 µg/kg/min	Start with 0.15 µg/kg/min

*Nesiritide can be initiated without bolus.

Vasodilators in Acute Heart Failure

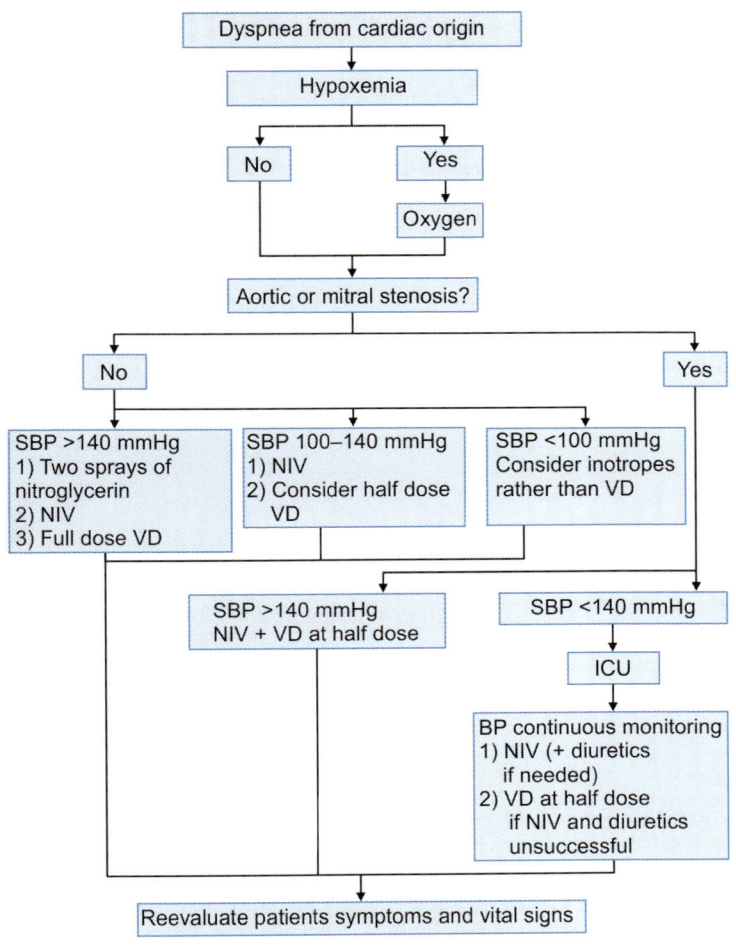

```
Dyspnea from cardiac origin
           ↓
      Hypoxemia
       ↓      ↓
      No     Yes
              ↓
           Oxygen
           ↓
Aortic or mitral stenosis?
       ↓              ↓
       No            Yes
```

| SBP >140 mmHg
1) Two sprays of nitroglycerin
2) NIV
3) Full dose VD | SBP 100–140 mmHg
1) NIV
2) Consider half dose VD | SBP <100 mmHg
Consider inotropes rather than VD |

- SBP >140 mmHg: NIV + VD at half dose
- SBP <140 mmHg → ICU
  - BP continuous monitoring
    1) NIV (+ diuretics if needed)
    2) VD at half dose if NIV and diuretics unsuccessful

Reevaluate patients symptoms and vital signs

SBP, systolic blood pressure; NIV, noninvasive ventilation; VD, vasodilators; ICU, intensive care unit; BP, blood pressure

ALGORITHM 1: Early management of patients with acute decompensated heart failure

IN CASE OF VASODILATORS INDUCED HYPOTENSION

All VDs have a possibility to cause hypotension. Patients with ADHF are treated with diuretics to alleviate volume overload. Blood pressure can drop abruptly after few hours. Excessive early drop of

Algorithms in Heart Failure

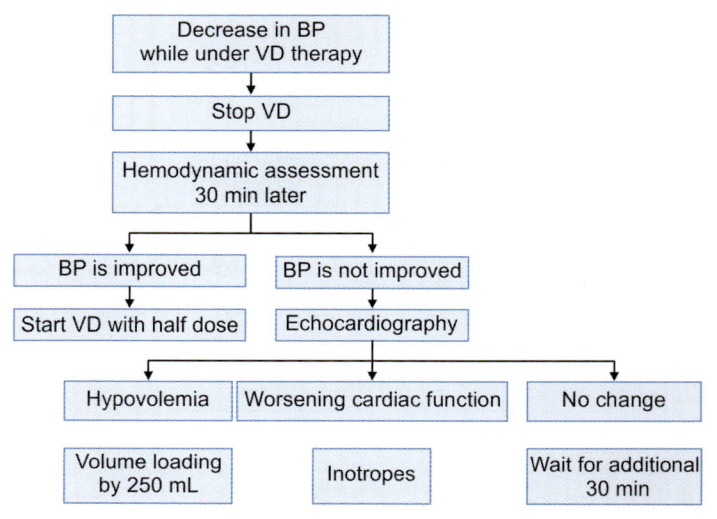

```
Decrease in BP
while under VD therapy
        ↓
     Stop VD
        ↓
Hemodynamic assessment
     30 min later
    ↓           ↓
BP is improved   BP is not improved
    ↓               ↓
Start VD with    Echocardiography
half dose       ↓        ↓         ↓
         Hypovolemia  Worsening   No change
                     cardiac function
         ↓              ↓           ↓
    Volume loading   Inotropes   Wait for additional
     by 250 mL                      30 min
```

BP, blood pressure; VD, vasodilators.

ALGORITHM 2: Management of vasodilators induced decrease in blood pressure

BP is known to worsen renal function. Management of decreased BP is seen in algorithm 2.

CONCLUSION

Although vasodilators have favorable effects on hemodynamic profile in patients with ADHF, including reduce preload and afterload and increase stroke volume, it should be avoided with patients with hypotension as excessive drop in systolic BP may affect organ perfusion.

KEY POINTS

- Vasodilators can unload the failing heart through reducing preload and afterload and increase cardiac output
- All vasodilators have a possibility to cause hypotension. When using vasodilators, careful attention should be paid to blood pressure.

SUGGESTED READINGS

1. McMurray JJ, Adamopoulos S, Anker SD, Auricchio A, Böhm M, Dickstein K, et al. ESC guidelines for the diagnosis and treatment of acute and chronic heart failure 2012: The Task Force for the Diagnosis and Treatment of Acute and Chronic Heart Failure 2012 of the European Society of Cardiology. Developed in collaboration with the Heart Failure Association (HFA) of the ESC. Eur Heart J. 2012;33(14):1787-847.
2. Mebazaa A, Gheorghiade M, Pina IL, Harjola VP, Hollenberg SM, Follath F, et al. Practical recommendations for prehospital and early in-hospital management of patients presenting with acute heart failure syndromes. Crit Care Med. 2008;36(1 Suppl):S129-39.
3. Publication Committee for the VMAC Investigators (Vasodilatation in the Management of Acute CHF). Intravenous nesiritide vs nitroglycerin for treatment of decompensated congestive heart failure: a randomized controlled trial. JAMA. 2002;287(12):1531-40.
4. Voors AA, Davison BA, Felker GM, Ponikowski P, Unemori E, Cotter G, et al. Early drop in systolic blood pressure and worsening renal function in acute heart failure: renal results of Pre-RELAX-AHF. Eur J Heart Fail. 2011;13(9):961-7.

CHAPTER 11

When and How to Use Inotropes?

John Parissis, Vasiliki Bistola

INTRODUCTION

Acute heart failure (AHF) encompasses a broad spectrum of clinical presentations, ranging from decompensation of chronic heart failure to low cardiac output; hypoperfusion syndromes with cardiogenic shock at the extreme end of this side. According to observational data from the Acute Decompensated Heart Failure National Registry (ADHERE), patients with low cardiac output-hypoperfusion comprise about 10% of the total AHF population and have the highest in-hospital mortality rates. Inotropes are pharmacological agents that enhance cardiac contractility, thereby, increasing cardiac output. Inotropes may be considered for the treatment of low cardiac output-hypoperfusion AHF patients to stabilize patient's hemodynamic condition and maintain or restore peripheral perfusion. However, they should be used with caution and only for short term because of their unfavorable adverse effect profile (tachyarrhythmias, hypotension or hypertension, and myocardial ischemia) and their association with increased medium and long-term mortality in heart failure (HF).

CLASSES OF INOTROPES AND MECHANISMS OF ACTION

Three major classes of inotropes are currently in clinical use with distinct mechanisms of action: (1) β-adrenergic agonists (dopamine, dobutamine, epinephrine, norepinephrine), (2) phosphodiesterase 3 inhibitors (PDE3Is) (milrinone) and (3) the calcium sensitizer levosimendan, (Table 1).

When and How to Use Inotropes?

TABLE 1: Pharmacological properties of inotropic agents and useful "tips" for their administration

Agents	Dobutamine	Dopamine	Norepinephrine	Epinephrine	Levosimendan	Milrinone
Mechanism of action	β1 > β2 > α	Dopaminergic > β; high dose α	β1 > α > β2	β1 = β2 > α	Calcium sensitizer; high dose PDE inhibitor	PDE inhibitor
Elimination t½ (min)	2.4	2.0	3.0	2.0	Active metabolite: 4800	150
Infusion dose	2–20 µg/kg/min	<3 µg/kg/min: renal effect 3–5 µg/kg/min: inotropic >5 µg/kg/min: vasoconstrictor	0.2–10 µg/kg/min	0.05–0.5 µg/kg/min	0.05–0.2 µg/kg/min	0.375–0.75 µg/kg/min
Bolus dose	No	No	No	1 mg can be given IV during resuscitation every 3–5 min	12 µg/kg/min over 10 min (optional)	25–75 µg/kg/min over 10–20 min
Inotropic effect	↑↑	↑↑	↑	↑↑	↑	↑
Arterial vasodilatation	↑	↑↑ (LD)	0	↑	↑↑	↑↑
Vasoconstriction	↑ (HD)	↑↑ (HD)	↑↑	↑ (HD)	0	0
Pulmonary vasodilatation	↑ or 0		↓ or 0 (at high PVR)	↓ or 0 (at high PVR)	↑↑	↑↑

Continued

Continued

Agents	Dobutamine	Dopamine	Norepinephrine	Epinephrine	Levosimendan	Milrinone
Chronotropic effect	↑	0 or ↑	↑	↑↑	0	0
Blood pressure effect	↑	↑ (HD)	↑	0 or ↑	↓	↓
Diuretic effect	0	↑↑ (LD)	↑	0	↑	0
Recommendation class						
ESC	IIa	IIb	IIb	IIb	IIb	IIb
ACC or AHA	IIb	IIb, I (CS)	I (CS)	I (CS)	Not licensed	IIb
Level of evidence	C	C	C	C	C	C
Adverse effects	Tachyarrhythmias, hypotension, headache, (rarely) eosinophilic myocarditis, peripheral eosinophilia	Tachyarrhythmias, hypertension, chest pain	Tachyarrhythmias, hypertension, headache	Tachyarrhythmias, headache, anxiety, cold extremities, cerebral hemorrhage, pulmonary edema	Hypotension, atrial and ventricular tachyarrhythmias, headache, nausea	Tachyarrhythmias, hypotension, headache

PDE, phosphodiesterase 3; IV, intravenous; HD, high dose; LD, low dose; PVR, pulmonary vascular resistances; CS, cardiogenic shock; ESC, European Society of Cardiology; ACC or AHA, American College of Cardiology Foundation or American Heart Association.

Beta Adrenergic Agonists

Beta adrenergic agonists mediate their cardiac inotropic effect through stimulation of sarcolemmal β1 adrenergic receptors of cardiac myocytes, which in turn activates the intracellular adenyl cyclase system resulting in increased cyclic adenosine monophosphate formation, release of intracellular Ca^{2+} from the sarcoplasmic reticulum, leading to increased strength of the actin-myosin-troponin interaction and enhanced myocardial contraction.

Dopamine

Dopamine is an endogenous molecule that acts through the dopaminergic type 1 and type 2 and β1 and α1 adrenergic receptors. At low doses (0.5–2.5 μg/kg/min), it causes renal and splanchnic vasodilation and leads to increased renal blood flow independently of the increase in cardiac output. At moderate doses (3–5 μg/kg/min), it has primarily inotropic and chronotropic effects, while at higher doses (>5 μg/kg/min), it causes vasoconstriction. Important side effects include tachyarrhythmias (more frequent at doses of ≥10 μg/kg/min) and hypertension.

Dobutamine

Dobutamine is a synthetic analog of dopamine that has primarily inotropic and weaker chronotropic effects. It can be administered at doses starting from 1–2 μg/kg/min up to 20 μg/kg/min (occasionally, up to 40 μg/kg/min). At low infusion doses (<5 μg/kg/min), it increases cardiac output with concomitant mild vasodilation. At high doses (>10 μg/kg/min), it exerts inotropic and vasoconstrictive effects. Main adverse effects are tachyarrhythmias at any infusion dose and hypotension at low infusion rates.

Norepinephrine

Norepinephrine is a potent vasoconstrictor and less a cardiac inotropic agent. In heart failure patients, it is used in conjunction with inotropic agents in cardiogenic shock or in patients treated with an inodilator to avoid hypotension. Norepinephrine is usually administered at doses of 0.01–0.03, but doses as high as 1 μg/kg/min may be required. Adverse effects include arrhythmias, myocardial ischemia, and hypertension.

Epinephrine

Epinephrine at low doses (<0.01 µg/kg/min) causes vasodilation, while doses more than 0.2 µg/kg/min produce a mixed inotropic and vasoconstrictor effect that overall increases peripheral vascular resistance and blood pressure. This agent is, especially, useful when combined inotropic or chronotropic and vasoconstrictor effects are urgently required. In HF patients, it is used in cardiogenic shock or in cardiac arrest. Epinephrine also causes pulmonary arterial and venous vasoconstriction, increasing pulmonary arterial and venous pressure through increased pulmonary blood flow. Infusion dose ranges from 0.01 to 0.03 µg/kg/min, but as high as 0.5 µg/kg/min may be reached. Adverse effects include myocardial ischemia, hypertension, ventricular tachyarrhythmias, pulmonary edema, and cerebral hemorrhage.

Milrinone

Milrinone is the PDE3I that is used most commonly for cardiovascular indications. It is approved for intravenous use in the United States and Europe. Milrinone is administered as short-term treatment in patients presenting with a low cardiac output state who are not severely hypotensive (e.g., systolic blood pressure >85 mmHg), especially when they were previously chronically treated with β-blockers, since these patients have been suggested to respond better to PDE3Is than to β-agonists. Side effects of milrinone include tachyarrhythmias and hypotension. Milrinone is infused at a rate of 0.375–0.75 µg/kg/min. Lower starting doses (0.1–0.375 µg/kg/min) may be given in patients at increased risk for hypotension or arrhythmias. Because of the long half-life (2.5 h) and its renal clearance, caution should be used when milrinone is administered in patients with impaired or changing renal function.

Levosimendan

Levosimendan exerts its inotropic effects through sensitization of cardiac troponin to the prevailing level of intracellular calcium, whereas at high doses, it also acts as a PDEI. Levosimendan also has a vasodilatory effect by opening adenosine triphosphate-sensitive potassium channels in the vascular smooth muscle cells. Levosimendan is available for clinical use only in Europe. It is indicated for AHF patients with vital organ hypoperfusion, who do not have significant hypotension, to reverse the effect of β-blockade if β-blockade is thought to be contributing to hypoperfusion. It is administered as an infusion at a rate of 0.05–0.2 μg/kg/min. Adverse effects include headache, hypotension, ventricular arrhythmias, atrial fibrillation, and hypokalemia.

WHEN TO USE INOTROPES IN ACUTE HEART FAILURE?

A proposed strategy for the use of inotropes in the management of patients with acutely decompensated chronic heart failure is presented in algorithm 1. A general rule when prescribing inotropes is to use them in the lowest possible doses and for the shortest necessary duration of time. In clinical practice, AHF patients who may be considered for inotropes are hypoperfused patients (clinically judged as "wet and cold") as contrasted to those who maintain adequate peripheral perfusion ("wet and warm") in whom vasodilators are appropriate. Detection of peripheral hypoperfusion can be assisted by laboratory findings, such as increased blood urea nitrogen and creatinine levels, increasing hepatic function markers (transaminases, γ-glutamyl transferase, and alkaline phosphatase) and hyponatremia, in cases where clinical assessment is not conclusive. Another patient population who may receive short-term inotropic support is those who initially present as "wet and warm" but during the course of treatment develop worsening cardiorenal syndrome indicating renal hypoperfusion. Intravenous diuretics are administered concomitantly with inotropes in patients with symptoms or signs of peripheral and/or pulmonary congestion. In patients with severe hypotension (SBP <85 mmHg) leading to high intracardiac filling pressures and vital organ hypoperfusion (evidenced as cold clam skin, low pulse volume, low or absent urine output, confusion, and myocardial ischemia), addition of a vasoconstrictor (such as dopamine or norepinephrine) to the therapeutic regimen is usually required. Additional therapeutic choices that can be administered concomitantly with inotropes include intra-aortic balloon counterpulsation (as a short-term mechanical ventricular unloading therapy, mainly in ischemic heart disease), and renal ultrafiltration in congested patients with diuretic resistance (patients nonresponsive to intense combination diuretic therapy). Post-inotropic therapy management depends on the patients' clinical and hemodynamic evolution. Stabilized and improving patients should be promptly weaned from inotropes, transitioned to an oral diuretic outpatient regimen and with

Algorithms in Heart Failure

Acutely decompensated chronic heart failure (on lifesaving medications and devices)

- **Well perfused (wet and warm)**
  - Intravenous vasodilators plus diuretics CPAP
    - Reinforce education (Na⁺/H₂O restriction), flexible diuretic regimens, continue β-blocker
    - Consider nitroglycerine, nitroprusside, ultrafiltration
  - Outcomes:
    - Stable outpatient
    - Recurrent hospitalizations and impaired functional capacity
    - Worsening cardiorenal syndrome (SBP <110 mmHg)
  - Consider digoxin

- **Hypoperfused (wet and cold)**
  - Inotropic support (dobutamine, levosimendan, milrinone)
    - Intravenous diuresis, reinforce education (Na⁺/H₂O restriction), flexible diuretic regimens
    - Consider vasoconstrictors, IABP, ultrafiltration
  - Outcomes:
    - Taper off and transition to stable outpatient regimen, restart β-blocker
    - Mechanical assist device or transplant
    - Palliative care (periodic inotropic support)

ALGORITHM 1: A proposed strategy on how to use inotropes in patients with acutely decompensated chronic heart failure

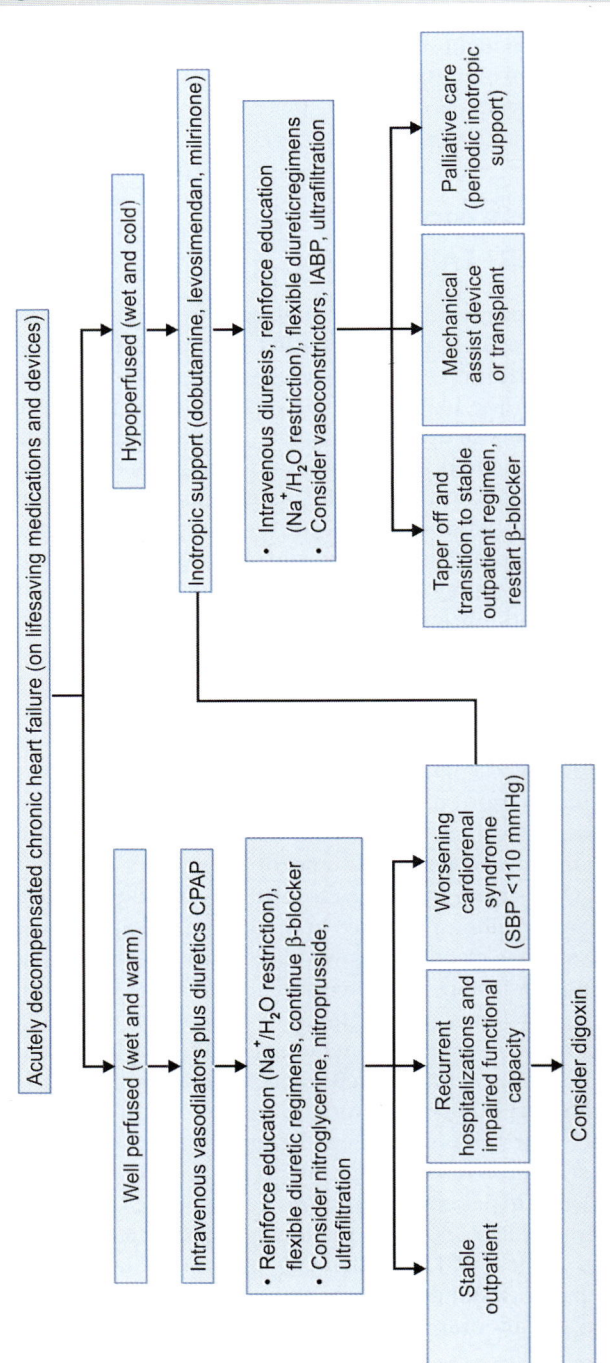

CPAP, continuous positive airway pressure; SBP, systolic blood pressure; IABP, Intra-aortic balloon pump.

β-blockers and other life saving HF medications properly reinstituted in case of in-hospital discontinuation. Unstable patients should be evaluated for candidacy for long-term mechanical circulatory support (MCS) and/or heart transplantation. Patients who are not candidates for MCS or heart transplantation should be considered for palliative long-term inotropic therapy.

SELECTION OF THE APPROPRIATE INOTROPE

Selection of the appropriate agent for each AHF patient depends on his/her clinical and hemodynamic characteristics. A proposed strategy for the selection of the appropriate inotrope is shown in algorithm 2. Patients with pulmonary arterial hypertension are more suitable for inodilators (milrinone, levosimendan) than for β-agonists, since inodilators exert vasodilatory effects in the pulmonary arterial vasculature. Such patients are those listed for cardiac transplantation who develop significantly elevated pulmonary vascular resistance (PVR) rendering them unsuitable for transplantation, in whom milrinone infusion has been effective to reduce PVR. Patients on chronic β-blockade therapy possibly respond better to levosimendan or milrinone, due to the independent mechanism of action of these agents of the β-adrenergic receptor pathway. However, this suggestion has recently been questioned after the publication of a small, double-blind, randomized trial, the best effectiveness after transition congestive heart failure, that showed no difference in the degree of improvement of pulmonary capillary wedge pressure and cardiac index at 24 hours after treatment with levosimendan or dobutamine in 60 AHF patients who were previously on β-blocker therapy. In patients with ischemic heart disease milrinone should rather be avoided due to its tendency to increase medium-term mortality and instead, levosimendan or dobutamine, should be used. Patients with primary renal insufficiency are better candidates for dobutamine due to its very short half-life (~2 min) compared to milrinone (half-life of 2.5 h) or levosimendan (half-life of the active metabolite ~80 h). However, in patients with acute cardiorenal syndrome, levosimendan may be the preferable drug as there is clinical evidence that this agent exert renoprotective effects by improving renal blood flow. Finally, patients with primary hepatic insufficiency are not suitable for levosimendan, because of its hepatic excretion. In contrast, patients with AHF and cardiohepatic dysfunction seem to be benefited by the use of levosimendan in comparison to dobutamine administration.

Algorithms in Heart Failure

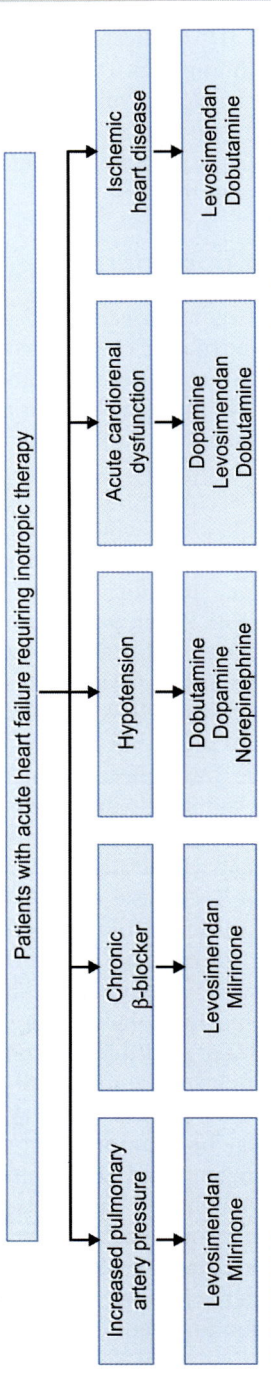

```
                    Patients with acute heart failure requiring inotropic therapy
                                              │
        ┌─────────────────────┬───────────────┼───────────────┬─────────────────────┐
        ▼                     ▼               ▼               ▼                     ▼
 Increased pulmonary      Chronic         Hypotension    Acute cardiorenal     Ischemic
   artery pressure       β-blocker                          dysfunction      heart disease
        │                     │               │               │                     │
        ▼                     ▼               ▼               ▼                     ▼
   Levosimendan         Levosimendan     Dobutamine        Dopamine           Levosimendan
    Milrinone            Milrinone        Dopamine       Levosimendan          Dobutamine
                                        Norepinephrine    Dobutamine
```

ALGORITHM 2: A proposed algorithm on how to choose the most appropriate inotropic agent according to the clinical and hemodynamic characteristics of the patient with acute heart failure

CONCLUSION

Despite their unfavorable adverse effect profile (tachyarrhythmias, myocardial ischemia, increase of medium and long-term mortality), inotropes represent "a necessary evil" for the hemodynamic stabilization and restoration of vital organ perfusion of patients with AHF presenting in a low cardiac output state. However, lowest possible doses and shortest necessary duration of inotropic therapy should be used, aiming to the earliest possible transition to either long-term oral therapies in stabilized patients or to mechanical circulatory support in non-responsive patients who are suitable candidates for such therapies. Periodic or continuous inotropic support may be considered as palliative care in patients who are deemed unsuitable candidates for advanced therapies. Selection of the appropriate inotrope among currently available agents (β-adrenergic agonists, phosphodiesterase III inhibitors and the calcium sensitizer levosimendan) should take into account patient's clinical and hemodynamic characteristics.

KEY POINTS

- Inotropes are indicated as a short-term therapy for patients with acute heart failure who present with signs of low cardiac output-hypoperfusion
- Caution is needed when inotropes are administered due to the frequent adverse effects and association with medium and long-term mortality. Lowest possible doses and shortest necessary duration of administration should be used
- Inotropes available for clinical use are β-adrenergic agonists, phosphodiesterase III inhibitors and the calcium sensitizer levosimendan
- Selection of the appropriate inotrope for each acute heart failure patient should take into account patient's clinical and hemodynamic characteristics.

SUGGESTED READINGS

1. Abraham WT, Adams KF, Fonarow GC, Costanzo MR, Berkowitz RL, LeJemtel TH, et al. In-hospital mortality in patients with acute decompensated heart failure requiring intravenous vasoactive medications: an analysis from the Acute Decompensated Heart Failure National Registry (ADHERE). J Am Coll Cardiol. 2005;46:57-64.
2. Bergh CH, Andersson B, Dahlstrom U, Forfang K, Kivikko M, Sarapohja T, et al. Intravenous levosimendan vs. dobutamine in acute decompensated heart failure patients on beta-blockers. Eur J Heart Fail. 2010;12:404-10.

3. Cuffe MS, Califf RM, Adams KF Jr., Benza R, Bourge R, Colucci WS, et al. Short-term intravenous milrinone for acute exacerbation of chronic heart failure: a randomized controlled trial. JAMA. 2002;287:1541-7.
4. Felker GM, Benza RL, Chandler AB, Leimberger JD, Cuffe MS, Califf RM, et al. Heart failure etiology and response to milrinone in decompensated heart failure: results from the OPTIME-CHF study. J Am Coll Cardiol. 2003;41:997-1003.
5. Filippatos G, Zannad F. An introduction to acute heart failure syndromes: definition and classification. Heart Fail Rev. 2007;12:87-90.
6. Fonarow GC, Adams KF Jr., Abraham WT, Yancy CW, Boscardin WJ, ADHERE Scientific Advisory Committee, Study Group, and Investigators. Risk stratification for in-hospital mortality in acutely decompensated heart failure: classification and regression tree analysis. JAMA. 2005;293:572-80.
7. Lowes BD, Tsvetkova T, Eichhorn EJ, Gilbert EM, Bristow MR. Milrinone versus dobutamine in heart failure subjects treated chronically with carvedilol. Int J Cardiol. 2001;81:141-9.
8. McMurray JJ, Adamopoulos S, Anker SD, Auricchio A, Böhm M, Dickstein K, et al. ESC Guidelines for the diagnosis and treatment of acute and chronic heart failure 2012: The Task Force for the Diagnosis and Treatment of Acute and Chronic Heart Failure 2012 of the European Society of Cardiology. Developed in collaboration with the Heart Failure Association (HFA) of the ESC. Eur Heart J. 2012;33:1787-847.
9. Nikolaou M, Parissis J, Yilmaz MB, Seronde MF, Kivikko M, Laribi S, et al. Liver function abnormalities, clinical profile, and outcome in acute decompensated heart failure. Eur Heart J. 2013;34:742-9.
10. Parissis JT, Farmakis D, Nieminen M. Classical inotropes and new cardiac enhancers. Heart Fail Rev. 2007;12:149-56.
11. Parissis JT, Rafouli-Stergiou P, Stasinos V, Psarogiannakopoulos P, Mebazaa A. Inotropes in cardiac patients: update 2011. Curr Opin Crit Care. 2010;16:432-41.

CHAPTER 12

Practical Approach to Hyponatremia in Heart Failure

Rajeev C Mohan, Hirsch S Mehta, JT Heywood

INTRODUCTION

Hyponatremia is defined as serum sodium of less than 136 mmol/L. It can be seen regardless of volume status. Severity of hyponatremia is based on serum sodium levels and clinical manifestations (Box 1).

In heart failure (HF) population, hyponatremia is generally dilutional and thus associated with increased total body volume. In dilutional hyponatremia, water is inappropriately reabsorbed resulting in a decreased sodium concentration even when total body sodium is elevated. This can also be seen in cirrhosis, nephrotic syndrome, and pregnancy.

Clinical manifestations of hyponatremia mainly involve the central nervous system. Severity is related to acute changes and absolute levels of serum sodium. Boxes 2 and 3 delineate the spectrum of signs and symptoms seen with hyponatremia.

Some patients with marked hyponatremia remain relatively asymptomatic, particularly when the onset is slow. However, rapidly developing hyponatremia can be life threatening. Prompt recognition and frequent monitoring are crucial as early treatment portends a more favorable prognosis.

Box 1: Definitions of hyponatremia

Hyponatremia severity defined by serum sodium
- Mild: 131–135 mmol/L
- Moderate: 125–130 mmol/L
- Severe: <125 mmol/L

> **Box 2: Symptoms of mild hyponatremia**
>
> **Symptoms of hyponatremia**
> - Headache
> - Nausea
> - Vomiting
> - Muscle cramping
> - Disorientation
> - Lack of coordination
> - Lethargy

> **Box 3: Signs of severe hyponatremia**
>
> **Signs of severe hyponatremia**
> - Seizure
> - Coma
> - Cerebral Edema
> - Brainstem herniation
> - Respiratory arrest

Hyponatremia (without hyperglycemia) has been associated with a poorer prognosis in HF patients. This has been demonstrated in both inpatient and outpatient settings and applies to those with preserved and depressed left ventricular function. Hyponatremia is both an independent predictor of increased rehospitalization rates as well as mortality. In cohort analysis, following HF patients with hyponatremia up to 7 years post index hospitalization, uncorrected hyponatremia remains the most significant risk factor for out of hospital mortality. This risk is reduced with correction of serum sodium levels.

MECHANISM

Mechanoreceptors in the left ventricle, carotid sinus, aortic arch, and afferent renal arterioles play an important role in the regulation of serum sodium. In patients with HF, the activation of these mechanoreceptors increases sympathetic tone and stimulation of the renin-angiotensin-aldosterone system. This increase persists despite increased total body fluid, facilitating sodium and water retention. These mechanisms cause Na^+ reception but not increased free water re-absorption which is mainly driven by increased vasopressin.

Role of Vasopressin

Regulation of total body water is directed by the hypothalamus, which controls thirst and the secretion of arginine vasopressin (AVP) from the posterior pituitary gland. Arginine vasopressin's primary functions include renal free water re-absorption, increasing peripheral vascular resistance, and regulation of both serum osmolality and blood volume. Additionally, it also indirectly affects myocardial contractile function.

Arginine vasopressin mediates its actions by three major receptors. Vasopressin 1a (V1a) receptors are found on vascular smooth muscle, platelets, and endometrium. Respectively, they are responsible for vasoconstriction and myocardial hypertrophy, platelet aggregation, and uterine contraction. Vasopressin 1b receptors are responsible for release of adrenocorticotropic hormone from the anterior pituitary. Vasopressin 2 (V2) receptors are found in the renal collecting duct which are responsible for free water resorption via aquaporins (proteins present in all cell membranes that regulate the flow of water into and out of cells) and in vascular endothelium where they release both von Willebrand factor and factor VII.

Increased secretion of AVP can occur two ways. Pressure receptors in blood vessels, particularly baroreceptors in carotid arteries, release AVP in response to decreased mechanical stimulation causing reduced plasma volume. This is referred to as nonosmotic release of vasopressin. Secretion of AVP in response to increased plasma osmotic pressure is mediated by osmoreceptors in the hypothalamus, and is referred to as osmotic release of AVP. These two pathways mediating AVP release are shown in algorithm 1.

Small changes in serum osmolality prompt changes in levels of serum AVP via a reflex arc aimed at maintaining salt and water homeostasis. Under usual circumstances, AVP release is prompted by a change in plasma tonicity, depletion of plasma volume, or reduction of blood pressure. Changes in plasma volume and blood pressure prompt arterial receptors to trigger the release of AVP from the nonosmotic pathway which can result water re-absorption despite hyponatremia. Among other factors, edematous states also tend to shift regulation toward nonosmotic regulation. This pathway is a more potent form of AVP regulation.

The primary mechanism of hyponatremia in hospitalized adults is AVP release via the nonosmotic pathway. When AVP is released, water re-absorption is inhibited by interactions with aquaporins in the collecting duct. The collecting duct accounts for approximately 5% of the body's re-absorption of both sodium and water but can adapt to resorb up to 25% of filtered water in times of dehydration. In the collecting duct, aquaporin V2 is crucial for water re-absorption in response to AVP. During times where AVP is abundant, aquaporins allow for robust re-absorption of water with resulting hyponatremia.

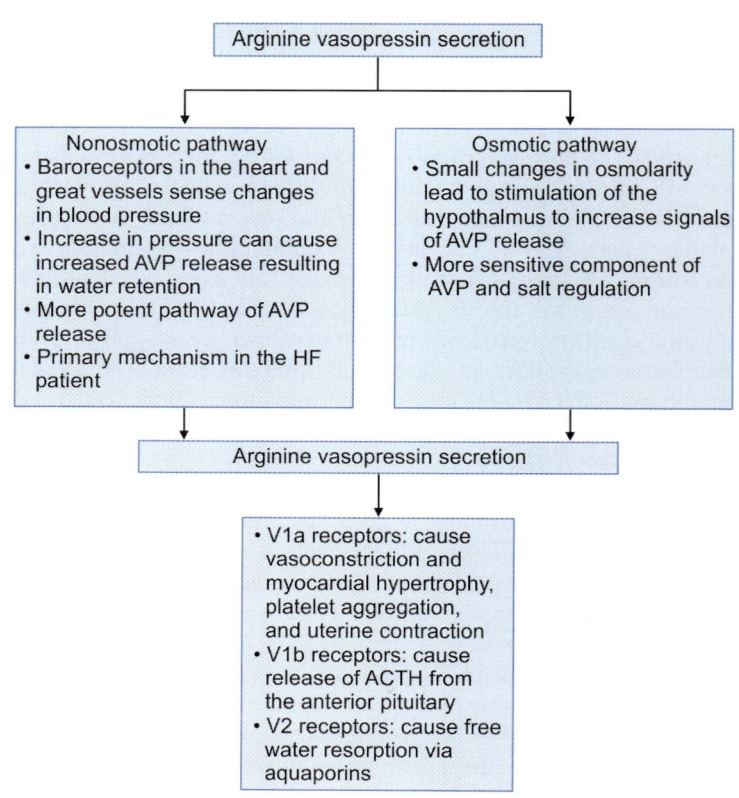

Algorithms in Heart Failure

```
                    ┌─────────────────────────────────┐
                    │ Arginine vasopressin secretion  │
                    └─────────────────────────────────┘
                         │                    │
            ┌────────────┘                    └────────────┐
            ▼                                              ▼
```

Nonosmotic pathway
- Baroreceptors in the heart and great vessels sense changes in blood pressure
- Increase in pressure can cause increased AVP release resulting in water retention
- More potent pathway of AVP release
- Primary mechanism in the HF patient

Osmotic pathway
- Small changes in osmolarity lead to stimulation of the hypothalamus to increase signals of AVP release
- More sensitive component of AVP and salt regulation

Arginine vasopressin secretion

- V1a receptors: cause vasoconstriction and myocardial hypertrophy, platelet aggregation, and uterine contraction
- V1b receptors: cause release of ACTH from the anterior pituitary
- V2 receptors: cause free water resorption via aquaporins

HF, heart failure; AVP, arginine vasopressin; ACTH, adrenocorticotropic hormone; V1a, vasopressin 1a; V1b, vasopressin 1b; V2, vasopressin 2.

ALGORITHM 1: Role of arginine vasopressin

Vasopressin and Heart Failure

Correlation between elevated plasma values of vasopressin with HF and left ventricular dysfunction have been shown in several studies. Substudies of the Studies of Left Ventricular Dysfunction trial showed that even asymptomatic patients with left ventricular dysfunction had higher levels of vasopressin compared to controls.

Vasopressin also possesses hemodynamic effects that are important in HF. Vasopressin increases systemic vascular resistance and pulmonary capillary wedge pressure via interactions with V1a receptors. Through this same mechanism, stroke volume, and cardiac output show a dose-dependent decrease in relation to levels of vasopressin.

Vasopressin directly effects salt and water balance via interactions with aquaporins and V2 receptors in the collecting duct. This is done via increased expression of aquaporin 2, which is inserted into cell membranes in the collecting duct. Aquaporin 2 facilitates free water absorption and an eventual decrease in serum sodium levels, which results in decreased osmolarity and fluid shifts leading to intravascular volume depletion. This process further stimulates vasopressin release resulting in worsening hyponatremia. This cyclic cascade of events is shown in figure 1.

Increased levels of vasopressin also retard the excretion of free water (without solute) in HF patients. Blocking aquaporin V2 receptors pharmacologically, on the other hand, leads to aquaresis. V2 receptor antagonism leads to a dose-related increase in solute-free water excretion, causing a rise in serum sodium and osmolality in HF patients.

Advanced HF patients are at risk for hyponatremia not only from mechanisms of water retention as outlined above, but also by aggressive diuresis leading to intravascular volume depletion despite an elevated total body fluid status. Diuretics cause a mechanistic water retention pathway similar to the inherent HF disease process.

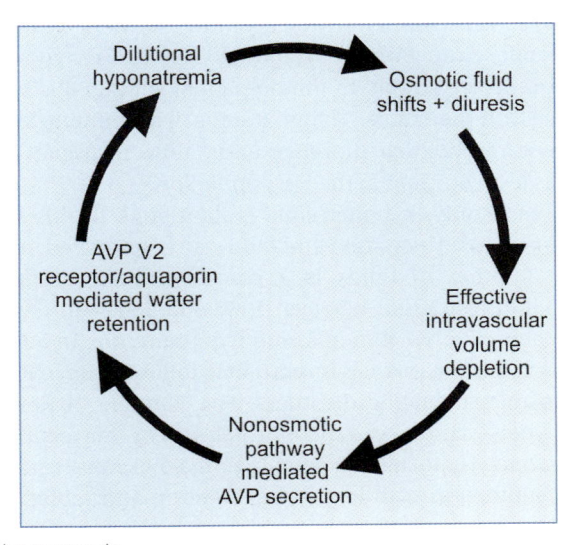

AVP, arginine vasopressin.

FIG. 1: Cyclical nature of hyponatremia in heart failure

Thiazide diuretics appear to have a role in hyponatremia as well. Retrospective analysis have shown that greater than 90% of diuretic induced hyponatremia in a hospitalized population can be attributed to thiazide diuretics, with greater than 95% of these being within recommended dosages.

EVALUATION AND TREATMENT OF HYPONATREMIA IN HEART FAILURE

Treatment of hyponatremia begins with optimizing therapy for HF. Recognition and treatment of hyponatremia can have prognostic implications for morbidity and mortality and is an important component in the overall management of HF patients.

A basic algorithm for the initial evaluation and management of HF patients with hyponatremia has been provided (Algorithm 2).

Although hyponatremia is common in HF patients, it is important to rule out non HF causes of low serum sodium. Endocrine disorders, such as syndrome of inappropriate antidiuretic hormone secretion, adrenal insufficiency, elevated blood sugars, and hypothyroidism, can all cause hyponatremia. Women of childbearing age should be evaluated for pregnancy and a complete history, including diet, fluid intake, and illicit substances should be questioned, as all can contribute to low serum sodium levels.

Careful consideration must be given to assess for symptoms of hyponatremia. Even without symptoms, significant hyponatremia in HF warrants treatment. In the outpatient setting, this begins by optimizing volume status. Hyponatremia with volume depletion simply requires holding diuretics and saline resuscitation. This scenario is less common in the HF population.

More commonly, hyponatremia is dilutional. In this scenario, diuretics need to be increased and fluid status optimized. Increased oral consumption of fluids is a common cause of depressed sodium. Fluid restriction between 1200 and 1500 mL/day should be implemented in HF patients with hyponatremia. In addition to correcting volume status, it is important to follow serum chemistries and to correct metabolic disorders. For example, hyponatremia due to hyperglycemia can be normalized by correcting blood glucose alone. Hypokalemia and hypomagnesemia can also be seen in conjunction with low serum sodium, and repleting these electrolytes are necessary in the management of hyponatremia.

Every patient evaluation for hyponatremia should include careful medicine reconciliation. It is important to remove any medications

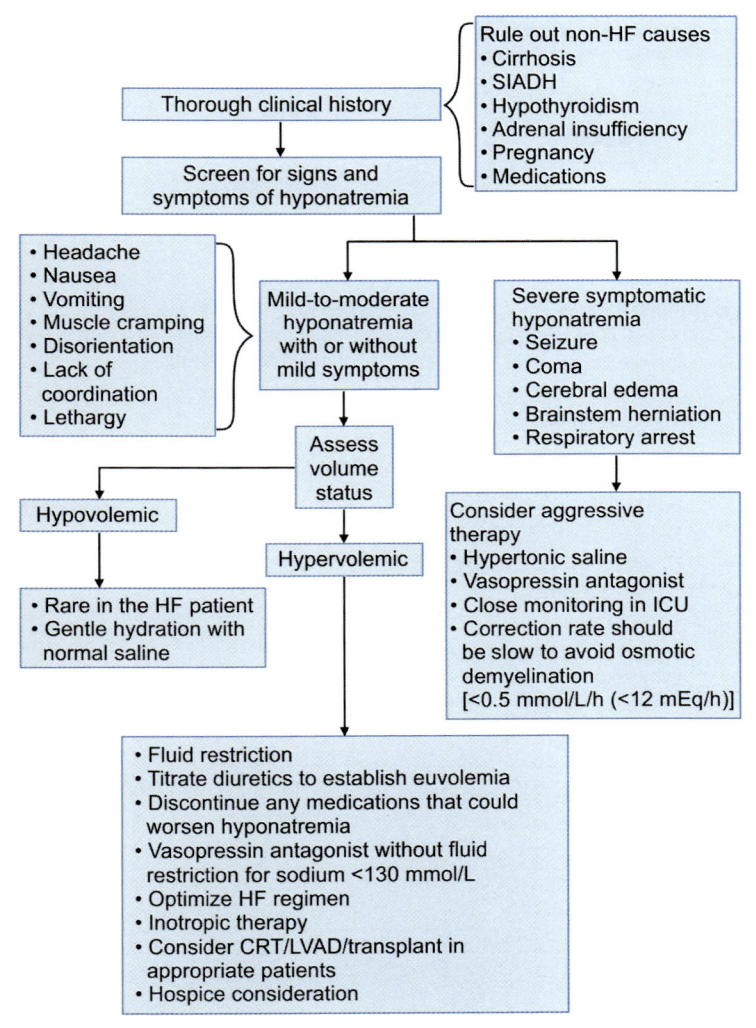

Practical Approach to Hyponatremia in Heart Failure

ALGORITHM 2: Evaluation of hyponatremia

```
Thorough clinical history
         │
         ▼
Screen for signs and
symptoms of hyponatremia
```

Rule out non-HF causes
- Cirrhosis
- SIADH
- Hypothyroidism
- Adrenal insufficiency
- Pregnancy
- Medications

- Headache
- Nausea
- Vomiting
- Muscle cramping
- Disorientation
- Lack of coordination
- Lethargy

→ Mild-to-moderate hyponatremia with or without mild symptoms

Severe symptomatic hyponatremia
- Seizure
- Coma
- Cerebral edema
- Brainstem herniation
- Respiratory arrest

Assess volume status → Hypovolemic / Hypervolemic

Hypovolemic:
- Rare in the HF patient
- Gentle hydration with normal saline

Severe: Consider aggressive therapy
- Hypertonic saline
- Vasopressin antagonist
- Close monitoring in ICU
- Correction rate should be slow to avoid osmotic demyelination [<0.5 mmol/L/h (<12 mEq/h)]

Hypervolemic:
- Fluid restriction
- Titrate diuretics to establish euvolemia
- Discontinue any medications that could worsen hyponatremia
- Vasopressin antagonist without fluid restriction for sodium <130 mmol/L
- Optimize HF regimen
- Inotropic therapy
- Consider CRT/LVAD/transplant in appropriate patients
- Hospice consideration

---

contributing to hyponatremia. A list of commonly prescribed medications that can worsen hyponatremia is shown in box 4. Thiazide diuretics are a common medication in a HF population that worsens hyponatremia. Replacing thiazide diuretics with loop diuretics can improve hyponatremia.

Optimization of HF medications can also improve serum sodium. Maximizing β-blockers, angiotensin converting enzyme

Box 4: Medications that exacerbate hyponatremia

- Diuretics
  - Loop Diuretics
    - Furosemide
    - Bumetanide
- Thiazide Diuretics
  - Hydrochlorothiazide
  - Chlorthalidone
  - Metolazone
- Antidepressants
  - Selective serotonin reuptake Inhibitors
  - Tricyclic antidepressants
    - Amitriptyline
    - Desipramine
  - Monoamine oxidase inhibitors
  - Bupropion
  - Duloxetine
- Antipsychotic drugs
  - Carbamazepine
  - Oxcarbazepine
  - Sodium valproate
  - Lamotrigine
- Antineoplastic Agents
  - Vinca alkaloids
    - Vincristine
    - Vinblastine
  - Platinum compounds
    - Cisplatin
    - Carboplatin
  - Alkylating agents
    - Cyclophosphamide
    - Melphalan
    - Ifosfamide
  - Other
    - Methotrexate
    - Interferon-α, γ
    - Levamisole
    - Pentostatin
    - Monoclonal antibodies
- Painkillers
  - Opiates
  - Nonsteroidal anti-inflammatory drugs
  - Acetaminophen
- ADH analogs
  - Desmopressin
  - Oxytocin
- Antihypertensives
  - ACE, angiotensin converting enzyme inhibitors
  - Amlodipine
- Antibiotics
  - Trimethoprim-sulfamethoxazole
  - Ciprofloxacin
  - Sulbactam
  - Rifabutin
- Anti-arrhythmic drugs
  - Amiodarone
  - Propafenone
- Miscellaneous
  - 3,4, methylenedioxymethamphetamine (ecstasy)
  - Intravenous immunoglobulin
  - Theophylline
  - Proton pump inhibitors
  - Bromocriptine

inhibitors, angiotensin receptor blockers (ARBs), and aldosterone antagonists (given normal potassium and creatinine levels) should be considered in hyponatremic patients. Angiotensin converting enzyme inhibitors have been shown to directly increase serum sodium levels. In addition to medications, advanced HF therapies should be considered in patients who have hyponatremia as a result of HF. Those with QRS duration of greater than 120 ms and left bundle branch morphology on electrocardiography should be offered cardiac resynchronization therapy. Hyponatremia in stage IV HF patients can be corrected with mechanical circulatory support and cardiac transplantation.

Patients with symptomatic or acute, severe hyponatremia require hospitalization. Correcting hyponatremia requires close monitoring of serum sodium, as levels should not increase by more than 0.5 mmol/L/h (<12 mEq/day) to minimize the risk of osmotic demyelination. Inpatient treatment of hyponatremia involves many of the same principles as outpatient management. However, despite adjusting diuretics and titrating medicines, hyponatremia may still persist. In such patients, more aggressive therapies, such as hypertonic saline infusion or vasopressin antagonists should be considered. In a HF population, hypertonic saline infusion becomes problematic due to the increased administration of solute. Because of this, the use of vasopressin antagonists, such as vaptan drugs, are a reasonable treatment approach.

Two major vaptan drugs approved for clinical use are conivaptan, which is selective for V1a and V2 receptors, and tolvaptan, which has its effect only on V2 receptors found in the renal collecting duct. While conivaptan can be taken both orally and intravenously, the more selective tolvaptan is only available in an oral form.

Both conivaptan and tolvaptan produce increased urine output and improve serum sodium levels. In HF patients, most trials show improvement in subjective and objective signs of congestion. Still, no independent benefit with regards to mortality or rehospitalization has been seen as a result of vaptan therapy amongst HF patients.

Vaptan therapy in HF patients should be used in cases of symptomatic hyponatremia with concentrations less than 130 mmol/L or in those patients with concentrations less than 125 mmol/L regardless of symptoms. These drugs should only be considered after conservative measures, such as fluid restriction and intravenous loop diuretics have been maximized and are refractory. Because of its selective nature toward the V2 receptor and robust oral bioavailability, tolvaptan is preferred as a first line agent over conivaptan.

The starting dose for tolvaptan is 15 mg daily. Once therapy is initiated, patients should not be fluid restricted and oral hydration limits should be liberalized due to a potent aquaresis that occurs with tolvaptan. The dose can be doubled daily until a desired

> **Box 5: Guidelines for initiating tolvaptan therapy**
> - Discontinue fluid restriction
> - Serial serum sodium measurements every 6 h until levels stabilize
> - Initial dose of 15 mg once daily
> - May double the dose based upon response
> - Max daily dose of 60 mg

response is achieved. The maximum suggested dose for tolvaptan is 60 mg daily. Once tolvaptan therapy has started, serum sodium should initially be checked every 6–8 hours for the first day, and can be checked once or twice daily after sodium levels and drug dosages have stabilized. Guidelines for the initiation of tolvaptan are shown in box 5.

Some patients may require chronic vaptan therapy to control hyponatremia as outpatient therapy. This cohort includes stage IV patients whose HF is advanced and the presence of persistent electrolyte abnormalities should be considered a marker for end stage disease. In addition to evaluating such patients for advanced stage D therapies, such as ventricular assist device or transplantation, chronic vaptan therapy may be required as an outpatient to keep serum sodium levels normalized. This should only be done after therapy is initiated and a safe dose is identified during hospitalization. Patients should have twice weekly metabolic panel evaluations while on outpatient tolvaptan and frequent clinic visits to ensure fluid status and medications are optimized. Often, tolvaptan can be stopped as HF treatment is optimized.

Hyponatremia in HF patients is a negative prognostic marker associated with a high mortality and rehospitalization rate. However, a keen clinical eye, prompt recognition, evaluation, and treatment can have prognostic implications in treating not only electrolyte disturbances, but overall HF as well.

CONCLUSION

Hyponatremia is simultaneously common and overlooked in the HF population. Moreover, the presence of hyponatremia has prognostic implications in outcomes for HF patients. Identification and treatment of sodium disturbances is not complex. The pathophysiology of hyponatremia has been briefly examined. Finally, a simplified approach to evaluation and treatment, complemented by tables featuring stepwise algorithms and common clinical scenarios are highlighted.

KEY POINTS

- Hyponatremia in heart failure patients is a negative prognostic marker associated with a higher mortality and rehospitalization rate
- Prompt recognition can have significant effects toward improving outcomes in this population
- Mechanistically, high levels of vasopressin are responsible for inappropriate natriuresis despite fluid overload, resulting in low serum sodium levels
- Treatment centers on reversing this cycle with fluid restriction, diuresis, and arginine vasopressin suppression with vaptan therapy
- Though most patients can have hyponatremia corrected during a hospital stay, stage IV patients may require chronic treatment for low serum sodium while awaiting advanced therapies.

SUGGESTED READINGS

1. Adrogue HJ and Madias NE. Hyponatremia. N Engl J Med. 2000;342:1581-89.
2. Agre, P. The aquaporin water channels. Proc Am Thorac Soc. 2006;3(1):5-13.
3. De Luca L, Klein L, Udelson JE, Orlandi C, Sardella G, Fedele F, et al. Hyponatremia in patients with heart failure. Am J Cardiol. 2005;96(12A):19L-23L.
4. Finley JJ 4th, Konstam MA, Udelson JE. Arginine vasopressin antagonists for the treatment of heart failure and hyponatremia. Circulation. 2008;118:410-21.
5. Francis GS, Benedict C, Johnstone DE, Kirlin PC, Nicklas J, Liang CS, et al. Comparison of neuroendocrine activation in patients with left ventricular dysfunction with and without congestive heart failure. A substudy of the Studies of Left Ventricular Dysfunction (SOLVD). Circulation. 1990;82:1724-9.
6. Goldsmith SR, Francis GS, Cowley AW Jr, Goldenberg IF, Cohn JN. Hemodynamic effects of infused arginine vasopressin in congestive heart failure. J Am Coll Cardiol. 1986;8:779-83.
7. Goldsmith SR, Francis GS, Cowley AW Jr Levine TB, Cohn JN. Increased plasma arginine vasopressin levels in patients with congestive heart failure. J Am Coll Cardiol. 1983;1:1385-90.
8. Jao GT and Chiong JR. Hyponatremia in acute decompensated heart failure: mechanisms, prognosis and treatment options. Clin. Cardiol. 2010;33(11):666-71.
9. Kalra PR, Anker SD, Coats AJ. Water and sodium regulation in chronic heart failure: the role of natriuretic peptides and vasopressin. Cardiovasc Res. 2001;51:495-509.
10. Lee DS, Austin PC, Rouleau JL, Liu PP, Naimark D, Tu JV. Predicting mortality among patients hospitalized for heart failure: derivation and validation of a clinical model. JAMA. 2003;290(19):2581-7.
11. Robertson GL. Vaptans for the treatment of hyponatremia. Nat Rev Endocrin. 2011;7:151-61.
12. Rusinaru D, Tribouilloy C, Berry C et al. Relationship of serum sodium concentration to mortality in a wide spectrum of heart failure patients with preserved and with reduced

ejection fraction: an individual patient data meta-analysis: Meta-Analysis Global Group in Chronic heart failure (MAGGIC). Eur J Heart Fail. 2012;14(10):1139-46.
13. Schrier RW, Abraham WT. Hormones and hemodynamics in heart failure. N Engl J Med. 1999;341:577-85.
14. Schrier RW, Berl T. Nonosmolar factors affecting renal water excretion (first of two parts). N Engl J Med. 1975;292:81-88 and 141-45.
15. Sonnenblick M, Friedlander Y, Rosin AJ. Diuretic-induced severe hyponatremia review and analysis of 129 reported patients. Chest. 1993;103:601-6.
16. Sterns RH, Cappuccio JD, Silver SM Cohen EP. Neurologic sequelae after treatment of severe hyponatremia: a multicenter perspective. J Am Soc Nephrol. 1994;4(8):1522-30.
17. Szatalowicz VL, Arnold PE, Chaimovitz C, Bichet D, Berl T, Schrier RW.Radioimmunoassay of plasma arginine vasopressin in hyponatremic patients with congestive heart failure. N Engl J Med. 1981;305:263-6.
18. Tribouilloy C, Buiciuc O, Leborgne L, et al. Relation of serum sodium level to long-term outcome after a first episode of heart failure: a prospective 7-year study. Int J Cardiol. 2010;140:309-14.
19. Udelson JE, Smith WB, Hendrix GH, Painchaud CA, Ghazzi M, Thomas I, et al. Acute hemodynamic effects of conivaptan, a dual V(1A) and V(2) vasopressin receptor antagonist, in patients with advanced heart failure. Circulation. 2001;104:2417-23.
20. Wong LL, Verbalis JG. Systemic diseases associated with diseases of water homeostasis. Endocrinol Metab Clin North Am. 2002;31:121-40.

13
CHAPTER

Heart Failure and Acute Coronary Syndrome

Kevin S Shah

INTRODUCTION

The most common cause of chronic heart failure in the United States is coronary artery disease (CAD). Furthermore, acute coronary syndrome (ACS) is noted to be a significant cause of acute decompensated heart failure as well, with CAD, hypertension, and atrial fibrillation continually identified as the most common underlying etiologies of new acute decompensated heart failure. Prognosis of patients with heart failure and CAD is considerably worse than that of patients without coronary disease and is related to the angiographic severity of coronary disease. Systematic evaluation for CAD is an essential part of the evaluation of patients with newly diagnosed or chronic heart failure.

CLINICAL APPROACH TO ACUTE CORONARY SYNDROME IN HEART FAILURE

History and Physical Examination

The evaluation for CAD in patients with heart failure (HF) follows the same approach for general screening in patient's initially presenting with symptoms concerning for ACS, beginning with a thorough history and a detailed physical examination. Essential features of the history include an accurate inquiry into prior histories of or current presentations of chest discomfort, including the severity, frequency, location, radiation, quality, alleviating and aggravating factors, and duration of any of these symptoms. The history and physical examination findings should be assessed in the context of the overall clinical status of the patient. Typical angina is described as pain that is substernal, occurs on exertion, and is relieved with rest. In patients with a reported history of CAD, an accurate characterization of the quality and frequency of any prior chest pain episodes is essential to determine whether a change in the angina pattern has occurred [i.e., a patient with chronic stable angina now has unstable angina (UA)] or if a noncardiac origin of pain is now present (i.e., a patient with chronic stable angina now with simply musculoskeletal pain).

In all patients with HF, cardiovascular risk factors should always be reviewed. Patients with a known diagnosis of chronic heart failure will likely have medical history that puts them at increased risk for CAD. Risk factors include a history of hypertension, hyperlipidemia, obesity, diabetes mellitus, cigarette smoking, and a family history of CAD. The physical examination in patients with ACS frequently is normal. Especially, concerning physical findings include a new murmur concerning for mitral regurgitation, hypotension, pulmonary rales, a new third heart sound (S3 gallop), and jugular venous distention. Patients with decompensated HF may have pre-existing exam findings including pulmonary rales, jugular venous distention, and S3 gallop.

Biomarkers

Laboratory testing, specifically for biomarkers, is critical and challenging in HF patients presenting with ACS. Cardiac biomarkers, troponin and the natriuretic peptides, will be specifically focused. Theoretically, the natriuretic peptides are markers of HF status while troponin is a marker of cardiac myocyte injury. However, the comorbidity of chronic heart failure confounds interpretation of the laboratory data in the setting of ACS. Troponins (T, I, and C) are found in cardiac and skeletal muscle. Historically, in the setting of ACS, a positive troponin test has been based on the 99th percentile rule. However, this cutoff does not imply that 1% of the normal population has active myocardial necrosis; this cutoff relies on, once again, a high pretest probability of ACS. Interpretation of troponin results is dependent on the assay used at the institution, as assays are being developed with higher and higher levels of sensitivity. While improving clinical sensitivity for the diagnosis of myocardial infarction (MI), the increased analytic sensitivity has come at the cost of reduced specificity. The interpretation of troponin levels in the setting of chronic heart failure becomes even more confounded as many patients have troponin levels elevated at baseline. These markers represent ongoing injury from multiple processes. Knowing a patient's baseline troponin level is crucial and the trends in the setting of possible ACS are more important as the leakage of enzymes may be from coronary plaque rupture causing myocardial necrosis, versus ongoing leakage from a failing heart. Routine assessment of troponin concentrations in chronic HF patients is not warranted, but in patients with the possibility of an ACS, it is critical.

The natriuretic peptides [brain natriuretic peptide (BNP) and N-terminal pro-brain natriuretic peptide, have played a pivotal role in the diagnosis and prognosis of patients with chronic heart failure. Their functions are physiological in response to ventricular wall stretch, dilatation, and pressure. They serve to counter-regulate the renin-angiotensin-aldosterone system via natriuresis, diuresis, and vasodilation. Multiple studies have demonstrated their ability to help diagnose HF in patients presenting with acute dyspnea. Their role in ACS are not as well elucidated as they are in patients with HF. Brain natriuretic peptide concentration rises rapidly over the first 24 hours after MI and then tends to stabilize; patients with a large infarct may have a second peak approximately 5 days later. When measured, 1–7 days after MI, elevation of BNP identifies patients at risk for left ventricular dysfunction, HF, and death. However, at this time, there is no recommendation for routine BNP testing in patients with ACS.

Screening

As depicted in algorithm 1, the process of screening for CAD or ACS in patients with HF begins with an assessment of the patient's likelihood of CAD. Patients at low risk for CAD based on initial assessment do not require further workup. However, patients deemed as moderate risk for having underlying CAD, should be further evaluated with a baseline electrocardiogram (ECG). The approach to picking a stress test for evaluation of CAD involves a linear line of questioning including: purpose of test, can the patient exercise, is the resting ECG normal, does body habitus pose problems to imaging, and cost effectiveness of the testing? Those with normal ECG's and with the capacity to safely engage in physical activity should undergo further evaluation with a stress ECG, with positively testing patients subsequently referred for a computed tomographic coronary angiogram (CTCA). Patients demonstrating

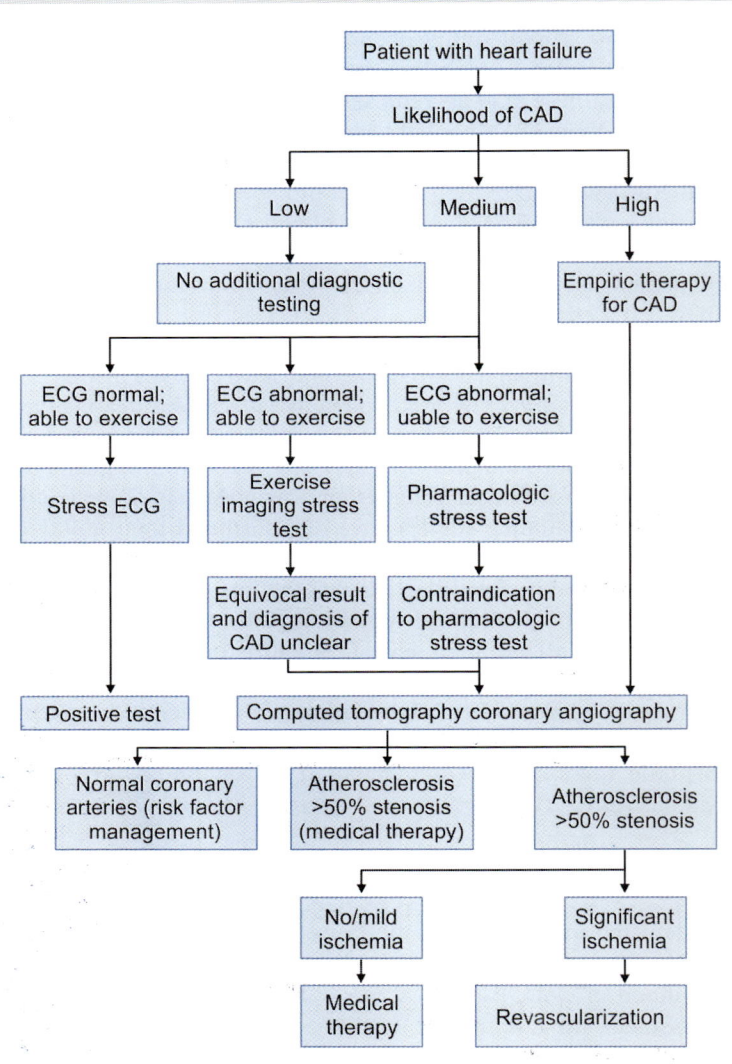

Algorithms in Heart Failure

```
Patient with heart failure
            │
    Likelihood of CAD
    ┌───────┼───────┐
   Low   Medium    High
    │       │        │
No additional       Empiric therapy
diagnostic testing  for CAD
```

- ECG normal; able to exercise → Stress ECG → Positive test
- ECG abnormal; able to exercise → Exercise imaging stress test → Equivocal result and diagnosis of CAD unclear → Computed tomography coronary angiography
- ECG abnormal; unable to exercise → Pharmacologic stress test → Contraindication to pharmacologic stress test → Computed tomography coronary angiography

Computed tomography coronary angiography:
- Normal coronary arteries (risk factor management)
- Atherosclerosis >50% stenosis (medical therapy)
- Atherosclerosis >50% stenosis
  - No/mild ischemia → Medical therapy
  - Significant ischemia → Revascularization

CAD, coronary artery disease; ECG, electrocardiogram.

ALGORITHM 1: Approach to screen for underlying coronary artery disease or acute coronary syndrome in patients with already established heart failure

an abnormal ECG (i.e., signs of current ischemia, prior ischemia, new axis deviation, hypertrophy, and rhythm blocks) and with a capacity to safely engage in exercise should be further evaluated with an exercise imaging stress test; patients with equivocal results and an unclear diagnosis of CAD should undergo a CTCA as well. It should also be noted that severe HF is an absolute contraindication to exercise stress testing.

Moderate risk patients demonstrating an abnormal ECG and unable to safely engage in exercise should be further evaluated for CAD with a pharmacologic stress test; if unable to tolerate such a test, these patients should directly undergo a CTCA. Heart failure patients deemed to be at high risk for underlying CAD should be immediately optimized with empiric therapy for their suspected CAD while being prepped for a CTCA. In both medium risk and high risk patients undergoing a coronary angiogram, patients should subsequently be further stratified based upon their coronary angiogram results. Patients with normal coronary arteries as evidence on their angiogram require only outpatient management of their CAD risk factors. On the other hand, patients with demonstrated atherosclerosis on angiogram, but less than 50% stenosis, require actual pharmaceutical medical therapy for treatment of their underlying CAD. Patients with demonstrated atherosclerosis on angiogram, with more than 50% stenosis, should be subcategorized into two further patient groups: those with evidence of significant ischemia and those with evidence of only mild or trace ischemia. Patients with significant ischemia should undergo coronary revascularization, where as those with only trace or mild evidence should be sufficiently treated if given medical therapy alone.

TREATMENT OF ACUTE CORONARY SYNDROME IN HEART FAILURE (BOX 2)

ST elevation Myocardial Infarction

Primary treatment of ACS involves categorizing patients into the category of UA or non-ST elevation myocardial infarction (NSTEMI) versus ST elevation myocardial infarction (STEMI). ST elevation myocardial infarction is defined as ST segment elevations of 1 mm (0.1 mV) in two anatomically contiguous leads or 2 mm (0.2 mV) in two contiguous precordial leads, or new left bundle branch block and presentation consistent with ACS. Initial interventions for patients with ACS include assessing airway or breathing or circulation and providing oxygen. Initial pharmacotherapy includes full dose aspirin, treatment of angina symptoms with sublingual nitroglycerin, followed by morphine sulfate depending on institutional preference or policy. If signs or symptoms of left HF are present, afterload reduction with sublingual nitroglycerin and/

or loop diuretic should be considered. Beta blocker therapy should be initiated as long as no contraindications are present (chronic obstructive pulmonary disease or asthma, cardiogenic shock, hypotension, symptomatic bradycardia, second or third degree heart block, or decompensated HF is present). Also, early delivery of statin therapy should be started preferably before percutaneous coronary intervention (PCI).

The acute management of STEMI typically involves the selection of reperfusion therapy (PCI versus fibrinolytic therapy). Percutaneous coronary intervention via cardiac catheterization is ideally performed within 90 minutes of patient's arrival to a hospital with capabilities. Thrombolytic therapy is indicated in the treatment of STEMI if it can be administered within 12 hours of onset of symptoms, patient eligibility based on specific inclusion or exclusion criteria, and if primary PCI is unavailable. Aside from reperfusion therapy, antiplatelet and anticoagulant therapies are essential in the management of STEMI. Antiplatelet therapy (after administration of aspirin) includes clopidogrel, ticagrelor, or prasugrel, depending on the reperfusion strategy. Anticoagulation, whether via unfractionated heparin, low molecular weight heparin, direct thrombin inhibitor, and/or glycoprotein IIb/IIIa inhibitor is also indicated in the management of STEMI. However, the selection of the specific agent is beyond the scope of this chapter.

Unstable Angina or Non-ST Elevation Myocardial Infarction

With respect to UA/NSTEMI, the specific definition of UA is angina which occurs at rest, or new onset angina that limits activity, or increasing angina that is more frequent, longer duration, or occurs with less exertion. Non-ST elevation myocardial infarction is distinguished by the presence of elevated markers of myocardial damage. Deciding on which strategy to pursue is primarily based on early invasive interventions in patients who are hemodynamically unstable, have refractory angina, or have high Thrombolysis in Myocardial Infarction (TIMI) scores (Table 1). Patients are considered to be at low risk with a score of 0–2; intermediate risk with a score of 3–4; and high risk with a score of 5–7. Initial management is similar to STEMI including oxygen, sublingual nitroglycerin, morphine (depending on institutional policy), β-blocker therapy, and statin therapy. Antiplatelet therapy includes aspirin and a P2Y12 receptor antagonist (ticagrelor, prasugrel, clopidogrel) should be given to all patients with NSTEMI. Decisions

TABLE 1: Thrombolysis in Myocardial Infarction Score for unstable angina or non-ST elevation myocardial infarction

Historical	Points
Age ≥65	1
≥3 CAD risk factors (FHx, HTN, cholesterol, DM, active smoker)	1
Known CAD (stenosis ≥50%)	1
Aspirin use in past 7 days	1
Presentation	
Recent (≤24 h) severe angina	1
Cardiac marker elevation	1
ST deviation ≥0.5 mm	1

CAD, coronary artery disease; FHx, family history; HTN, hypertension; DM, diabetes mellitus.

> **Box 1: When to start heparin in patient with unstable angina (who is at high risk)**
>
> - Electrocardiogram changes such as ST segment changes ≥1 mm or T wave changes
> - Ongoing chest pain >20 min
> - Angina with new pulmonary edema, S3, rales, worsening mitral regurgitation, or hypotension

between antiplatelet therapies are made primarily based on risk of bleeding and cost to patient. Decision with respect to use of a glycoprotein IIb/IIIa inhibitor (eptifibatide, tirofiban, abciximab) will be determined based on which approach is being pursued. All UA/NSTEMI patients should also receive anticoagulation therapy. Indications to start heparin in intermediate or high risk UA are listed in box 1. Bivalirudin or unfractionated heparin should be used in patients undergoing an early invasive strategy while patients on track for a conservative approach, fondaparinux or enoxaparin should be given over unfractionated heparin or bivalirudin. In addition to antiplatelet and anticoagulation, all UA/NSTEMI patients should receive β-blockers, angiotensin-converting enzyme inhibitor, aldosterone antagonist (acute MI and left ventricular ejection fraction <40%). Selection of a management strategy for UA/NSTEMI is often made based on a patient's TIMI score. Patients with high and intermediate risk scores (3 and greater) benefit from an early invasive strategy (immediate coronary arteriography and revascularization). Patients with lower scores can undergo a conservative approach.

> **Box 2: Medications indicated in acute coronary syndrome**
>
> - Anti-ischemic
>   - Nitroglycerin
>   - Morphine sulfate
>   - β-blocker*
>   - Nondihydropyridine calcium channel blocker
>   - Angiotensin converting enzyme inhibitor*
> - Antiplatelet
>   - Aspirin
>   - Clopidogrel
>   - PDY12 adenosine diphosphate receptor antagonists
>   - Glycoprotein IIb/IIIa inhibitors
> - Anticoagulant
>   - Unfractionated heparin
>   - Low molecular weight heparin
>   - Direct thrombin inhibitors
>   - Factor Xa inhibitors
> - Lipid lowering therapy
>   - Statin
>
> *Indicated in congestive heart failure
> CAD, coronary artery disease; ECG, electrocardiogram.

CONCLUSION

Patients with a history of HF should be closely screened for ACS risk factors. The evaluation for ACS will involve history and assessment of risk factors, physical examination, lab work, and risk stratification via imaging. Ultimately, the management of ACS has little variation in the setting of concomitant HF and its mainstays remain revascularization therapy and medical management.

KEY POINTS

- Acute coronary syndrome (ACS) is a significant cause of acute decompensated heart failure (HF)
- The evaluation for coronary artery disease in patients with HF is primarily based on risk factor assessment
- Troponin and brain natriuretic peptide are critically integrated in the evaluation of ACS and HF respectively, but also have complementary roles in both syndromes
- Management of ACS in the setting of HF is still primarily based on antiplatelet therapy, anticoagulation, anti-anginals, and reperfusion strategy.

Heart Failure and Acute Coronary Syndrome

SUGGESTED READINGS

1. Anderson JL, Adams CD, Antman EM, Bridges CR, Califf RM, Casey DE Jr, et al. ACC/AHA 2007 guidelines for the management of patients with unstable angina/non-ST-elevation myocardial infarction: a report of the American College of Cardiology/American Heart Association Task Force on Practice Guidelines (Writing Committee to revise the 2002 Guidelines for the Management of Patients with Unstable Angina/Non-ST-Elevation Myocardial Infarction) developed in collaboration with the American College of Emergency Physicians, American College or Physicians, Society for Academic Emergency Medicine, Society for Cardiovascular Angiography and Interventions, and Society of Thoracic Surgeons. J Am Coll Cardiol. 2007.
2. Bart BA, Shaw LK, McCants CB, Fortin DF, Lee KL, O'Connor CM. The clinical and angiographic diagnosis of ischemic cardiomyopathy: a need to reassess our diagnostic criteria. Circulation. 1996;94(suppl I):I-338.
3. Bourassa MG, Gurne' O, Bangdiwala SI, Ghali JK, Young JB, Rousseau M, et al. Natural history and patterns of current practice in heart failure. The Studies of Left Ventricular Dysfunction (SOLVD) Investigators. J Am Coll Cardiol. 1993;22(4 suppl A):14A-19A.
4. Braunwald E. Application of current guidelines to the management of unstable angina and non-ST-elevation myocardial infarction. Circulation. 2003;108(16 Suppl 1):III28-37.
5. de Lemos JA, Morrow DA. Brain natriuretic peptide measurement in acute coronary syndromes : ready for clinical application? Circulation. 2002;106:2868-70.
6. Gaggin HK, Januzzi JL Jr. Natriuretic peptides in heart failure and acute coronary syndrome. Clin Lab Med. 2014;34(1):43-58, vi.
7. Gheorghiade M, Bonow RO. Chronic heart failure in the United States: a manifestation of coronary artery disease. Circulation. 1998;97:282-9.
8. Jneid H, Anderson JL, Wright RS, Adams CD, Bridges CR, Casey DE Jr, et al. 2012 ACCF/AHA focused update of the guideline for the management of patients with unstable angina/non-ST-elevation myocardial infarction (updating the 2007 guideline and replacing the 2011 focused update): a report of the American College of Cardiology Foundation/American Heart Association Task Force on practice guidelines. J Am Coll Cardiol. 2012; 60(7):645-81.
9. Jneid H, Anderson JL, Wright RS, Adams CD, Bridges CR, Casey DE Jr, et al. 2012 ACCF/AHA focused update of the guideline for the management of patients with unstable angina/Non-ST-elevation myocardial infarction (updating the 2007 guideline and replacing the 2011 focused update): a report of the American College of Cardiology Foundation/American Heart Association Task Force on practice guidelines. Circulation. 2012;126(7):875-910.
10. Larsen AI, Dickstein K. BNP in acute coronary syndromes: the heart expresses its suffering. Eur Heart J. 2004;25(15):1284-6.
11. Mahajan VS, Jarolim P. How to interpret elevated cardiac troponin levels. Circulation. 2011;124(21):2350-4.
12. O'Gara PT, Kushner FG, Ascheim DD, Casey DE Jr, Chung MK, de Lemos JA, et al. 2013 ACCF/AHA guideline for the management of ST-elevation myocardial infarction: executive summary: a report of the American College of Cardiology Foundation/American Heart Association Task Force on Practice Guidelines: developed in collaboration with the American College of Emergency Physicians and Society for Cardiovascular Angiography and Interventions. Catheter Cardiovasc Interv. 2013;82(1):E1-27.
13. O'Gara PT, Kushner FG, Ascheim DD, Casey DE Jr, Chung MK, de Lemos JA, et al. 2013 ACCF/AHA guideline for the management of ST-elevation myocardial infarction: a report of the American College of Cardiology Foundation/American Heart Association Task Force on Practice Guidelines. Circulation. 2013;127(4):e362-425.

14. Peacock WF 4th, De Marco T, Fonarow GC, Diercks D, Wynne J, Apple FS, et al. Cardiac troponin and outcome in acute heart failure. N Engl J Med. 2008;358:2117-26.
15. Potluri S, Ventura HO, Mulumudi M, Mehra MR. Cardiac troponin levels in heart failure. Cardiol Rev. 2004;12(1):21-5.
16. Tatum JL, Jesse RL, Kontos MC, Nicholson CS, Schmidt KL, Roberts CS, et al. Comprehensive strategy for the evaluation and triage of the chest pain patient. Ann Emerg Med. 1997;29:116-25.
17. Wang TJ. Significance of circulating troponins in heart failure: if these walls could talk. Circulation. 2007;116:1217-20.

SECTION 3

Chronic Heart Failure Patients in the Outpatient Setting

14
CHAPTER

Echocardiography: Getting It Right

Nicholas A Marston, Daniel G Blanchard, Jeremy Egnatios

INTRODUCTION

Echocardiography is a useful non-invasive tool that can assess cardiac function, structure, and volume status in patients with suspected cardiac pathology. When performed at the bedside it can quickly augment the physical exam and aid in narrowing the differential diagnosis. The information gained from an echocardiogram can provide insight into many cardiac pathologies including cardiogenic shock, heart failure, ischemic disease, valvular disease, pericardial disease, cardiomyopathies, and right heart disease. This chapter will review how an echocardiogram can be useful in each of these conditions and ultimately guide the appropriate management decisions.

HEMODYNAMIC INSTABILITY/SHOCK

Echocardiography can be enormously helpful in assessing several critical parameters in a patient with shock of unclear etiology (Algorithm 1).

Ventricular Systolic Function

A normal or hyperdynamic left ventricular ejection fraction (LVEF) would strongly suggest that the shock is not cardiogenic, but rather septic, hypovolemic, or vasodilatory. On the other hand, a depressed LVEF does not conclusively mean the shock is cardiogenic, but it dramatically increases the likelihood (especially if the left venticular

Algorithms in Heart Failure

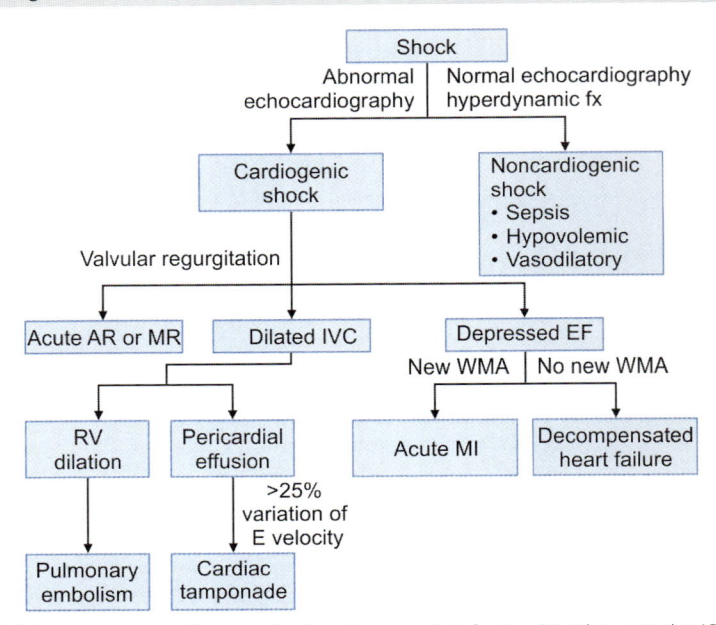

```
                        Shock
              Abnormal  │  Normal echocardiography
         echocardiography │  hyperdynamic fx
                    │       │
                    ▼       ▼
              Cardiogenic   Noncardiogenic
                shock           shock
                              • Sepsis
                              • Hypovolemic
                              • Vasodilatory

   Valvular regurgitation
        │
   ┌────┴────────────┬──────────────────┐
   ▼                 ▼                  ▼
Acute AR or MR   Dilated IVC        Depressed EF
                                  New WMA │ No new WMA
                 ┌────┴────┐         ▼         ▼
                 ▼         ▼      Acute MI  Decompensated
               RV      Pericardial              heart failure
            dilation    effusion
                         >25%
                      variation of
                       E velocity
                ▼          ▼
            Pulmonary   Cardiac
            embolism   tamponade
```

IVC, inferior vena cava; EF, ejection fraction; MI, myocardial infarction, RV, right ventricular; AR, aortic regurgitation; MR, mitral regurgitation; WMA, wall motion abnormalities.

ALGORITHM 1: Algorithm for assessing shock

dysfunction is new). If right ventricular function is depressed in the setting of shock, one should strongly consider a large pulmonary embolus or right ventricular infarction.

Valvular Function

In most settings, echocardiography can diagnose severe valve dysfunction (e.g., severe aortic and mitral regurgitation and/or stenosis). A sudden onset of hemodynamic instability is more likely due to acute aortic or mitral regurgitation, as valvular stenosis is a more gradual process. Color Doppler imaging is diagnostic in most cases, but transesophageal echocardiography (TEE) is occasionally necessary.

Regional Wall Motion Abnormalities

Echocardiography can also identify regional abnormalities of left ventricular function which occur in myocardial infarction (MI). In cases of acute MI, nonaffected areas of the left ventricular often become hyperdynamic to maintain a near-normal ejection fraction (EF). Echocardiography can also detect mechanical complications that may lead to shock, such as ventricular septal rupture, severe mitral regurgitation, and left ventricular free wall rupture. Intravenous injection of echocardiography contrast can be used to opacify the left ventricular cavity and make wall motion abnormalities more apparent.

Estimation of Intracardiac Pressures

Echocardiography can be used to estimate right atrial pressure (RAP), pulmonary artery pressure (PAP), and left ventricular filling pressure. Right atrial (central venous) pressure can be estimated by assessing the diameter of the inferior vena cava (IVC) and its response to inspiration. Normally, the IVC diameter is less than 2 cm, and it collapses more than 50% with inspiration (this corresponds to a RAP no greater than 5 mmHg). If the IVC is dilated, but its diameter still decreases more than 50% with inspiration, the RAP is likely around 10 mmHg. However, when the IVC is markedly dilated and decreases in diameter during inspiration by less than 10%, the RAP is probably in the range of 15–20 mmHg (Algorithm 2). Unfortunately, this method is not accurate in an intubated patient, due to positive pressure ventilation.

Pulmonary artery pressure can be estimated using the modified Bernoulli's equation. This states that the pressure in the right ventricle is directly related to the velocity of tricuspid regurgitation blood flow. Most people have mild tricuspid regurgitation, and the velocity of this flow can be measured with Doppler echocardiography. The

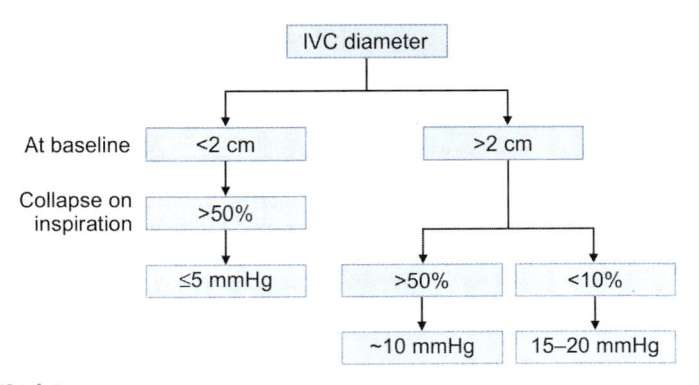

IVC, inferior vena cava.

ALGORITHM 2: Algorithm for assessing right atrial pressure

pressure gradient across the tricuspid valve is equal to four times the velocity of the tricuspid regurgitant velocity (TRV) squared, plus the RAP. If there is no pulmonic stenosis, then the right ventricular systolic pressure is essentially the same as the systolic PAP:

$$\text{Systolic PAP} = 4 \times (\text{TRV})^2 + \text{RAP}$$

When the TRV exceeds 3 m/s, pulmonary hypertension is usually present.

Left ventricular filling pressures can be measured using diastolic flow patterns discussed in the following section.

HEART FAILURE

Echocardiography provides valuable information about systolic and diastolic function in patients presenting with dyspnea and possible congestive heart failure (CHF). In the past several years, CHF patients have been classified as having either reduced left ventricular systolic function (HFrEF) or preserved systolic function (HFpEF). In HFrEF, the echocardiography findings are straightforward and primarily consist of a reduced EF. Further analysis of left ventricular size, thickness, wall motion, and aortic or mitral valves may help determine the etiology of the systolic dysfunction (Algorithm 3).

Findings in HFpEF are less obvious, but left atrial enlargement can often be the first clue to elevated left ventricular filling pressures and diastolic dysfunction. Further analysis includes diastolic flow

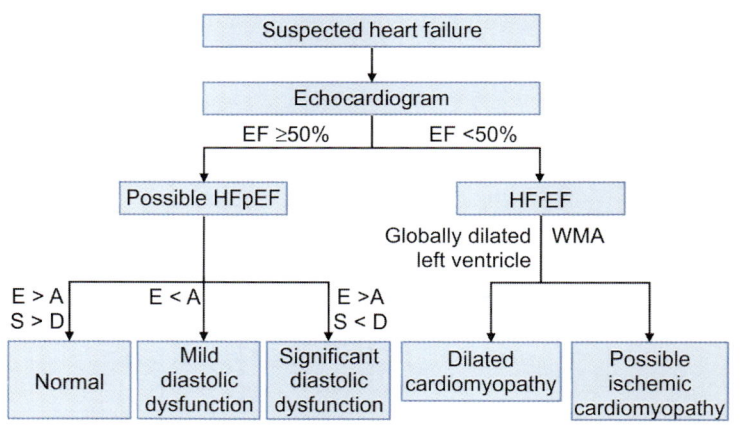

EF, ejection fraction; HFpEF, heart failure with preserved ejection fraction; HFrEF, heart failure with reduced ejection fraction; WMA, wall motion abnormalities.

ALGORITHM 3: Algorithm for determining the type of heart failure patterns through the mitral valve and the pulmonary vein. In a normal individual, about two-thirds of left ventricular filling occurs early during diastole (the early rapid filling or E wave), and one-third during late diastole (the atrial contraction or A wave). Similarly, the majority of flow from the pulmonary vein into the left atrium occurs during diastole (the D wave), and less during ventricular systole (the S wave). As humans age, a pattern of mild diastolic dysfunction occurs, where the transmitral E wave velocity is less than that of the A wave (and the pulmonary venous S wave becomes greater than the D wave). Though technically abnormal, this change in diastolic filling is expected with aging, and predicts a normal mean left ventricular diastolic pressure.

In patients with HFpEF, moderate-to-severe diastolic left ventricular dysfunction is often present. In these cases, the transmitral E velocity is greater than the A velocity, but the pulmonary venous S velocity is less than the D velocity. As opposed to people with normal diastolic function, however, the mitral annular diastolic velocity is also markedly reduced. This suggests abnormally elevated left ventricular filling pressure.

ISCHEMIC HEART DISEASE

Although ischemic heart disease is often diagnosed with electrocardiography (ECG), stress testing, and cardiac catheterization, visualization of wall motion abnormalities on echocardiography may be the first clue of a prior MI. In the acute evaluation of chest pain, echocardiography can be especially useful in patients with left bundle branch block or pre-existing ST-T wave abnormalities, as the ECG may not be completely diagnostic of ischemia or injury. A new left ventricular wall motion abnormality will direct the care toward acute intervention, whereas unchanged or normal left ventricular systolic function is reassuring. Additionally, echocardiography can evaluate right ventricular systolic function, which is especially important in cases of inferior MI (where right ventricular involvement portends a worse prognosis and mandates an aggressive approach).

VALVULAR HEART DISEASE

Two-dimensional echocardiography is very useful for diagnosing valvular disease, but Doppler echocardiography is necessary to assess its severity. Doppler echocardiography measures velocity of blood within the heart and vasculature, and color Doppler can quickly screen for the presence of valvular regurgitation. In general, stenotic lesions are easier to quantify than regurgitant lesions. For aortic stenosis, the continuity equation is used:

$$A_1 \times V_1 = A_2 \times V_2$$

where A_1 and V_1 are the cross-sectional area and maximum systolic velocity through the left ventricular outflow tract, respectively and V_2 is the maximum velocity through the aortic valve. These three variables can be measured with echocardiography and then used to solve for aortic valve area. Aortic valve area less than 1.5 cm^2 is considered moderate and less than 1.0 cm^2 is generally considered severe.

Mitral stenosis is quantified using the pressure half-time method, which measures how quickly the pressure gradient between the left atrium and left ventricle decreases during diastole. If the gradient decreases quickly between the two chambers, then the stenosis is relatively mild; if the gradient decreases slowly, the stenosis is more severe.

The quantification of valvular regurgitation is more challenging. Color Doppler is an essential part of the examination, and in general shows color "jets" in the chamber proximal to the valve (e.g., the left atrium in mitral regurgitation and the left ventricle in aortic regurgitation). The size of the color jet has been used to estimate severity with some success, but regurgitant jets are not always central and may be quite eccentric. In these cases, the jet may be "wall-hugging" and lead to underestimation of the regurgitation severity.

Doppler echocardiography measurements can also be used to calculate the effective regurgitant orifice (ERO) size. For cases of mitral regurgitation, an ERO of less than 0.2 cm^2 is generally mild, while approximately 0.4 cm^2 is more likely moderate, and approximately 0.6 cm^2 is usually severe. In cases of aortic regurgitation, the pressure half-time method can also be used. If the pressure gradient between the aorta and the left ventricle decreases quickly, the aortic regurgitation is likely severe. A pressure half-time less than 250 ms almost always signifies severe aortic regurgitation.

In the setting of positive blood cultures and possible infective endocarditis, transthoracic echocardiography should be ordered. Transthoracic echocardiogram (TTE) is reasonably good at detecting valvular vegetations and even better at diagnosing regurgitation due to leaflet destruction. However, TEE has much better diagnostic accuracy, especially for visualizing valvular abscesses and small vegetations.

Echocardiography can help evaluate the function of both bioprosthetic and mechanical prosthetic heart valves. Because prosthetic valves (especially mechanical ones) block ultrasound waves and cause "shadowing" posterior to the valve, TEE may be necessary to evaluate a prosthesis more completely.

PERICARDIAL DISEASE

Acute Pericarditis

The diagnosis of pericarditis is a clinical one, based on history, physical examination, and the ECG. An echocardiogram should be ordered for all patients thought to have pericarditis (to make sure they do not have a pericardial effusion with cardiac tamponade), but the absence of an effusion does not rule out pericarditis. It is important to remember that even raging pericarditis can be present without a pericardial effusion.

Pericardial Effusion

Echocardiography is extremely accurate in detecting pericardial effusions, even if only trivial. Small pericardial effusions tend to be posterior, especially if the patient is supine. Larger effusions can be circumferential or loculated, and may contain clot, fibrinous strands, or tumor. Purulent effusions tend to be loculated. This distinction between loculated effusions and nonloculated effusions is clinically important, as loculated effusions are harder to drain completely via pericardiocentesis. In these cases, surgical drainage or debridement and creation of a pericardial window may be required.

Cardiac Tamponade

Echocardiography now plays a major in the diagnosis of cardiac tamponade. The most important echocardiography findings in tamponade are: distension of the vena cava, diastolic compression of the right ventricle, and abnormal mitral inflow pattern. Distension in the vena cave is nonspecific, but represents elevated central venous pressure. More specific is the diastolic right ventricular compression and septal "buckling" that occurs due to ventricular interdependence and near-fixed volumes throughout the cardiac cycle. The most specific finding is the abnormal mitral flow pattern with inspiration. During normal inspiration, venous return increases more on the right side of the heart than the left. This leads to a mild (<10%) increase in peak transtricuspid blood flow velocity and a reciprocal mild decrease in transmitral blood flow velocity. Several important studies have shown that a respiratory variation in the mitral "E" velocity of more than 25% strongly suggests cardiac tamponade when a pericardial effusion is present.

CARDIOMYOPATHIES

Echocardiography can help distinguish the three primary cardiomyopathies: (1) dilated, (2) restrictive, and (3) hypertrophic. Patients with dilated cardiomyopathy usually have global left ventricular (and sometimes right ventricular) enlargement with global systolic dysfunction. Diastolic dysfunction is also often present. Regional left ventricular dysfunction, however, is suggestive of ischemic heart disease.

Restrictive cardiomyopathy can be completely idiopathic, but is most commonly caused by an infiltrative process. Echocardiography evaluation often shows increased left ventricular wall thickness, valvular thickening, marked biatrial enlargement, and moderate-to-severe left ventricular diastolic dysfunction. Severe diastolic dysfunction by echocardiography is a sign of poor prognosis in these patients. Magnetic resonance imaging should be performed in suspected amyloidosis.

In the setting of hypertrophic cardiomyopathy (HCM), echocardiography can detect asymmetric septal hypertrophy, one of the cardinal findings of HCM. In cases of hypertrophic obstructive cardiomyopathy (HOCM), echocardiography can identify systolic anterior motion (SAM) of the mitral valve leaflet ("SAM," which causes left ventricular outflow tract obstruction), elevated late systolic blood flow velocity through the left ventricular outflow tract and late systolic partial closure of the aortic valve. Taken together, the presence of all these findings are diagnostic of HOCM in the majority of cases.

RIGHT HEART DISEASE

Echocardiography is reasonably good at detecting right heart enlargement and right ventricular dysfunction. Doppler Echocardiography is excellent in estimating right ventricular and pulmonary artery systolic pressure, and color Doppler imaging can assess severity of tricuspid and pulmonic regurgitation. Echocardiography is indicated in cases of pulmonary embolism, as residual thrombi are occasionally seen in the right atrium or ventricle. In cases of severe pulmonary hypertension, the right ventricle is markedly enlarged, and the interventricular septum is flattened by the high right ventricular pressure. By measuring peak TRV, echocardiography can assess the responses to treatment for pulmonary hypertension.

TRANSESOPHAGEAL ECHOCARDIOGRAPHY

Transesophageal echocardiography provides superior views of the heart, but should be reserved for the following situations: suboptimal TTE images, suspected endocarditis, *Staphylococcus aureus* bacteremia, unclear source of embolus, and valvular disease when considering surgery (especially for mitral valve disease).

CONCLUSION

Echocardiography plays an instrumental role in the clinical assessment of cardiac disease. It can be utilized in the inpatient or outpatient setting, at the bedside or in the laboratory, and may be transthoracic or transesophageal. An understanding of when an echocardiogram is clinically indicated and how to interpret the results are key skills for any provider caring for patients with cardiac disease. The information obtained from the echocardiogram can significantly aid the physician in diagnosis and guide management of both acute and chronic cardiac pathologies.

KEY POINTS

- Echocardiography is the most commonly used cardiac imaging technique, and is extremely useful in multiple clinical settings, including shock, heart failure, coronary heart disease, valvular disease, pericardial disease, and cardiomyopathy
- Echocardiography can be used to estimate right atrial (central venous) pressure, pulmonary artery pressure, and left ventricular filling pressure
- Doppler flow patterns are used to diagnose diastolic dysfunction and determine severity
- Color Doppler is useful in assessing valvular abnormalities, especially regurgitation
- Transesophageal echocardiogram provides superior imaging and may be warranted in cases with suspected endocarditis, unclear source of systemic embolus, and valvular heart disease.

SUGGESTED READINGS

1. DeMaria AN, Blanchard DG. Echocardiography. In: Fuster V, Walsh RA, Harrington RA (Eds). Hurst's The Heart, 13th ed. New York: McGraw-Hill; 2011. pp. 411-89.
2. Yancy CW, Jessup M, Bozkurt B, Butler J, Casey DE, Drazner MH,et al. 2013: ACCF/AHA guidelines for the diagnosis and management of heart failure: A report of the American College of Cardiology Foundation/American Heart Association task force on practice guidelines. J Am Coll Cardiol 2013;62(16):e147-239.
3. Bonow RO, Carabello BA, Chatterjee K, de Leon AC Jr, Faxon DP, Freed MD, et al. 2008 Focused update incorporated into the ACC/AHA 2006 guidelines for the management of patients with valvular heart disease: A report of the American College of Cardiology/American Heart Association task Force on practice guidelines endorsed by the Society of Cardiovascular Anesthesiologists, Society for Cardiovascular Angiography and Interventions, and Society of Thoracic Surgeons. J Am Coll Cardiol. 2008;52:e1-e142.
4. Khandaker MH, Espinosa RE, Nishimura RA, Sinak LJ, Hayes SN, Melduni RM, et al. Pericardial Disease: Diagnosis and Management. Mayo Clin Proc. 2010;85(6):572-93.
5. Hoen B, Duval X. Infective endocarditis. N Engl J Med. 2013;368:1425-33.
6. Maron BJ. Contemporary insights and strategies for risk stratification and prevention of sudden death in hypertrophic cardiomyopathy. Circulation. 2010;121:445-56.

CHAPTER 15

Initiation of Angiotensin Converting Enzyme Inhibitors and Beta-blockers in Heart Failure: Putting Evidence into Practice

Boris Arbit, Alan S Maisel

INTRODUCTION

Decades of well-designed, large scale, randomized clinical trials have produced a wealth of knowledge regarding efficacy and implementation of medical treatments for heart failure (HF). However, the actual uptake of these evidence-based treatments into real clinical practice has been variable. This has resulted in HF patients being denied the benefit of proven treatments. Therefore, this chapter serves the purpose of providing practical guidance on the appropriate and safe use of treatments of proven benefit in the management of patients with HF.

GENERAL FOUR-STEP APPROACH TO MEDICATION INITIATION (ALGORITHM 1)

The first step involves establishing a clinical diagnosis of HF and initiating appropriate diuretic treatment. The second step involves verifying the presence of left ventricular dysfunction (typically defined as an ejection fraction <0.4) via echocardiography, radionuclide ventriculography, radiological left ventricular angiography, or cardiac magnetic resonance. The third step is the initiation of first line therapy for all patients with HF due to left ventricular dysfunction, namely an angiotensin converting enzyme inhibitor (ACEI) and a β-blocker unless contraindications are present. Angiotensin converting enzyme inhibitor generally should be initiated first at a low dose and quickly followed by a

Algorithms in Heart Failure

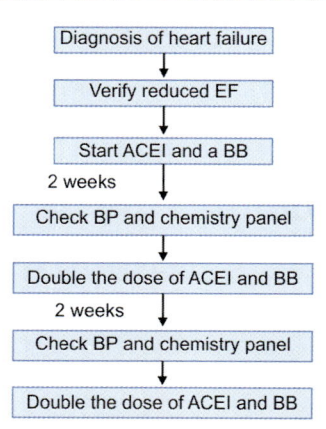

```
Diagnosis of heart failure
          ↓
   Verify reduced EF
          ↓
   Start ACEI and a BB
2 weeks   ↓
Check BP and chemistry panel
          ↓
Double the dose of ACEI and BB
2 weeks   ↓
Check BP and chemistry panel
          ↓
Double the dose of ACEI and BB
```

ACEI, angiotensin converting enzyme inhibitor; BB, β-blockers; BP, blood pressure; EF, ejection fraction.

ALGORITHM 1: Approach for clinical diagnosis of heart failure

β-blocker once the patient is considered no longer decompensated. In situations where the ACEI is not tolerated, such as situations of coughing, angiotensin receptor blockers should be utilized. The last step involves the implementation of additional pharmacologic therapy for patients with persisting signs and symptoms of HF, specifically the use of spironolactone in patients with New York Heart Association (NYHA) class III/IV after optimization of ACEIs and β-blockers and the addition of eplerenone in situations where unpleasant antiandrogenic side effects of spironolactone become too bothersome.

APPROACH TO INITIATE ANGIOTENSIN CONVERTING ENZYME INHIBITOR IN HEART FAILURE

The justification for initiating ACEI in patients with HF stems from a multitude of studies supporting their use. Clinical trials alongside multiple meta-analyses demonstrated that ACEIs increased survival, reduced hospital admissions, and improved NYHA class and quality of life in patients with all grades of symptomatic HF.

Absolute contraindications to ACEIs and situations requiring caution are listed in table 1. The general strategy is to start at a low dose and double the dose at 2 week intervals till the optimum target dose is achieved (Table 2). Blood pressure and blood chemistry, specifically the blood urea nitrogen, serum creatinine and serum

TABLE 1: Contraindications for angiotensin converting enzyme inhibitors in heart failure

Contraindications	Cautions
• History of angioedema • Bilateral renal artery stenosis	• Hyperkalemia • Cr >2.5 mg/dL • Symptomatic or severe asymptomatic hypotension (SBP <90 mmHg)

Cr, creatinine; SBP, systolic blood pressure.

TABLE 2: Angiotensin converting enzyme inhibitors and proper dosing

ACEIs	Starting dose	Target dose
Captopril	6.25 mg TID	50 mg TID
Enalapril	2.5 mg BID	10–20 mg BID
Lisinopril	2.5–5 mg QD	20–35 mg QD
Ramipril	2.5 mg QD	10 mg QD

ACEIs, angiotensin converting enzyme inhibitors; BID, twice a day; TID, thrice a day; QD, four times a day..

potassium levels should be monitored 1–2 weeks following initiation of ACEI and additionally monitored again 1–2 weeks after the final titration dose adjustment. Symptomatic hypotension should prompt consideration of decreasing the patient's diuretic dose, if there are no signs of volume overload. One should reconsider the use of nitrates and calcium channel blockers and other vasodilators, if the patient complains of dizziness, light headedness, or confusion. An increase in creatinine up to 50% above baseline or 3 mg/dL (whichever is smaller) is acceptable. In situations where the increase in creatinine or potassium exceeds these boundaries, the dose of the ACEI should be halved and repeat blood chemistries should be assessed in 1–2 weeks after the dosage adjustment.

Patients should be advised to report primarily principal adverse side effects including dizziness, symptomatic hypotension and cough, and to avoid nonsteroidal anti-inflammatory drugs not prescribed by a physician and salt substitutes high in potassium to avoid hyperkalemia.

APPROACH TO INITIATE BETA-BLOCKERS IN HEART FAILURE

Several major randomized controlled clinical trials have convincingly demonstrated that specific β-blockers increase survival, reduce

Algorithms in Heart Failure

TABLE 3: Contraindications for β-blockers in heart failure

Contraindications	Cautions
• Asthma	• NYHA IV HF • Heart block/heart rate <60 beats/min • Persisting sign of volume overload • Current exacerbation of HF

HF, heart failure; NYHA, New York Heart Association.

TABLE 4: Beta-blockers and proper dosing

Beta-blockers	Starting dose	Target dose
Bisoprolol	1.25 mg QD	10 mg QD
Carvedilol	3.125 mg BID	25–50 mg BID
Metoprolol CR/XL	1.25–25 mg QD	200 mg QD

BID, twice a day; CR, controlled release; QD, four times a day; XL, extended release.

hospital admissions, and improve NYHA class and quality of life in patients with stable mild, moderate, and even severe HF.

The primary absolute contraindication to initiating β-blocker therapy is asthma (Table 3). However, precaution should also be taken before initiating β-blockers in patients with severe NYHA IV HF, ongoing or recent (<4 weeks) congestive heart failure exacerbation, heart block, bradycardia, persisting signs of congestion, and hypotension (SBP <90 mmHg).

Specific β-blockers that should be considered are tabulated in table 4. As with ACEI, β-blockers should be started at low doses, with a goal of doubling the dose at 2 week intervals till the target dose shown to yield proven clinical benefit. As with ACEIs, blood chemistry should also be checked 1–2 weeks after starting the treatment, and again 1–2 weeks immediately after making the final titration changes in dose. Patients should be advised to immediately report any worsening dyspnea, fatigue, however, should not decrease their β-blocker dose without consulting their physician. If increasing volume status is observed, diuretic dosing should be increased or the β-blocker dose should be halved, if increased dieresis does not result in improvement. Increased fatigue or bradycardia should be managed with a reduction in the β-blocker dose as well. Asymptomatic hypotension does not warrant any change in the β-blocker dose; symptomatic hypotension, in conjunction with euvolemic volume status, warrants consideration for reducing the patient's diuretic or ACEI dose.

CONCLUSION

The clinical short- and long-term benefit of β-blockers and ACEI in patients with HF is well known. However, underprescribing and underdosing of these proven beneficial medications is a problem. This chapter's concise clinical recommendations for administering clinically proven medical therapies provides the clear framework for easily implementing proven evidence based therapies appropriately and effectively.

KEY POINTS

- A remarkable number of randomized double-blinded clinical trials have been conducted on patients with heart failure (HF). However, the actual uptake of these evidence based treatments into real clinical practice has been variable
- Underprescribing and underdosing of these proven beneficial medications is a persistent problem
- The chapter describes concise clinical recommendations for administering these two clinically proven medical therapies and also provides the clear framework for easily implementing angiotensin converting enzyme inhibitors and β-blockers effectively in HF.

SUGGESTED READINGS

1. Boyles PJ, Peterson GM, Bleasel MD, Vial JH. Undertreatment of congestive heart failure in an Australian setting. J Clin Pharm Ther. 2004;29(1):15-22.
2. Bungard TJ, McAlister FA, Johnson JA, Tsuyuki RT. Underutilization of ACE inhibitors in patients with congestive heart failure. Drugs. 2001;61(14): 2021-33.
3. Cleland JG, Cohen-Solal A, Aguilar JC, Dietz R, Eastaugh J, Follath F, et al. Management of heart failure in primary care (the IMPROVEMENT of Heart Failure Programme): an international survey. Lancet. 2002;360(9346):1631-9.
4. Digitalis Investigation Group. The effect of digoxin on mortality and morbidity in patients with heart failure. N Engl J Med. 1997;336(8):525-33.
5. Effect of metoprolol CR/XL in chronic heart failure: Metoprolol CR/XL Randomised Intervention Trial in Congestive Heart Failure (MERIT-HF). Lancet. 1999;353(9169):2001-7.
6. Effects of enalapril on mortality in severe congestive heart failure. Results of the Cooperative North Scandinavian Enalapril Survival Study (CONSENSUS). The CONSENSUS Trial Study Group. N Engl J Med. 1987;316(23):1429-35.
7. Effects of enalapril on survival in patients with reduced left ventricular ejection fractions and congestive heart failure. The SOLVD Investigators. N Engl J Med. 1991;325(5):293-302.
8. Heart Failure Society of America (HFSA) practice guidelines. HFSA guidelines for management of patients with heart failure caused by left ventricular systolic dysfunction—pharmacological approaches. J Card Fail. 1999;5(4):357-82.

Algorithms in Heart Failure

9. Hobbs FD, Jones MI, Allan TF, Wilson S, Tobias R. European survey of primary care physician perceptions on heart failure diagnosis and management (Euro-HF). Eur Heart J. 2000;21(22):1877-87.
10. Hoppe UC, Erdmann E, Kommission Klinische Kardiologie. Guidelines for the treatment of chronic heart failure. Issued by the executive committee of the German society of cardiology—heart and circulation research, compiled on behalf of the commission of clinical cardiology in cooperative with pharmaceutic commission of the German physicians' association. Z Kardiol. 2001;90:218-37.
11. Houghton AR, Cowley AJ. Why are angiotensin converting enzyme inhibitors underutilised in the treatment of heart failure by general practitioners? Int J Cardiol. 1997;59(1):7-10.
12. Hunt SA, Baker DW, Chin MH, Cinquegrani MP, Feldman AM, Francis GS, et al. ACC/AHA guidelines for the evaluation and management of chronic heart failure in the adult: executive summary. A report of the American College of Cardiology/American Heart Association Task Force on Practice Guidelines (Committee to Revise the 1995 Guidelines for the Evaluation and Management of Heart Failure). J Am Coll Cardiol. 2001;104:2996-3007.
13. Komajda M, Follath F, Swedberg K, Cleland J, Aguilar JC, Cohen-Solal A, et al. The EuroHeart Failure Survey programme—a survey on the quality of care among patients with heart failure in Europe. Part 2: treatment. Eur Heart J. 2003;24(5):464-74.
14. Konstam MA, Dracup K, Baker DW, Bottorff MB, Brooks NH, Dacey RA, et al. Heart failure: evaluation and care of patients with left ventricular systolic dysfunction. J Card Fail. 1995;1(2):183-7.
15. Krum H, Jelinek MV, Stewart S, Sindone A, Atherton JJ; National Heart Foundation of Australia, et al. 2011 update to National Heart Foundation of Australia and Cardiac Society of Australia and New Zealand Guidelines for the prevention, detection and management of chronic heart failure in Australia, 2006. Med J Aust. 2011;194(8):405-9.
16. Krum H, Tonkin AM, Currie R, Djundjek R, Johnston CI. Chronic heart failure in Australian general practice. The Cardiac Awareness Survey and Evaluation (CASE) Study. Med J Aust. 2001;174(9):439-44.
17. Liu P, Arnold JM, Belenkie I, Demers C, Dorian P, Gianetti N, et al. Canadian Cardiovascular Society. The 2002/3 Canadian Cardiovascular Society consensus guideline update for the diagnosis and management of heart failure. Can J Cardiol. 2003;19:347-56.
18. Mair FS, Crowley TS, Bundred PE. Prevalence, aetiology and management of heart failure in general practice. Br J Gen Pract. 1996;46(403):77-9.
19. Masoudi FA, Rathore SS, Wang Y, Havranek EP, Curtis JP, Foody JM, et al. National patterns of use and effectiveness of angiotensin-converting enzyme inhibitors in older patients with heart failure and left ventricular systolic dysfunction. Circulation. 2004;110(6):724-31.
20. McMurray J, Gyarfas I, Wenger NK, Al Nozha MM, Boskis B, Bristow M, et al. Concise guide to the management of heart failure. Am J Geriatr Cardiol. 1996;5:13-30.
21. Mosterd WL, Rosier PF. Guideline 'chronic heart failure'. Tijdschr Geneeskd. 2004;148:609-14.
22. Muntwyler J, Cohen-Solal A, Freemantle N, Eastaugh J, Cleland JG, Follath F. Relation of sex, age and concomitant diseases to drug prescription for heart failure in primary care in Europe. Eur J Heart Fail. 2004;6(5):663-8.
23. Murphy NF, Simpson CR, McAlister FA, Stewart S, MacIntyre K, Kirkpatrick M, et al. National survey of the prevalence, incidence, primary care burden, and treatment of heart failure in Scotland. Heart. 2004;90(10):1129-36.
24. National Institute for Health and Clinical Excellence. (2010). Chronic heart failure: Management of chronic heart failure in adults in primary and secondary care. NICE clinical guideline 108. [online] Available from www.nice.org.uk/nicemedia/live/13099/50517/50517.pdf. [Accessed Jan, 2016].

25. Packer M, Bristow MR, Cohn JN, Colucci WS, Fowler MB, Gilbert EM, et al. The effect of carvedilol on morbidity and mortality in patients with chronic heart failure. U.S. Carvedilol Heart Failure Study Group. N Engl J Med. 1996;334(21):1349-55.
26. Pitt B, Zannad F, Remme WJ, Cody R, Castaigne A, Perez A, et al. The effect of spironolactone on morbidity and mortality in patients with severe heart failure. Randomized Aldactone Evaluation Study Investigators. N Engl J Med. 1999;341(10):709-17.
27. Roman-Sanchez P, Conthe P, Garcia-Alegria J, Forteza-Rey J, Montero M, Montoto C. Factors influencing medical treatment of heart failure patients in Spanish internal medicine departments: a national survey. QJM. 2005;98(2):127-38.
28. The Cardiac Insufficiency Bisoprolol Study II (CIBIS-II): a randomised trial. Lancet. 1999;353(9146):9-13.
29. The National Heart Foundation of New Zealand, Cardiac Society of Australia and New Zealand, the Royal New Zealand College of General Practitioners Working Party. New Zealand guidelines for management of chronic heart failure. N Z Med J. 1997;110:99-107.

16 CHAPTER

Atrial Fibrillation Done Right

Amir A Schricker, David E Krummen

INTRODUCTION

Atrial fibrillation (AF) is the most common sustained arrhythmia and thus frequently encountered in clinical practice. Although a wide array of treatment options exist, optimal AF management encompasses the following general principles: prevention of thromboembolism; appropriate heart rate control; and maintenance of sinus rhythm, if significant symptoms are present after achieving adequate rate control.

EPIDEMIOLOGY

Atrial fibrillation is the most common sustained arrhythmia, occurring in approximately 1% of the population, and increasing steadily with age. The risk of AF reaches almost 10% in patients over the age of 80. In general, AF is not acutely dangerous (except in the presence of a rapidly conducting accessory pathway), but is associated with increased risks of stroke, heart failure, hospitalization, dementia, and premature death.

In addition to well-established risk factors of advanced age, hypertension and ischemic heart disease, other AF risk factors include transient reversible causes and underlying heart disease (Table 1).

TABLE 1: Additional risk factors for atrial fibrillation

Transient reversible risk factors	Underlying heart disease risk factors
<ul><li>Thyrotoxicosis</li><li>Alcohol ingestion</li><li>Acute MI</li><li>Pericarditis</li><li>Pulmonary disease</li><li>Obstructive sleep apnea (increasingly recognized as independent AF risk factor[6]</li></ul>	<ul><li>Recent cardiac surgery</li><li>Congestive heart failure</li><li>Recent MI</li></ul>

AF, atrial fibrillation; MI, myocardial infarction.

CLASSIFICATION

Many terms have been used to classify AF. Currently, guidelines propose the following classification scheme for AF:
- First detected AF: the term to describe AF at first diagnosis
- Paroxysmal AF: recurrent AF episodes that terminate spontaneously in 7 days or less
- Persistent AF: characterized as AF with episodes that last longer than 7 days and typically require pharmacologic or electrical cardioversion to restore sinus rhythm
- Long-standing AF: refers to AF that has lasted for 1 year or more
- Permanent AF: AF in which cardioversion has failed, or AF patients in whom sinus rhythm restoration is no longer pursued or deemed futile.

This classification scheme applies to recurrent episodes of AF lasting more than 30 seconds that are unrelated to reversible causes.

CLINICAL PRESENTATION

Atrial fibrillation can be asymptomatic or symptomatic, regardless of the heart rate. A significant proportion with asymptomatic AF may present with stroke as their first symptom. Symptoms due to AF vary, are often due to the degree of heart rate elevation, and can commonly include the following:
- Palpitations
- Shortness of breath
- Weakness
- Fatigue
- Chest pain (less common)
- Syncope (less common).

CLINICAL EVALUATION

A complete history and physical examination is an essential part of the AF workup. Comprehensive baseline laboratory testing should be performed to assess for electrolyte abnormalities, renal dysfunction, and other potentially reversible causes. The electrocardiogram (ECG) is an essential tool in the diagnosis and management of AF, as is an echocardiogram. Important aspects of each are listed below:

History and Physical Examination

- Determine symptoms timeline, frequency, duration, and severity of AF episodes
- Identify precipitating factors (if any)
- Determine presence of existing cardiovascular disease, hypertension, diabetes, history of stroke and vascular disease
- Vital signs, in particular during AF
- Detailed cardiac examination, including evaluation for valvular disease and evidence of heart failure.

Laboratory Tests

- Chemistry panel
- Renal function
- Complete blood count (CBC)
- Thyroid function tests.

Electrocardiogram

- Characterized by absence of clear P waves, coarse or undulating baseline, and irregularly irregular RR interval (Fig. 1)
- Evaluate for prior myocardial infarction, left ventricular hypertrophy, Wolff-Parkinson-White syndrome, and evidence for pericarditis, all of which are associated with AF
- Distinguish from sinus rhythm with frequent premature atrial complexes, multifocal atrial tachycardia and atrial flutter with variable atrioventricular (AV) block.

Echocardiogram

- Assess structural disease, including cardiomyopathy and valvular disease

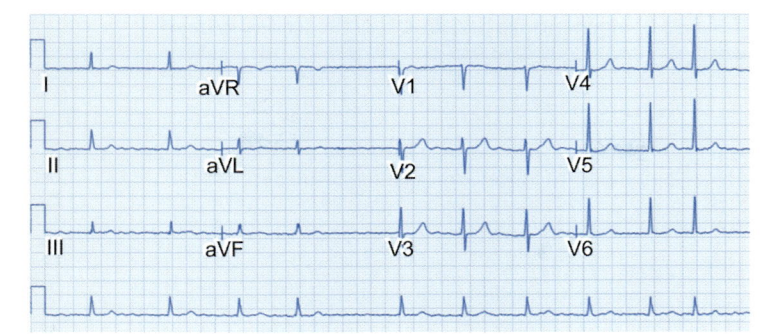

FIG. 1: Electrocardiogram example showing AF. Note the lack of P waves and irregularly irregular rhythm

- Left ventricular wall thickness should be noted if antiarrhythmic medications are being considered
- Transesophageal echocardiogram (TEE) may be necessary to assess for a left atrial appendage thrombus, if cardioversion is considered.

TREATMENT

The treatment of an unstable patient in AF is immediate direct current (DC) cardioversion. For patients who are tolerant of AF, the three central goals of AF management are:
1. Anticoagulation for prevention of systemic embolization
2. Control of ventricular heart rate
3. Restoring sinus rhythm, if symptoms are present.

An important decision in the management of AF is to decide upon a treatment strategy for the patient. In general, there are two management strategies: (1) rate control or (2) rhythm control. Notably, several large studies compared the rate and rhythm control strategies, and neither was associated with a significant difference in long arm morbidity and mortality. However, more recent studies have shown benefit for rhythm control in younger and healthier patients with significant symptoms.

Anticoagulation

Regardless of management strategy, all patients require protection from systemic embolization, as determined by the CHA_2DS_2-VASc scoring system (Table 2).

TABLE 2: Components of the CHA_2DS_2–VASc scoring system[3,10]

	Condition	Points
C	Congestive heart failure (or left ventricular systolic dysfunction)	1
H	Hypertension, or treated hypertension on medications	1
A_2	Age ≥75 years	2
D	Diabetes mellitus	1
S_2	Prior stroke or transient ischemic attack	2
V	Vascular disease (e.g., peripheral artery disease)	1
A	Age 65–74 years	1
Sc	Sex category (i.e., female gender)	1

- CHA_2DS_2-VASc score more than or equal to 2 require long-term oral anticoagulation, either with:
  - Warfarin, with goal international normalized ratio (INR) of 2.0–3.0
  - Novel oral anticoagulants, including dabigatran, rivaroxaban, or apixaban
- CHA_2DS_2-VASc score 1 may be treated with either aspirin or oral anticoagulation therapy
- CHA_2DS_2-VASc score 0 may be managed with aspirin therapy alone.

For new onset AF, patients who have been in AF for longer than 48 hours should be anticoagulated.

Ventricular Rate Control

- For asymptomatic patients, it is appropriate to proceed with a rate control strategy (i.e., anticoagulation and medications to control ventricular heart rate)
- Medications include AV nodal blocking agents with or without digoxin (Table 3) to achieve target heart rate less than 110 beats per minute. However, if symptoms of tachycardia persist, more aggressive heart rate control is required
- For symptomatic and refractory AF where ventricular rate is unable to be controlled, a long-term option is AV node ablation followed by permanent pacemaker implantation; long-term anticoagulation is still required.

TABLE 3: Medications to achieve ventricular rate control in atrial fibrillation

Drugs	Intravenous doses	Oral maintenance doses
Beta-blockers		
Metoprolol	2.5–5 mg bolus every 5 min, up to 3 doses	25–100 mg bid (metoprolol succinate ER: 50–200 mg daily)
Esmolol	Bolus: 500 µg/kg Continuous: 50–200 µg/kg/min	NA
Carvedilol	NA	3.125–25 mg bid (up to 50 mg bid if >85 kg)
Calcium channel blockers		
Diltiazem	Bolus: 0.25 mg/kg (average 20 mg) every 5 min. Continuous: 5–15 mg/h	120–480 mg daily
Verapamil	0.075–0.15 mg/kg	120–480 mg daily (slow-release available)
Digitalis		
Digoxin	Load: 500 µg, followed every 6 h by 250 µg twice	0.125–0.375 µg daily (depending on renal function)
Other		
Amiodarone	150 mg over 10 min, then 0.5–1 mg/min	200 mg daily

bid, twice daily.

Restoring and Maintaining Sinus Rhythm

For persistent AF patients, typically at least one attempt to restore sinus rhythm is made, accomplished using the algorithm in algorithm 1.

For patients with significant symptoms due to AF, a rhythm control strategy is appropriate. In this strategy, the patient is placed on appropriate anticoagulation, and attempts are made to restore and maintain sinus rhythm, either via cardioversion (pharmacologic or DC) or ablation. Although several older studies have shown no benefit to the rhythm control strategy, more recent studies have shown benefit in younger and healthier patients with significant symptoms.

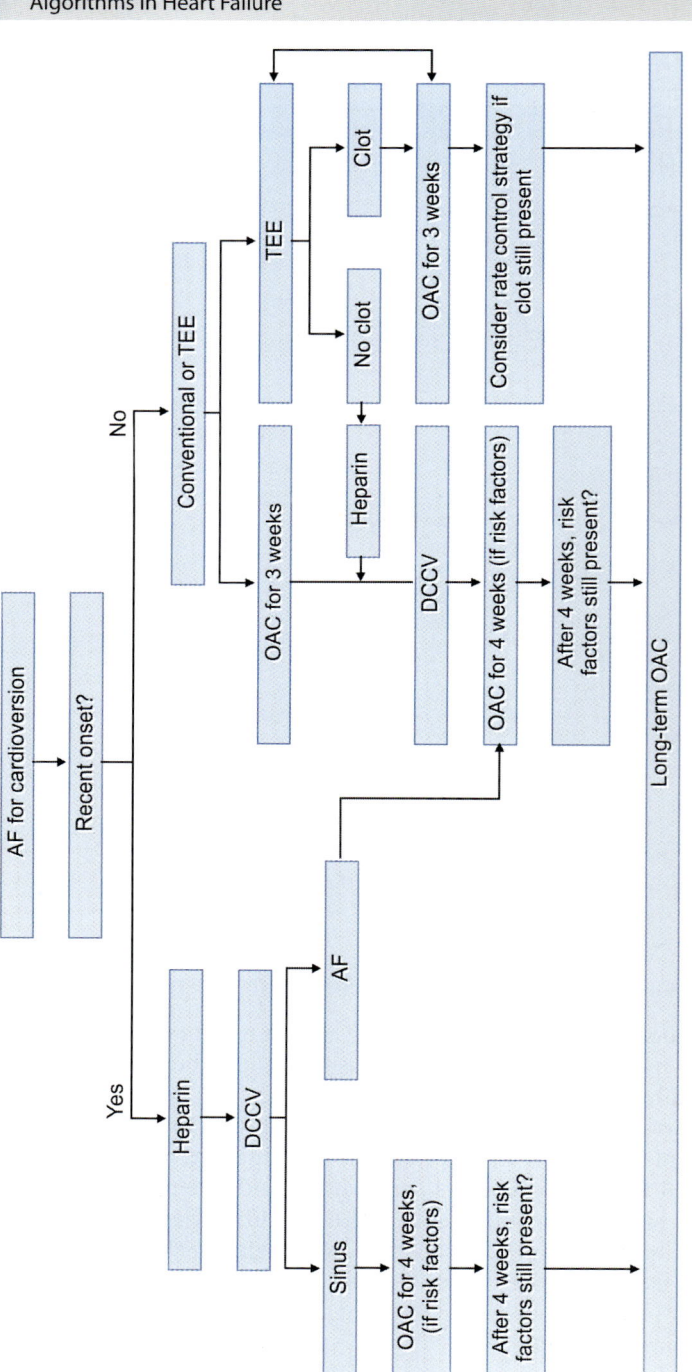

Algorithms in Heart Failure

ALGORITHM 1: Algorithm to guide cardioversion of hemodynamically stable AF

AF, atrial fibrillation; DCCV, direct current cardioversion; OAC, oral anticoagulation; TEE, transesophageal echocardiogram.

Options for achieving rhythm control include DC cardioversion, antiarrhythmic medications, and catheter ablation, as discussed below.

Direct Current Cardioversion

- Effective more than 75% of the time (depending on AF duration and left atrium size)
- Success rate is approximately 90%, if AF duration is less than 1 year; approximately 50%, if more than 5 years
- Must first ensure no left atrial appendage thrombus (as outlined in algorithm 1).

Antiarrhythmic Medications

- Typically require cardiologist or electrophysiologist to monitor side effects and safety profile. Common options include:
  - Class IC antiarrhythmic drugs: in patients without structural or ischemic heart disease, these agents may be safely used to prevent AF. Flecainide and propafenone are commonly used agents in this class
  - Class III antiarrhythmic drugs: sotalol and dofetilide may be safely used in patients with CHF, however, patients must be closely monitored for QT prolongation during initiation of these medications; dofetilide must be administered in hospital for the first five doses. Amiodarone is the most effective antiarrhythmic drug but also has significant and often irreversible side effects when used in long term. Dronedarone, the newest class III agent, is contraindicated in patients with CHF
- Algorithm 2 outlines the selection criteria for antiarrhythmic medications.

Catheter Ablation

- Typically reserved for symptomatic patients who have failed one or more antiarrhythmic medications
- Performed by electrophysiologists but may also be performed by cardiothoracic surgeons during concomitant open heart surgery
- Ablation goals traditionally include electrical isolation of pulmonary veins, which have been identified as common sources of AF-triggering ectopy. More recent data indicate localized sources such as rotors and focal drivers may be successfully targeted to improve ablation success.

Algorithms in Heart Failure

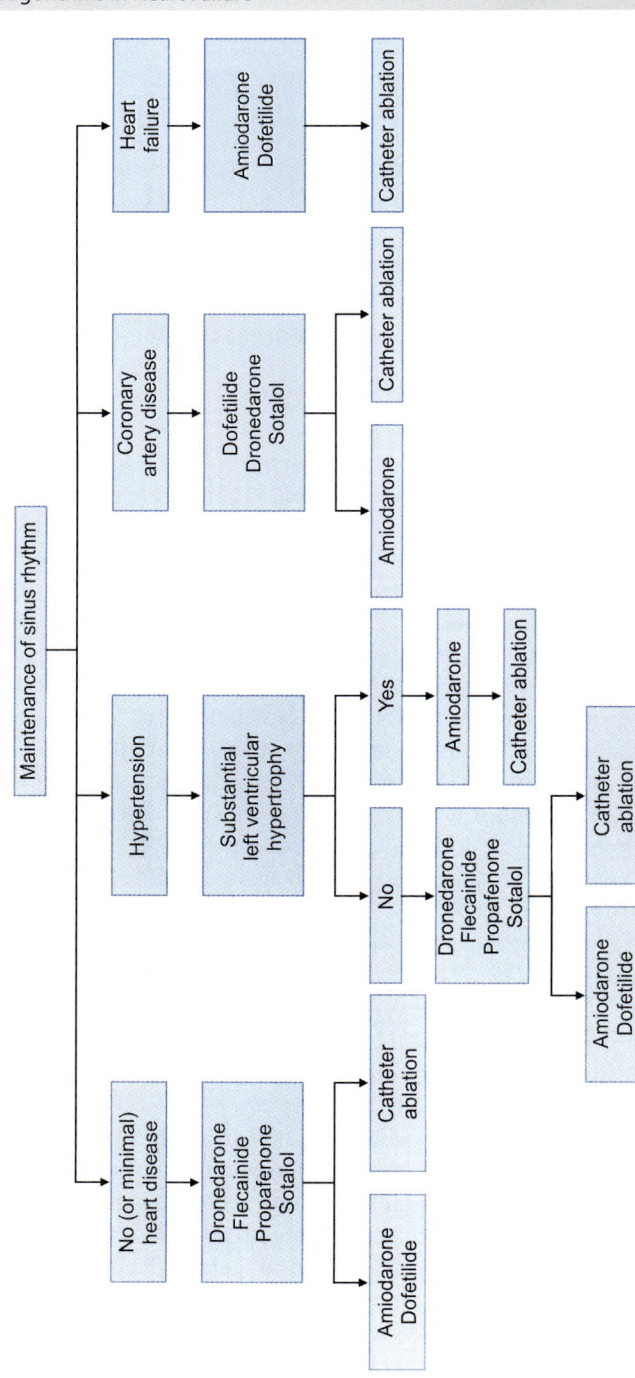

ALGORITHM 2: Antiarrhythmic algorithm based upon concomitant heart disease

```
Maintenance of sinus rhythm
├── No (or minimal) heart disease
│     └── Dronedarone / Flecainide / Propafenone / Sotalol
│           ├── Amiodarone / Dofetilide
│           └── Catheter ablation
├── Hypertension
│     └── Substantial left ventricular hypertrophy
│           ├── No → Dronedarone / Flecainide / Propafenone / Sotalol
│           │        ├── Amiodarone / Dofetilide
│           │        └── Catheter ablation
│           └── Yes → Amiodarone → Catheter ablation
├── Coronary artery disease
│     └── Dofetilide / Dronedarone / Sotalol
│           ├── Amiodarone
│           └── Catheter ablation
└── Heart failure
      └── Amiodarone / Dofetilide
            └── Catheter ablation
```

ATRIAL FIBRILLATION AND HEART FAILURE

Overall, patients with CHF should receive the same care for their AF as patients without CHF. However, there are important caveats to keep in mind:

- Beta-blockers are typically recommended first for rate control, as CHF patients require this medication for long-term management
- Digoxin should be strongly considered if a second agent is needed
- Antiarrhythmic therapy for CHF patients is predominantly limited to dofetilide, amiodarone, and occasionally sotalol
- Patients who fail medical rate control may be candidates for AV node ablation and biventricular pacing.

SPECIAL SITUATION: ATRIAL FIBRILLATION AND WOLFF-PARKINSON-WHITE SYNDROME

Occasionally, AF occurs in conjunction with an accessory pathway, which presents an increased risk to the patient of sudden death. In the setting of pre-excited AF, therapy should begin with an antiarrhythmic drug, such as intravenous procainamide or ibutilide rather than a pure AV nodal blocking agent, which may paradoxically increase the ventricular rate, and lead to ventricular fibrillation. Such patients should also be referred for electrophysiology evaluation and possible electrophysiology study and ablation of the accessory pathway.

PROGNOSIS

Patient with AF are at a significantly increased risk of stroke, CHF, and mortality, however, appropriate rate control and anticoagulation significantly reduce these complications. In patients with significant symptoms despite adequate rate control, restoration of sinus rhythm may improve quality of life.

CONCLUSION

In conclusion, AF is a frequently-encountered condition whose adverse events may be significantly reduced by guideline-based therapy as described in this chapter. AF may asymptomatic in many patients, and clinicians should have a low threshold for screening of high-risk patients. Fortunately, there are an increasing number of options for monitoring, anticoagulation, and procedural management which continue to reduce the burden of this arrhythmia.

> **KEY POINTS**
>
> ❏ Atrial fibrillation is the most common sustained arrhythmia and is commonly encountered in patients with heart failure
> ❏ Atrial fibrillation patients are at increased risk of stroke, congestive heart failure, and mortality, but appropriate evidence-based treatment significantly reduce these complications
> ❏ The mainstay of treatment includes: thromboembolism prevention, heart rate control, and maintenance of sinus rhythm (if rate control is insufficient).

SUGGESTED READINGS

1. Calkins H, Kuck KH, Cappato R, Brugada J, Camm AJ, Chen SA, et al. 2012 HRS/EHRA/ECAS expert consensus statement on catheter and surgical ablation of atrial fibrillation: recommendations for patient selection, procedural techniques, patient management and follow-up, definitions, endpoints, and research trial design: a report of the Heart Rhythm Society (HRS) Task Force on Catheter and Surgical Ablation of Atrial Fibrillation. Developed in partnership with the European Heart Rhythm Association (EHRA), a registered branch of the European Society of Cardiology (ESC) and the European Cardiac Arrhythmia Society (ECAS); and in collaboration with the American College of Cardiology (ACC), American Heart Association (AHA), the Asia Pacific Heart Rhythm Society (APHRS), and the Society of Thoracic Surgeons (STS). Endorsed by the governing bodies of the American College of Cardiology Foundation, the American Heart Association, the European Cardiac Arrhythmia Society, the European Heart Rhythm Association, the Society of Thoracic Surgeons, the Asia Pacific Heart Rhythm Society, and the Heart Rhythm Society. Heart rhythm. 2012;9:632-696 e21.
2. European Heart Rhythm Association; European Association for Cardio-Thoracic Surgery, Camm AJ, Kirchhof P, Lip GY, Schotten U, Savelieva I, et al. Guidelines for the management of atrial fibrillation: the Task Force for the Management of Atrial Fibrillation of the European Society of Cardiology (ESC). Eur Heart J. 2010;31:2369-429.
3. European Heart Rhythm Association and Heart Rhythm Society, Fuster V, Rydén LE, Cannom DS, Crijns HJ, Curtis AB, et al. ACC/AHA/ESC 2006 guidelines for the management of patients with atrial fibrillation--executive summary: a report of the American College of Cardiology/American Heart Association Task Force on Practice Guidelines and the European Society of Cardiology Committee for Practice Guidelines (writing committee to revise the 2001 guidelines for the management of patients with atrial fibrillation). J Am Coll Cardiol. 2006;48:854-906.
4. Fuster V, Ryden LE, Cannom DS, Crijns HJ, Curtis AB, Ellenbogen KA, et al. ACC/AHA/ESC 2006 guidelines for the management of patients with atrial fibrillation: a report of the American College of Cardiology/American Heart Association Task Force on Practice Guidelines and the European Society of Cardiology Committee for Practice Guidelines (writing committee to revise the 2001 guidelines for the management of patients with atrial fibrillation): developed in collaboration with the European Heart Rhythm Association and the Heart Rhythm Society. Circulation. 2006;114:e257-354.

5. Gami AS, Hodge DO, Herges RM, Olson EJ, Nykodym J, Kara T, et al. Obstructive sleep apnea, obesity, and the risk of incident atrial fibrillation. J Am Coll Cardiol. 2007;49:565-71.
6. Go AS, Hylek EM, Phillips KA, Chang Y, Henault LE, Selby JV, et al. Prevalence of diagnosed atrial fibrillation in adults: national implications for rhythm management and stroke prevention: the AnTicoagulation and Risk Factors in Atrial Fibrillation (ATRIA) Study. JAMA. 2001;285:2370-5.
7. Miyasaka Y, Barnes ME, Gersh BJ, Cha SS, Bailey KR, Abhayaratna WP, et al. Secular trends in incidence of atrial fibrillation in Olmsted County, Minnesota, 1980 to 2000, and implications on the projections for future prevalence. Circulation. 2006;114:119-25.
8. Narayan SM, Krummen DE, Shivkumar K, Clopton P, Rappel WJ, Miller JM. Treatment of atrial fibrillation by the ablation of localized sources: CONFIRM (conventional ablation for atrial fibrillation with or without focal impulse and rotor modulation) Trial. J Am Coll Cardiol. 2012;60:628-36.
9. Ogawa S, Yamashita T, Yamazaki T, Aizawa Y, Atarashi H, Inoue H, et al. Optimal treatment strategy for patients with paroxysmal atrial fibrillation: J-RHYTHM study. Circulation. 2009;73:242-8.
10. Van Gelder IC, Groenveld HF, Crijns HJ, Tuininga YS, Tijssen JGP, Alings M, et al. Lenient versus strict rate control in patients with atrial fibrillation. N Eng J Med. 2010;362:1363-73.
11. Wann LS, Curtis AB, January CT, Ellenbogen KA, Lowe JE, Estes NAM, et al. 2011 ACCF/AHA/HRS focused update on the management of patients with atrial fibrillation (updating the 2006 guideline): a report of the American College of Cardiology Foundation/American Heart Association Task Force on Practice Guidelines. Circulation. 2011;123:104-23.
12. Wyse DG, Waldo AL, DiMarco JP, Domanski MJ, Rosenberg Y, Schron EB, et al. A comparison of rate control and rhythm control in patients with atrial fibrillation. N Engl J Med. 2002;347:1825-33.

17
CHAPTER

Ventricular Tachycardia Done Right

Gautam G Lalani, David E Krummen

INTRODUCTION

Ventricular tachycardia (VT) is a common, life-threatening arrhythmia with a high prevalence in patients with heart failure. Because of the high risk of morbidity and mortality, rapid identification and initiation of proper management are of paramount importance. For VT survivors, a thorough patient evaluation is essential to determine the specific etiology. Fortunately, advances in both short- and long-term therapies for VT can significantly improve patient survival. In this chapter, we have discussed about the clinical presentation, evaluation, diagnosis, and acute treatment, and then focus on further workup and chronic management of VT. This section is based upon current guidelines and clinical experience with a focus on efficient diagnosis and initial workup and management strategies.

CLINICAL PRESENTATION

The presentation of VT can vary widely, and depends on the characteristics of the tachycardia such as rate, duration, and extent of structural or ischemic heart disease. Episodes can be nonsustained (nonsustained ventricular tachycardia; <30 seconds), sustained with hemodynamic stability, or unstable potentially resulting in severe palpitations, chest pain, syncope, and sudden death.

INITIAL EVALUATION

The clinical evaluation of VT revolves around history, physical examination, and testing which may provide insight to potential etiology of VT. Among the most important determinants are a history of coronary or structural heart disease and signs or symptoms of ischemia or heart failure. Comprehensive laboratory testing, including electrolytes and cardiac biomarkers, will also aid in the patient's diagnostic evaluation.

Electrocardiogram

The electrocardiogram (ECG) is the most important tool in establishing the diagnosis of VT. The diagnosis of VT requires three or more consecutive ventricular beats which exceeds an average rate of 100 beats per minute.

Several algorithms have been developed to aid in the differentiation of VT versus other wide complex tachycardias (WCT), such as supraventricular (SVT) with aberrant conduction. The Brugada criteria (Algorithm 1A) has a stepwise approach to the assessment of WCT. If any of the criteria are satisfied, VT is diagnosed. The aVR criteria (Algorithm 1B) utilizes only lead aVR in a sequential approach to differentiate WCT. The complete morphology criteria has been described by Baman TS et al.

Independent atrial and ventricular activation [atrioventricular (AV)] is one of the key features of VT, and can manifest in several ways: lack of AV relationship and fusion beats or capture beats. In figure 1, complexes 4, 17, and 25 are narrower than others, and represent capture beats, consistent with AV dissociation and VT in this WCT in a patient with severe palpitations and presyncope. However, in the setting of 1:1 ventriculoatrial (VA) conduction or lack of discernible P waves, this may not be clear.

The ECG can also give information of potential VT etiology including ischemia, electrolyte abnormalities, prior infarcts, abnormal QT intervals, epsilon waves, and J-point elevation.

Imaging

A transthoracic echocardiogram is essential in the evaluation for structural heart disease, including assessment of left ventricular function, hypertrophy, and signs of cardiomyopathy. Computed tomography and cardiac magnetic resonance imaging (MRI) may

Algorithms in Heart Failure

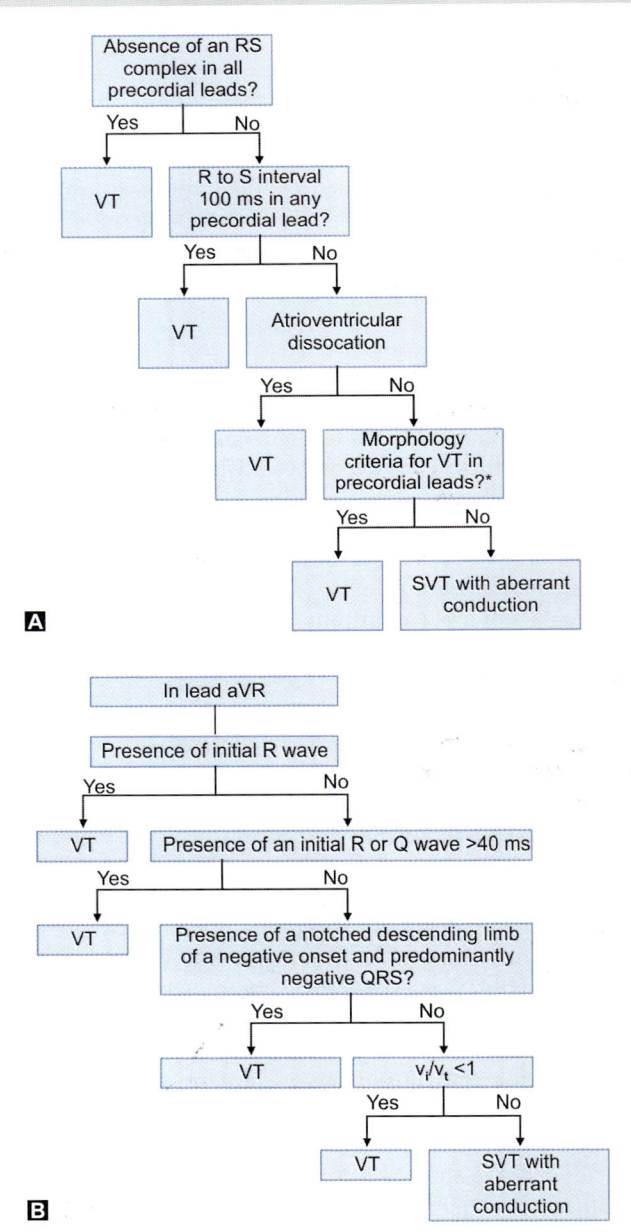

A

```
Absence of an RS complex in all precordial leads?
├── Yes → VT
└── No → R to S interval 100 ms in any precordial lead?
        ├── Yes → VT
        └── No → Atrioventricular dissocation
                ├── Yes → VT
                └── No → Morphology criteria for VT in precordial leads?*
                        ├── Yes → VT
                        └── No → SVT with aberrant conduction
```

B

```
In lead aVR
Presence of initial R wave
├── Yes → VT
└── No → Presence of an initial R or Q wave >40 ms
        ├── Yes → VT
        └── No → Presence of a notched descending limb of a negative onset and predominantly negative QRS?
                ├── Yes → VT
                └── No → $v_i/v_t < 1$
                        ├── Yes → VT
                        └── No → SVT with aberrant conduction
```

ALGORITHMS 1: Differentiating ventricular tachycardia from other wide complex tachycardias

*Morphology criteria as described in Brugada P, Brugada J, Mont L, Smeets J, Andries EW. A new approach to the differential diagnosis of a regular tachycardia with a wide QRS complex. Circulation. 1991;83:1649-59.

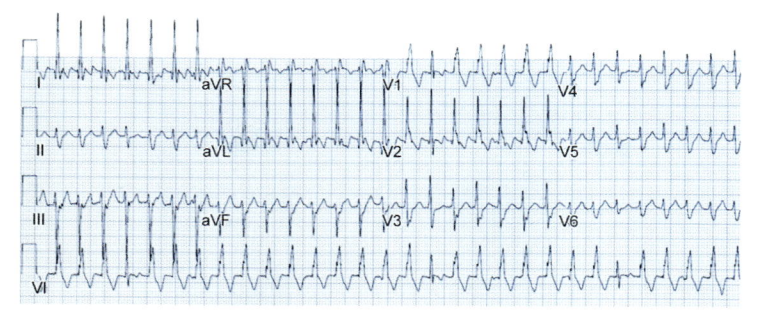

FIG. 1: Examples of atrioventricular dissociation

provide information about ventricular size and scar distribution. Cardiac MRI may also be useful in the evaluation of arrhythmogenic right ventricular cardiomyopathy/dysplasia or hypertrophic cardiomyopathy.

Ischemic Evaluation

An ischemic etiology of VT should always be considered. If suspicion remains high, patients should undergo ischemic evaluation, either by perfusion imaging, or more commonly by coronary angiography. Identified ischemia may then be referred for potential revascularization.

TREATMENT

Acute

Acute treatment strategy is first determined by patient stability (Algorithm 2). In hemodynamically stable patients, initial medical therapy should be implemented, which include amiodarone, lidocaine, and procainamide (usually given as bolus, followed by infusion). In contrast, if there is any evidence of hemodynamic instability, patient should proceed directly to direct current cardioversion, synchronized at 200 J with biphasic wave form, which can be followed with an antiarrhythmic medication to prevent recurrence.

Patients with incessant VT or ventricular fibrillation (VF) or VT storm should be evaluated promptly for ischemia and may need additional mechanical circulatory support. Emergent ablation for electrical storms can also be considered at experienced centers.

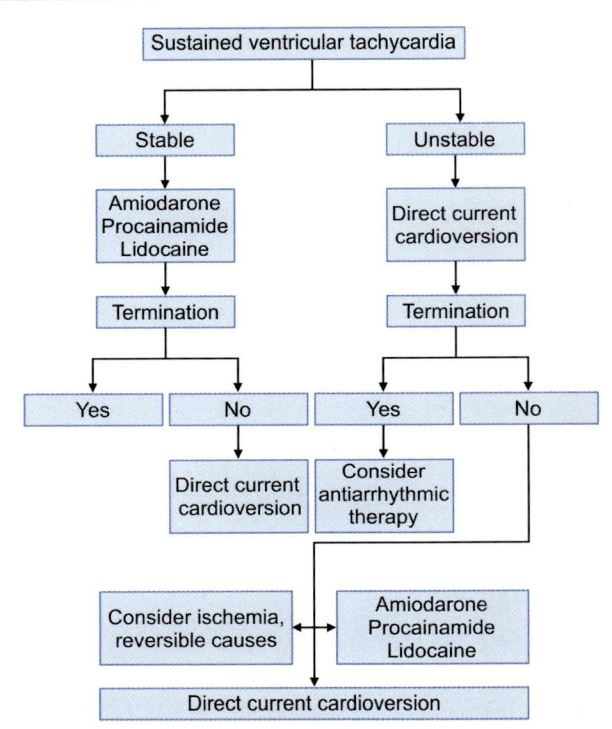

```
Sustained ventricular tachycardia
                │
        ┌───────┴───────┐
      Stable          Unstable
        │                │
   Amiodarone      Direct current
   Procainamide    cardioversion
   Lidocaine            │
        │                │
   Termination      Termination
    ┌───┴───┐       ┌────┴───┐
   Yes     No      Yes      No
            │       │
    Direct current  Consider
    cardioversion   antiarrhythmic
                    therapy
```

ALGORITHM 2: Stepwise approach the acute treatment of sustained ventricular tachycardia

Examples of tailored acute therapies for specific types of VT:
- Patients with fascicular VT, characterized by right bundle branch block (QRS duration 120–140 ms) and a superior axis, may be particularly responsive to verapamil
- In electrical storm associated with inferolateral early repolarization or long QT syndrome (LQTS), isoproterenol can be used for VT/VF suppression and prevention of recurrence
- Transvenous pacing at higher rates can also be effective in suppressing VT/VF recurrence in LQTS.

Once the patient has been stabilized, a complete evaluation as listed above should be performed in order to determine the presence of any reversible causes. Identified reversible causes should be promptly treated.

Chronic

In the absence of structural heart disease, treatment should focus on idiopathic VT suppression, where medical therapy is often

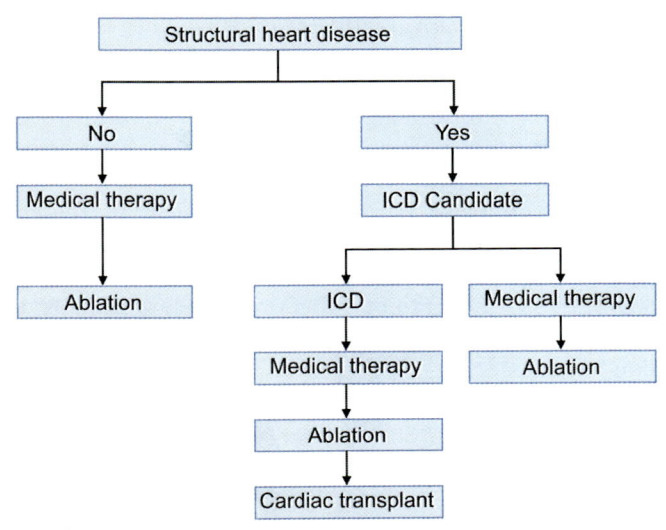

```
Structural heart disease
├── No
│   └── Medical therapy
│       └── Ablation
└── Yes
    └── ICD Candidate
        ├── ICD
        │   └── Medical therapy
        │       └── Ablation
        │           └── Cardiac transplant
        └── Medical therapy
            └── Ablation
```

ICD, implantable cardioverter defibrillator.

ALGORITHM 3: Chronic treatment of ventricular tachycardia is based largely upon the presence or absence of structural heart disease and focuses on prevention of recurrence arrhythmias and sudden cardiac death

the first line of therapy (Algorithm 3). Although not technically VT, a high burden of premature ventricular contractions (PVCs) (>15,000 PVCs per 24 h) may be a risk factor for the development of cardiomyopathy, and should be considered for suppressive therapy as well. Beta-blockers are typically used as first line agents in this setting. If ineffective, sotalol, dofetilide, and amiodarone may be considered.

Sotalol and dofetilide require baseline renal function assessment and monitoring for QTc prolongation, both at initiation and at regular follow-up. Amiodarone, while not requiring ongoing QTc monitoring, does require semiannual thyroid, liver, pulmonary function, and ophthalmologic evaluation to monitor for side effects.

Examples of tailored chronic medical therapy for specific types of VT:
- Verapamil may be considered for long-term suppression of fascicular VT in patients in whom ablation is not an option or is not desired
- Recently, quinidine (class IA) has been shown to be useful in patients with early repolarization syndrome.

Frequently, idiopathic VT subtypes, such as left or right ventricular outflow tract VTs, are amenable to ablation, which may be considered early in the treatment strategy. A cardiac electrophysiology consultation should be obtained for a detailed discussion of all treatment options.

The presence, nonsustained VT/VF in the setting structural heart disease (ejection fraction <40%) is associated with a high risk of mortality, and patients should be considered for implantable cardioverter defibrillator (ICD) therapy for primary prevention of sudden cardiac death (Algorithm 3). For secondary prevention of sustained VT in patients with structural ischemic heart disease, ICD therapy has been shown to be superior to medical therapy, with the greatest benefit in the patients with depressed left ventricular ejection fraction.

Patients with recurrent ICD shocks benefit from suppression of their ventricular arrhythmias with antiarrhythmics or ablation. Specifically, β-blockers, sotalol, dofetilide, and amiodarone are commonly used in this setting, tailored to patients' response, tolerance, and side effects. Sotalol, in particular, should be used with caution in patients with depressed left ventricular function.

Patients who are not responsive to medical therapy or ablation with frequent ventricular arrhythmias should be considered for sympathectomy or cardiac transplant.

Ablation in the Chronic Management of Ventricular Tachycardia

Studies have shown the utility of ablation for the chronic management of VT, including reducing appropriate ICD shocks. Consultation with electrophysiologist is recommended to allow a thorough discussion with the patient of all the risks, benefits, and probability of success in each case.

PROGNOSIS

The prognosis for patients with ventricular arrhythmias is dependent upon both the specific etiology and the presence of structural heart disease. For patients with idiopathic VT and normal ventricular function, the prognosis is relatively benign. In contrast, patients with inherited channelopathies, such as LQTS, or those with VT and structural heart disease, may be at higher risk and require further stratification and ICD implantation, based upon current guidelines.

CONCLUSION

The presentation of VT can vary from asymptomatic, nonsustained episodes to unstable events precipitating VF. Initial evaluation and treatment should be based on patient stability, with urgent intervention in the presence of hemodynamic compromise. Further workup is needed to determine etiology and long-term treatment plan. Management should be directed at arrhythmia suppression or elimination and risk reduction with ICD implantation, when appropriate. With the advent of advanced electrophysiology care, timely initiation of optimal management has the potential to dramatically improve the survival of patients with ventricular tachycardia.

KEY POINTS

- Initial evaluation should confirm the diagnosis of ventricular tachycardia
- Acute treatment is based on hemodynamic stability
- Long-term treatment is largely based on the presence of structural heart disease or inherited conditions.

SUGGESTED READINGS

1. A comparison of antiarrhythmic-drug therapy with implantable defibrillators in patients resuscitated from near-fatal ventricular arrhythmias. The antiarrhythmics versus implantable defibrillators (AVID) investigators. N Engl J Med. 1997;337:1576-83.
2. Baman TS, Lange DC, Ilg KJ, Gupta SK, Liu TY, Alguire C, et al. Relationship between burden of premature ventricular complexes and left ventricular function. Heart Rhythm. 2010;7:865-9.
3. Bardy GH, Lee KL, Mark DB, Poole JE, Packer DL, Boineau R, et al. Amiodarone or an implantable cardioverter-defibrillator for congestive heart failure. N Engl J Med. 2005;352:225-37.
4. Brugada P, Brugada J, Mont L, Smeets J, Andries EW. A new approach to the differential diagnosis of a regular tachycardia with a wide QRS complex. Circulation. 1991;83:1649-59.
5. Buxton AE, Lee KL, Fisher JD, Josephson ME, Prystowsky EN, Hafley G. A randomized study of the prevention of sudden death in patients with coronary artery disease. Multicenter unsustained tachycardia trial investigators. N Engl J Med. 1999;341:1882-90.
6. Connolly SJ, Gent M, Roberts RS, Dorian P, Green MS, Klein GJ, et al. Canadian implantable defibrillator study (CIDS): Study design and organization. CIDS Co-Investigators. Am J Cardiol. 1993;72:103F-108F.
7. Epstein AE, DiMarco JP, Ellenbogen KA, Estes NA, Freedman RA, Gettes LS, et al. 2012 ACCF/AHA/HRS focused update incorporated into the ACCF/AHA/HRS 2008 guidelines for device-based therapy of cardiac rhythm abnormalities: A report of the american college

of cardiology foundation/american heart association task force on practice guidelines and the heart rhythm society. Circulation. 2013;127:e283-352.
8. Epstein AE, DiMarco JP, Ellenbogen KA, Estes NA, Freedman RA, Gettes LS, et al. ACC/AHA/HRS 2008 guidelines for device-based therapy of cardiac rhythm abnormalities: A report of the american college of cardiology/american heart association task force on practice guidelines (writing committee to revise the ACC/AHA/NASPE 2002 guideline update for implantation of cardiac pacemakers and antiarrhythmia devices) developed in collaboration with the american association for thoracic surgery and society of thoracic surgeons. Circulation. 2008;117:e350-408.
9. Haissaguerre M, Sacher F, Nogami A, Komiya N, Bernard A, Probst V, et al. Characteristics of recurrent ventricular fibrillation associated with inferolateral early repolarization role of drug therapy. J Am Coll Cardiol. 2009;53:612-9.
10. Hayase J, Patel J, Narayan SM, Krummen DE. Percutaneous stellate ganglion block suppressing VT and VF in a patient refractory to VT ablation. J Cardiovasc Electrophysiol. 2013;24:926-8.
11. Issa Z, Miller J. Clinical Arrhythmology and Electrophysiology: A Companion to Braunwald's Heart Disease, 2nd edition. Saunders; 2012.
12. Kadish A, Dyer A, Daubert JP, Quigg R, Estes NA, Anderson KP, et al. Prophylactic defibrillator implantation in patients with nonischemic dilated cardiomyopathy. N Engl J Med. 2004;350:2151-8.
13. Maisel AS, Filippatos GS. Heart Failure: The Expert's Approach, 1st edition. New Delhi: Jaypee Brothers Medical Publishers (P) Ltd; 2014.
14. Moss AJ, Zareba W, Hall WJ, Klein H, Wilber DJ, Cannom DS, et al. Prophylactic implantation of a defibrillator in patients with myocardial infarction and reduced ejection fraction. N Engl J Med. 2002;346:877-83.
15. Reddy VY, Reynolds MR, Neuzil P, Richardson AW, Taborsky M, Jongnarangsin K, et al. Prophylactic catheter ablation for the prevention of defibrillator therapy. N Engl J Med. 2007;357:2657-65.
16. Siebels J, Cappato R, Ruppel R, Schneider MA, Kuck KH. Preliminary results of the Cardiac Arrest Study Hamburg (CASH). CASH investigators. Am J Cardiol. 1993;72:109F-113F.

18
CHAPTER

Management of the Patient with Heart Failure with Preserved Ejection Fraction

Alan S Maisel, Gerasimos S Filippatos, Kevin S Shah, Jeffrey Chan

INTRODUCTION

Patients with heart failure with preserved ejection fraction (HFpEF) constitute a large proportion of heart failure patients. In fact, epidemiologic studies have shown that roughly 30–55% of heart failure patients with acute decompensation have in fact normal or near normal left ventricular function. Heart failure with preserved ejection fraction has emerged as the predominant form of heart failure in the elderly and in women, and may in fact eventually emerge as the predominant form of heart failure in the general population as well. Yet, despite this growing prevalence, HFpEF has been largely understudied because of the difficulty in its diagnosis and lack of clarity in management as guidelines are still currently being discussed and modified. In the past, HFpEF was frequently referred to as "diastolic" heart failure as opposed to "systolic" heart failure, which corresponded with heart failure with reduced ejection fraction (HFrEF). However, because diastolic left ventricular dysfunction was also observed in patients with reduced left ventricular ejection fractions (LVEF), the term "diastolic" heart failure was eventually replaced by HFpEF.

Heart failure with preserved ejection fraction has been defined, according to Framingham criteria, as heart failure with a LVEF greater than 45% and the absence of mitral stenosis, pericardial disease, or noncardiac causes of dyspnea, edema, and fatigue. It is a broad classification that essentially encompasses patients with left ventricular diastolic HFpEF.

PATHOPHYSIOLOGY

Though similar in many ways to HFrEF, HFpEF demonstrates a variety of distinct disease characteristics that uniquely distinguish it. Patients with HFpEF, generally, exhibit a concentric pattern of left ventricular remodeling, normal or near normal end-diastolic volume, increased wall thickness, and a high ratio of mass to volume with a high ratio of wall thickness to chamber radius. Cardiomyocytes often exhibit an increased diameter and collagen content, and changes in calcium homeostasis contribute to impaired cardiomyocyte relaxation and increased stiffness. This stiff ventricle is the driving force behind much of the signs and symptoms demonstrated in HFpEF exacerbations.

The actual pathogenesis of HFpEF, however, is far more complex and currently sits embedded in a broad spectrum of inter-related diseases and comorbidities. Hypertension is believed to be the main foundation from which the majority of cardiovascular changes occur that ultimately lead to HFpEF. In fact, compared to healthy patients, those with HFpEF have been noted to have markedly increased rest brachial pulse pressure and systolic blood pressure. In theory, prolonged elevations in blood pressure would facilitate microvascular remodeling that would in time induce arterial stiffness and thus, a decreased ability of the vasculature to accommodate large volumes of blood ejected from the left ventricle. The resulting increased systolic blood pressure and LV afterload ultimately induce compensatory processes of myocardial hypertrophy, increased myocardial oxygen consumption, and LV hypertrophy that perpetuate an ongoing cycle of organ damage and progressively worsening heart failure. Other theories behind HFpEF include the thought that comorbidities such as obesity, diabetes mellitus, chronic obstructive pulmonary disease (COPD), contribute to a pro-inflammatory state. This state may also lead to endothelial inflammation and downstream hypertrophy and fibrosis of cardiomyocytes. Figure 1 demonstrates multiple comorbidities, and their interplay with the development of HFpEF.

DIAGNOSIS

In general, the process of diagnosing HFpEF is a two-step process. The first step should be to verify the presence of clinical signs and symptoms of heart failure such as dyspnea, reduced exercise capacity, orthopnea, edema, or ascites. The second step focuses on verifying the presence of a preserved LVEF via an echocardiogram.

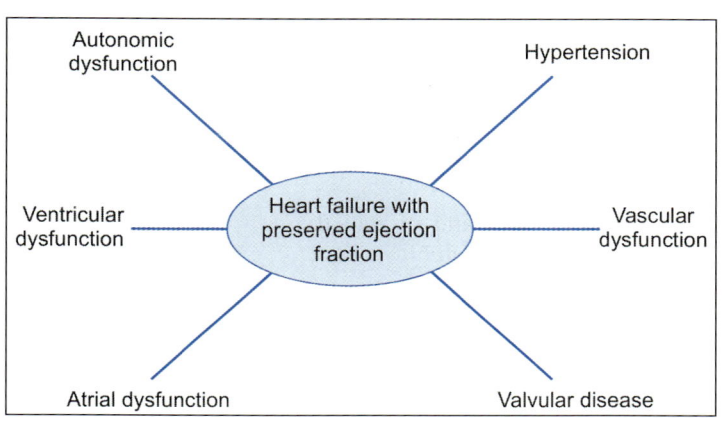

FIG. 1: Comorbidities associated with heart failure with preserved ejection fraction

> **Box 1: European Society of Cardiology heart failure guidelines 2012**
> - Diagnostic criteria for heart failure with preserved ejection fraction (all four must be met)
> - Symptoms of heart failure
> - Signs typical of heart failure
> - Noemal or only mildly reduced left ventricular ejection fraction and left ventricular
> - Relevant sturcture heart disease

Particular emphasis, however, should initially be placed on appropriately diagnosing heart failure in general and excluding other explanations for the observed clinical symptoms as other conditions including obesity, respiratory disease, and myocardial ischemia can present similarly to heart failure. Once these alternative diagnoses have been ruled out, a diagnosis of HFpEF can then be presumed in patients with symptoms of heart failure, normal LVEF, and no valvular abnormalities. The general approach described above for making the official diagnosis of HFpEF in accordance with European Society of Cardiology (ESC) guidelines is illustrated in box 1.

While the approach described above appears quite simplistic, the actual details of diagnosing HFpEF with regards to echocardiography are much more intricate. Four sets of guidelines for the diagnosis of HFpEF have been published in current studies. They all require the simultaneous presence of signs or symptoms of heart failure, evidence of normal systolic left ventricular function, and evidence of diastolic left ventricular dysfunction or surrogate markers of diastolic left ventricular dysfunction (left ventricular hypertrophy, left atrial enlargement, atrial fibrillation), or elevated plasma natriuretic peptide levels. The various guidelines include the working group on myocardial function of the ESC, the National Heart, Lung, and Blood Institute (NHLBI) Framingham Heart Study, and the Lahey Clinic. The fourth set of guidelines, which is the selected approach in this chapter, comes from the Heart Failure and Echocardiography Associations of the European Society of Cardiology. In accordance to this last set of guidelines, the diagnosis of HFpEF requires signs or symptoms of heart failure and the following echocardiographic findings: LVEF more than 50%, a left ventricular end-diastolic volume index (LVEDVI) less than 97 mL/m^2, evidence of diastolic left ventricular dysfunction, left ventricular end-diastolic pressure more than 16 mmHg, pulmonary capillary wedge pressure more than 12 mmHg, and/or early mitral valve flow velocity to early tissue. Doppler lengthening velocity ratio more than 15 if there is sufficient evidence of diastolic left ventricular dysfunction and more than 8 if there is supportive evidence with natriuretic peptides [brain natriuretic peptide (BNP >200 pg/mL)]; also, a mitral flow velocity Doppler signal demonstrating a ratio of the early to late mitral flow velocity less than 0.5, and a pulmonary vein flow velocity signal showing a duration of reverse pulmonary vein atrial systole flow. A detailed flow sheet illustrating this guideline is depicted in algorithm 1.

The use of cardiac biomarkers in the diagnosis of HFpEF remains controversial. While BNP or N-terminal proBNP (NT-proBNP) levels have been firmly established as markers of heart failure, the use of such markers to specifically identify HFpEF is less clear. In the current guideline for diagnosing HFpEF, an NT-proBNP more than 220 pg/mL or a BNP more than 200 pg/mL are factored into the algorithm for making the diagnosis. In current literature, levels of NT-pro-BNP and BNP are known to be higher in patients with HFpEF than normal, but lower than in patients with HFrEF. Exact cutoffs to help the diagnosis of HFpEF have yet to be determined.

TREATMENT

The management of HFpEF has been extremely challenging primarily due to very limited clinical trial data thus far. The current heart failure guidelines recommend blood pressure monitoring, low sodium diet, and diuresis to improve signs and symptoms of volume overload. The primary approach to management of HFpEF involves symptomatic relief of dyspnea and clinical volume overload with

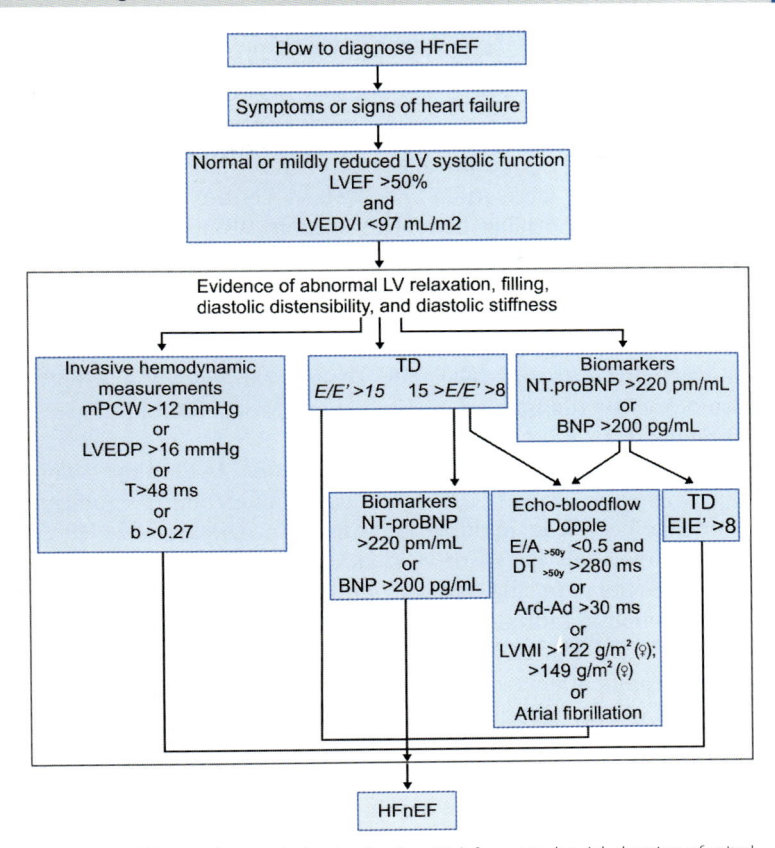

Management of the Patient with Heart Failure with Preserved Ejection...

```
How to diagnose HFnEF
        ↓
Symptoms or signs of heart failure
        ↓
Normal or mildly reduced LV systolic function
           LVEF >50%
              and
        LVEDVI <97 mL/m2
              ↓
Evidence of abnormal LV relaxation, filling,
diastolic distensibility, and diastolic stiffness
```

- Invasive hemodynamic measurements: mPCW >12 mmHg or LVEDP >16 mmHg or τ >48 ms or b >0.27
- TD: E/E' >15 | 15 > E/E' >8
  - Biomarkers NT-proBNP >220 pm/mL or BNP >200 pg/mL
  - Echo-bloodflow Dopple: $E/A_{>50y}$ <0.5 and $DT_{>50y}$ >280 ms or Ard-Ad >30 ms or LVMI >122 g/m² (♀); >149 g/m² (♂) or Atrial fibrillation
- Biomarkers: NT-proBNP >220 pm/mL or BNP >200 pg/mL
  - TD E/E' >8

→ HFnEF

HFnEF, Heart failure with normal ejection fraction; LV, left ventricular; Ad, duration of mitral valve atrial wave flow; Ard, duration of reverse pulmonary vein atrial systole flow; b, constant of left ventricular chamber stiffness; BNP, brain natriuretic peptide; DT, deceleration time; E, early mitral valve flow velocity; E', early TD lengthening velocity; E/A, ratio of early (E) to late (A) mitral valve flow velocity; LAVI, left atrial volume index; LVEDP, left ventricular end-diastolic pressure; Echo, echocardiography; LVEDVI, left ventricular end-diastolic volume index; LVEF, left ventricular ejection fraction; LVMI, left ventricular mass index; mPCW, mean pulmonary capillary wedge pressure; NT-proBNP = N-terminal pro-brain natriuretic peptide; τ = time constant of left ventricular relaxation; TD = tissue Doppler.

ALGORITHM 1: Diagnosis of heart failure with preserved ejection fraction incorporating echocardiography and biomarkers

aggressive use of diuretics. In the inpatient setting, IV loop diuretics are the preferred agent of choice. Evidence has demonstrated that diuretic therapy improves symptoms and quality of life in HFpEF. Similarly, to HFrEF, goals of diuresis include symptomatic relief of dyspnea or congestion and return to baseline dry weight. Low sodium diet and blood pressure management are also important in the chronic management to prevent fluid retention and worsening of diastolic dysfunction in the case of chronic elevated blood pressure.

Beta-blockers (specifically carvedilol and long-acting metoprolol), in large scale randomized controlled trials, have demonstrated mortality benefit in chronic systolic heart failure. However, no trials have yet to show a mortality benefit for β-blocker use in acute or chronic HFpEF. Despite no mortality benefit, β-blockers have shown ability to slow heart rate and regression of left ventricular hypertrophy, and even improvement of left ventricular filling and relaxation on echocardiogram. Currently, β-blockers should be used in HFpEF to control comorbidities such as tachyarrhythmias and hypertension.

Angiotensin converting enzyme inhibitors (ACEIs) and angiotensin receptor blocker (ARBs) have also demonstrated a significant mortality benefit in multiple large trials in patients with HFrEF. Three large trials have not yielded similar results in the HFpEF patient population. The Candesartan in Heart Failure: Assessment of Reduction in Mortality and Morbidity (CHARM)-preserved trial demonstrated a moderate impact in preventing admissions for CHF among patients with HFpEF. The ACEI perindopril has also shown a similar ability to prevent re-admissions, but fell short of a mortality benefit in HFpEF. The ARB irbesartan was also trialed against placebo in against patients with HFpEF (ejection fraction >45%) and there was no benefit in mortality, heart failure death, or rehospitalization. The recently Treatment of Preserved Cardiac Function Heart Failure With an Aldosterone Antagonist (TOPCAT) trial demonstrated spironolactone providing a signal of benefit in HFpEF with elevated natriuretic peptides in a geographical subset for heart failure rehospitalization, but this class of medication has not shown significant a mortality benefit.

Alternative pharmacological approaches to HFpEF have been studied with similarly negative results. The calcium channel blocker, verapamil, has demonstrated improvement of exercise capacity in small studies. Digoxin has also shown no morbidity or mortality benefit. Retrospective data has shown some mortality benefit in HFpEF. One novel therapy has yielded recent positive results with respect to symptomatic relief in decompensated HFpEF. This is serelaxin, a recombinant drug of human relaxin 2. In patients with HFpEF randomized to serelaxin administration, significant improvement in symptoms of dyspnea was observed in one trial. Once again, no mortality benefit was seen. However, this is a novel

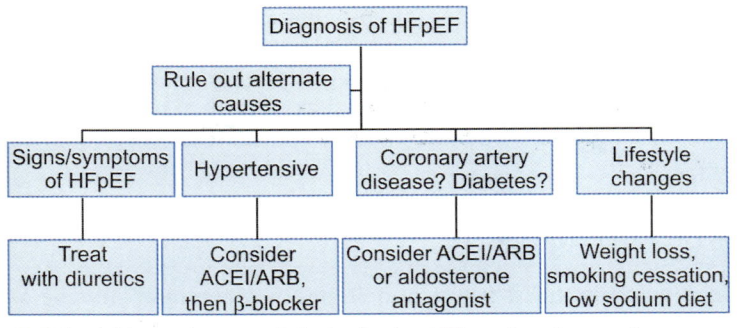

Management of the Patient with Heart Failure with Preserved Ejection...

```
                    Diagnosis of HFpEF
                            │
                   Rule out alternate
                        causes
        ┌───────────────┬───┴───────────────┬───────────────┐
  Signs/symptoms    Hypertensive      Coronary artery      Lifestyle
    of HFpEF                         disease? Diabetes?     changes
        │                │                   │                │
     Treat          Consider         Consider ACEI/ARB    Weight loss,
  with diuretics   ACEI/ARB,          or aldosterone    smoking cessation,
                  then β-blocker        antagonist       low sodium diet
```

HFpEF, heart failure with preserved ejection fraction; ACEIs, angiotensin converting enzyme inhibitors; ARB, angiotensin receptor blocker

ALGORITHM 2: Treatment of heart failure with preserved ejection fraction

drug and future trials utilizing it in acute and chronic heart failure will be developed in the future.

In conclusion, no single therapy has proven to demonstrate a mortality benefit in HFpEF. However, diuretics, β-blockers, ACEI, and ARB all have small roles in terms of improving other indicators of disease (Algorithm 2). In patients with other indications for these medications (i.e., tachyarrhythmias, hypertension in the setting of diabetes mellitus), institution of these medications is still warranted to help with management of comorbidities that are integral players in the pathophysiology of HFpEF.

PROGNOSIS

The overall prognosis of HFpEF has somewhat conflicting data. Some studies have shown a 5-year survival rate after a first episode of 43% with similar mortality rates as in HFrEF. Other meta-analyses have shown that mortality among patients with HFpEF was half that observed in those with HFrEF. Once again, comorbidities are numerous amongst these populations and it can be difficult to discern what disease entity is the major player in terms of mortality. Nevertheless, heart failure in general portends a poor prognosis, regardless of ejection fraction.

FUTURE DIRECTIONS

The future direction of HFpEF management includes multiple novel therapies targeting different pathophysiologic mechanisms.

Therapies such as ranolazine (an anti-anginal), phosphodiesterase-5 inhibitors, xanthine oxidase inhibitors (anti-inflammatories), and heart rate control through devices are all being considered. Promising basic science research has shown a role for these therapies in HFpEF, but translation to clinical results are yet to be seen.

CONCLUSION

In conclusion, heart failure and HFpEF is a common subtype of congestive heart failure. Heart failure with preserved ejection fraction is difficult to diagnose and associated with multiple comorbidities. Approach to the management of HFpEF has not demonstrated as many therapies with as strong mortality benefits as in heart failure with HFrEF, but treatment of comorbidities and management of symptoms are current recommendations to help improve outcomes and quality of life in those suffering with this prevalent condition.

KEY POINTS

- Heart failure with preserved ejection fraction (HFpEF) is a significant subset of people diagnosed with heart failure
- The pathophysiology behind HFpEF is primarily driven by hypertension promoting remodeling and stiffness of the left ventricle
- The diagnosis of HFpEF hinges on a clinical diagnosis of heart failure and echocardiogram demonstrating the presence of preserved ejection fraction as well as signs of diastolic dysfunction
- Management of acute decompensated HFpEF is based on diuretics for symptom control and management of comorbidities including hypertension and tachyarrhythmias.

SUGGESTED READINGS

1. Ahmed J, Rich MW, Flegl JL, Zile MR, Young JB, Kitzman DW, et al. Effects of digoxin on morbidity and mortality of diastolic heart failure: the ancillary digitalis investigation group trial. Circulation. 2006;114:397-403.
2. Andersen MJ, Borlaug BA. Heart failure with preserved ejection fraction: current understandings and challenges. Curr Cardiol Rep. 2014;16(7):501.
3. Basaraba JE, Barry AR. Pharmacotherapy of heart failure with preserved ejection fraction. Pharmacotherapy. 2015;35(4):351-60.

4. Bergström A, Andersson B, Edner M, Nylander E, Persson H, Dahlström U. Effect of carvedilol on diastolic function in patients with diastolic heart failure and preserved systolic function. Results of the Swedish Doppler-echocardiographic study (SWEDIC). Eur J Heart Fail. 2004;6(4):453-61.
5. Bhatia RS, Tu JV, Lee DS, Austin PC, Fang J, Haouzi A, et al. Outcome of heart failure with preserved ejection fraction in a population-based study. N Engl J Med. 2006;355(3):260-9.
6. Borlaug BA. The pathophysiology of heart failure with preserved ejection fraction. Nat Rev Cardiol. 2014;11(9):507-15.
7. Bursi F, Weston SA, Redfield MM, Jacobsen SJ, Pakhomov S, Nkomo VT, et al. Systolic and diastolic heart failure in the community. JAMA. 2006;296(18):2209-16.
8. Carson P, Massie BM, McKelvie R, McMurray J, Komajda M, Zile M, et al. The irbesartan in heart failure with preserved systolic function (I-PRESERVE) trial: rationale and design. J Card Fail. 2005;11(8):576-85.
9. Chatterjee K, Massie B. Systolic and diastolic heart failure: differences and similarities. J Card Fail. 2007;13(7):569-76.
10. Cleland JG, Swedberg K, Follath F, Komajda M, Cohen-Solal A, Aguilar JC, et al. The EuroHeart Failure survey programme – a survey on the quality of care among patients with heart failure in Europe. Part 1: patient characteristics and diagnosis. Eur Heart J. 2003;24(5):442-63.
11. Cleland JG, Tendera M, Adamus J, Freemantle N, Polonski L, Taylor J; PEP-CHF Investigators. The perindopril in elderly people with chronic heart failure (PEP-CHF) study. Eur Heart J. 2006;27(19):2338-45.
12. Effect of metoprolol CR/XL in chronic heart failure: Metoprolol CR/XL Randomised Intervention Trial in Congestive Heart Failure (MERIT-HF). Lancet. 1999;353:2001-7.
13. Flather MD, Shibata MC, Coats AJ, van Veldhuisen DJ, Parkhomenko A, Borbola J, et al. Randomized trial to determine the effect of nebivolol on mortality and cardiovascular hospital admission in elderly patients with heart failure (SENIORS). Eur Heart J. 2005;26:215-25.
14. Gutierrez C, Blanchard DG. Diastolic heart failure: challenges of diagnosis and treatment. Am Fam Physician. 2004;69(11): 2609-16.
15. Heart Failure Society of America, Lindenfeld J, Albert NM, Boehmer JP, Collins SP, Ezekowitz JA, et al. HFSA 2010 Comprehensive Heart Failure Practice Guideline. J Card Fail. 2010;16(6):e1-194.
16. Heidenreich PA, Lee TT, Massie BM. Effect of beta-blockade on mortality in patients with heart failure: a meta-analysis of randomized clinical trials. J Am Coll Cardiol. 1997;30:27-34.
17. Hogg K, Swedberg K, McMurray J. Heart failure with preserved left ventricular systolic function; epidemiology, clinical characteristics, and prognosis. J Am Coll Cardiol. 2004;43(3):317-27.
18. How to diagnose diastolic heart failure. European Study Group on Diastolic Heart Failure. Eur Heart J. 1998;19:990-1003.
19. Hundley WG, Kitzman DW, Morgan TM, Hamilton CA, Darty SN, Stewart KP, et al. Cardiac cycle-dependent changes in aortic area and distensibility are reduced in older patients with isolated diastolic heart failure and correlate with exercise intolerance. J Am Coll Cardiol. 2001;38(3):796-802.
20. Hunt SA, Abraham WT, Chin MH, Feldman AM, Francis GS, Ganiats TG, et al. ACC/AHA 2005 Guideline Update for the Diagnosis and Management of Chronic Heart Failure in the Adult: a report of the American College of Cardiology/American Heart Association Task Force on Practice Guidelines (Writing Committee to Update the 2001 Guidelines

for the Evaluation and Management of Heart Failure): developed in collaboration with the American College of Chest Physicians and the International Society for Heart and Lung Transplantation: endorsed by the Heart Rhythm Society. Circulation. 2005;112(12):e154-235.
21. Lechat P, Packer M, Chalon S, Cucherat M, Arab T, Boissel JP. Clinical effects of beta-adrenergic blockade in chronic heart failure: a meta-analysis of double-blind, placebo-controlled, randomized trials. Circulation. 1998;98:1184-91.
22. Masoudi FA, Havranek EP, Smith G, Fish RH, Steiner JF, Ordin DL, et al. Gender, age, and heart failure with preserved left ventricular systolic function. J Am Coll Cardiol. 2003;41(2):217-23.
23. Massie BM, Carson PE, McMurray JJ, Komajda M, McKelvie R, Zile MR, et al. Irbesartan in patients with heart failure and preserved ejection fraction. N Engl J Med. 2008;359(23):2456-67.
24. McMurray J, Pfeffer MA. New therapeutic options in congestive heart failure: Part II. Circulation. 2002;105:2223-8.
25. McMurray JJ, Carson PE, Komajda M, McKelvie R, Zile MR, Ptaszynska A, et al. Heart failure with preserved ejection fraction: clinical characteristics of 4133 patients enrolled in the I-PRESERVE trial. Eur J Heart Fail. 2008;10(2):149-56.
26. Oghlakian GO, Sipahi I, Fang JC. Treatment of heart failure with preserved ejection fraction: Have we been pursuing the wrong paradigm? Mayo Clin Proc. 2011;86(6):531-9.
27. Owan TE, Hodge DO, Herges RM, Jacobsen SJ, Roger VL, Redfield MM. Trends in prevalence and outcome of heart failure with preserved ejection fraction. N Engl J Med. 2006;355(3):251-9.
28. Packer M, Bristow MR, Cohn JN, Colucci WS, Fowler MB, Gilbert EM, et al. The effect of carvedilol on morbidity and mortality in patients with chronic heart failure. US. Carvedilol Heart Failure Study Group. N Engl J Med. 1996;334:1349-55.
29. Packer M, Fowler MB, Roecker EB, Coats AJ, Katus HA, Krum H, et al. Effect of carvedilol on the morbidity of patients with severe chronic heart failure: results of the carvedilol prospective randomized cumulative survival (COPERNICUS) study. Circulation. 2002; 106:2194-9.
30. Paulus WJ, Tschöpe C. A novel paradigm for heart failure with preserved ejection fraction: comorbidities drive myocardial dysfunction and remodeling through coronary microvascular endothelial inflammation. J Am Coll Cardiol. 2013;pii: S0735-1097(13)01890-1.
31. Pitt B, Pfeffer MA, Assmann SF, Boineau R, Anand IS, Claggett B, et al. Spironolactone for heart failure with preserved ejection fraction. N Engl J Med. 2014;370(15):1383-92.
32. Setaro JF, Zaret BL, Schulman DS, Black HR, Soufer R. Usefulness of verapamil for congestive heart failure associated with abnormal left ventricular diastolic filling and normal left ventricular systolic performance. Am J Cardiol 1990;66:981-6.
33. Somaratne JB, Berry C, McMurray JJ, Poppe KK, Doughty RN, Whalley GA. The prognostic significance of heart failure with preserved left ventricular ejection fraction: a literature-based meta-analysis. Eur J Heart Fail. 2009;11(9):855-62.
34. Teerlink JR, Cotter G, Davison BA, Felker GM, Filippatos G, Greenberg BH, et al. Serelaxin, recombinant human relaxin-2, for treatment of acute heart failure (RELAX-AHF): a randomised, placebo-controlled trial. Lancet. 2013;381(9860):29-39.
35. Tehrani F, Morrissey R, Phan A, Chien C, Schwarz ER. Statin therapy in patients with diastolic heart failure. Clin Cardiol. 2010;33(4):E1-5.
36. The Cardiac Insufficiency Bisoprolol Study II (CIBIS-II): a randomised trial. Lancet. 1999; 353:9-13.

37. Tribouilloy C, Rusinaru D, Mahjoub H, Soulière V, Lévy F, Peltier M, et al. Prognosis of heart failure with preserved ejection fraction: a 5 year prospective population-based study. Eur Heart J. 2008;29(3):339-47.
38. van Veldhuisen DJ, Linssen GC, Jaarsma T, van Gilst WH, Hoes AW, Tijssen JG, et al. B-type natriuretic peptide and prognosis in heart failure patients with preserved and reduced ejection fraction. J Am Coll Cardiol. 2013;61(14):1498-506.
39. Vasan RS, Levy D. Defining diastolic heart failure: a call for standardized diagnostic criteria. Circulation. 2000;101:2118-21.
40. Vasan RS, Levy D. The role of hypertension in the pathogenesis of heart failure. A clinical mechanistic overview. Arch Intern Med. 1996;156(16):1789-96.
41. Yip GW, Wang M, Wang T, Chan S, Fung JW, Yeung L, et al. The Hong Kong diastolic heart failure study: a randomised controlled trial of diuretics, irbesartan and ramipril on quality of life, exercise capacity, left ventricular global and regional function in heart failure with a normal ejection fraction. Heart. 2008;94(5):573-80.
42. Yturralde RF, Gaasch WH. Diagnostic criteria for diastolic heart failure. Prog Cardiovasc Dis. 2005;47:314-9.
43. Yusuf S, Pfeffer MA, Swedberg K, Granger CB, Held P, McMurray JJ, et al. Effects of candesartan in patients with chronic heart failure and preserved left-ventricular ejection fraction: the CHARM-Preserved Trial. Lancet. 2003;362(9386):777-81.
44. Zile MR, Baicu CF, Bonnema DD. Diastolic heart failure: definitions and terminology. Prog Cardiovasc Dis. 2005;47(5):307-13.

19
CHAPTER

Implantable Cardioverter Defibrillator and Cardiac Resynchronization Therapy in Heart Failure Patients: How to Choose the Right Device?

Khwaja S Alim, Erik A Green

INTRODUCTION

There has been continuing and expanding indications for device therapy in patients with heart failure (HF) who can be at an increased risk for sudden cardiac death (SCD). As the number of patients with cardiac implantable electronic devices increases, and as our understanding of HF and HF therapy develops and grows, the indications of implantable cardioverter defibrillator (ICD) and cardiac resynchronization therapy (CRT) are continuously being modified.

Landmark trials were performed like Multicenter Automatic Defibrillator Implantation Trial II (MADIT II), Comparison of Medical Therapy, Pacing, and Defibrillation in Heart Failure (COMPANION) trial, Defibrillators in Nonischemic Cardiomyopathy Treatment Evaluation (DEFINITE) trial, sudden death in heart failure (SCD-HeFT) trial. Based on the studies, the recommendations for ICD placement are listed in table 1.

INDICATIONS FOR IMPLANTABLE CARDIOVERTER-DEFIBRILLATOR IN HYPERTROPHIC CARDIOMYOPATHY

Hypertrophic cardiomyopathy (HCM) is the disease of the myocardium in which a portion of the myocardium is hypertrophied.

TABLE 1: Recommendations for implantable cardioverter defibrillator placement

Recommendation	Medical Conditions
IA	• Survivors of cardiac arrest due to VF or hemodynamically unstable sustained VT after evaluation to define the cause of the event and to exclude any completely reversible causes • LVEF ≤35% due to prior MI who are at least 40 days post-MI and are in NYHA functional class II or III • Left ventricular dysfunction due to prior MI who are at least 40 days post-MI, have an LVEF ≤30%, and are in NYHA functional class I
IB	• Patients with structural heart disease and spontaneous sustained VT, whether hemodynamically stable or unstable • Syncope of undetermined origin with clinically relevant, hemodynamically significant sustained VT or VF induced at electrophysiological study • Nonischemic DCM who have an LVEF ≤35% and who are in NYHA functional class II or III • Non-sustained VT due to prior MI, LVEF ≤40%, and inducible VF or sustained VT at electrophysiological study
IIaB	• ICD implantation is reasonable to reduce SCD in patients with long-QT syndrome who are experiencing syncope and/or VT while receiving β-blockers
IIaC	• Patients with unexplained syncope, significant left ventricular dysfunction, and nonischemic DCM • Patients with sustained VT and normal or near-normal ventricular function • ICD implantation is reasonable for patients with HCM who have one or more major risk factors for SCD • Patients with arrhythmogenic right ventricular dysplasia or cardiomyopathy who has one or more risk factors for SCD • Patients awaiting transplantation • Patients with Brugada syndrome who have had syncope • Patients with Brugada syndrome who have documented VT that has not resulted in cardiac arrest • Patients with catecholaminergic polymorphic VT who have syncope and/or documented sustained VT while receiving β-blockers • Patients with cardiac sarcoidosis, giant cell myocarditis, or Chagas disease
IIbB	• ICD therapy may be considered for patients with long-QT syndrome and risk factors for SCD

Continued

Algorithms in Heart Failure

Continued

Recommendation	Medical Conditions
IIbC	• ICD therapy may be considered in patients with nonischemic heart disease who have an LVEF of ≤35% and who are in NYHA functional class I • Patients with syncope and advanced structural heart disease in whom thorough invasive and noninvasive investigations have failed to define a cause • Patients with a familial cardiomyopathy associated with sudden death • Patients with left ventricular noncompaction

Note: All primary SCD prevention ICD recommendations apply only to patients who are receiving optimal medical therapy and have reasonable expectation of survival with good functional capacity for more than 1 year.

VT, ventricular tachycardia; LVEF, left ventricular ejection fraction; MI, myocardial infarction; NYHA, New York Heart Association; VF, ventricular fibrillation; DCM, dilated cardiomyopathy; ICD, implantable cardioverter defibrillator; SCD, sudden cardiac death; HCM, hypertrophic cardiomyopathy.

Hence, the SCD risk stratification-recommendations are as follows:
- CLASS I
  - All patients with HCM should undergo comprehensive SCD risk stratification at initial evaluation to determine the presence of the following: (level of evidence: B):
    - A personal history for ventricular fibrillation, sustained ventricular tachycardia, or SCD events, including appropriate ICD therapy for ventricular tachyarrhythmias
    - A family history for SCD events, including appropriate ICD therapy for ventricular tachyarrhythmias
    - Unexplained syncope
    - Documented nonsustained ventricular tachycardia defined as three or more beats at greater than or equal to 120 beats per minute on ambulatory (Holter) electrocardiogram
    - Maximal left ventricular wall thickness greater than or equal to 30 mm.
- CLASS IIa
  - It is reasonable to assess blood pressure response during exercise as part of SCD risk stratification in patients with HCM. (level of evidence: B)
  - Sudden cardiac death risk stratification is reasonable on a periodic basis (every 12–24 months) for patients with HCM who have not undergone ICD implantation but would otherwise be eligible in the event that risk factors are identified (12–24 months).
- CLASS III
  - Invasive electrophysiologic testing as routine SCD risk stratification for patients with HCM should not be performed.

CARDIAC RESYNCHRONIZATION THERAPY

Cardiac resynchronization therapy in selected patients improves exercise capacity as measured by maximal oxygen uptake, left ventricular ejection fraction, New York Heart Association (NYHA) class, and overall mortality benefit (Algorithm 1).

Biventricular pacing has been found to be superior to right ventricular pacing in patients with atrioventricular block and left ventricular systolic dysfunction with NYHA class I, II, or III HF. The beneficial impact of CRT comes from the interventricular and intraventricular synchrony. This results not only in the improvement

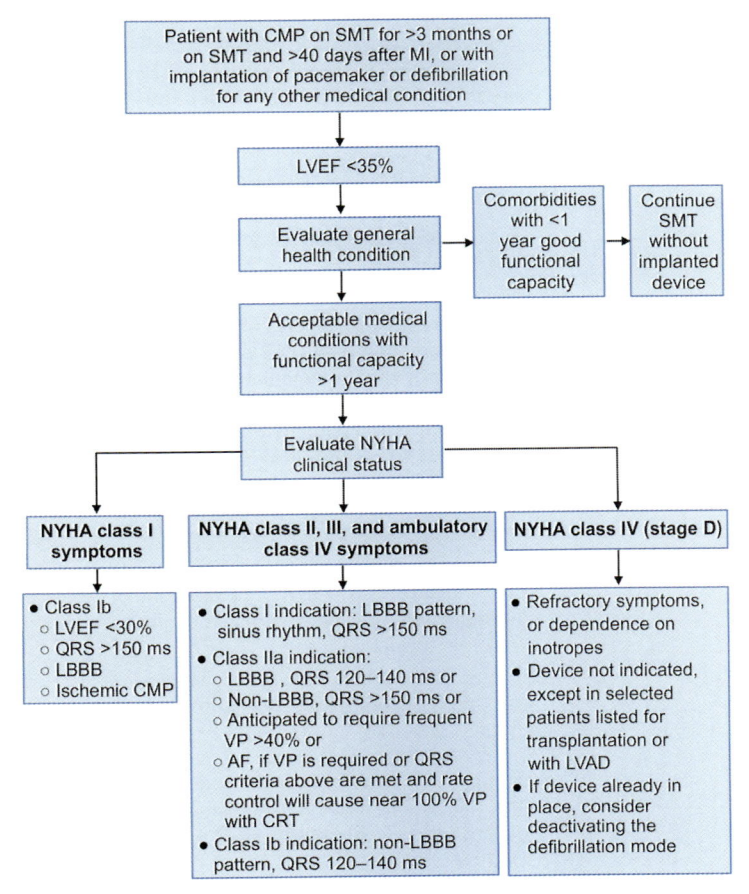

```
Patient with CMP on SMT for >3 months or
on SMT and >40 days after MI, or with
implantation of pacemaker or defibrillation
for any other medical condition
                │
                ▼
           LVEF <35%
                │
                ▼
      Evaluate general  ──→  Comorbidities  ──→  Continue
      health condition       with <1              SMT
                             year good            without
                             functional           implanted
                             capacity             device
                │
                ▼
      Acceptable medical
      conditions with
      functional capacity
      >1 year
                │
                ▼
       Evaluate NYHA
       clinical status
```

NYHA class I symptoms	NYHA class II, III, and ambulatory class IV symptoms	NYHA class IV (stage D)

• Class Ib
  ○ LVEF <30%
  ○ QRS >150 ms
  ○ LBBB
  ○ Ischemic CMP
	• Class I indication: LBBB pattern, sinus rhythm, QRS >150 ms
	• Class IIa indication:
	  ○ LBBB, QRS 120–140 ms or
	  ○ Non-LBBB, QRS >150 ms or
	  ○ Anticipated to require frequent VP >40% or
	  ○ AF, if VP is required or QRS criteria above are met and rate control will cause near 100% VP with CRT
	• Class Ib indication: non-LBBB pattern, QRS 120–140 ms
		• Refractory symptoms, or dependence on inotropes
		• Device not indicated, except in selected patients listed for transplantation or with LVAD
		• If device already in place, consider deactivating the defibrillation mode

CMP, cardiomyopathy; MI, myocardial infarction; LVEF, left ventricular ejection fraction; SMT, standard medical therapy; NYHA, New York Heart Association; LBBB, left bundle branch block; LVAD, left ventricular assist device; VP, ventricular pacing; AF, atrial fibrillation.

ALGORITHM 1: Indications for cardiac resynchronization therapy

of the left ventricular geometry but also in the mechanical function, contractility, and performance. According to the Combined Cardiac Resynchronization and Implantable Cardioversion Defibrillation in Advanced Chronic Heart Failure: the Multicenter InSync ICD Randomized Clinical Evaluation (MIRACLE ICD) trial, CRT improved quality of life, functional status, and exercise capacity in patients with moderate-to-severe HF, and significant reduction of ventricular arrhythmias in patients with left bundle branch block. Based on several other studies, the recommendation for the CRT is listed in table 2.

TABLE 2: Recommendation for the cardiac resynchronization therapy

Recommendation	Medical Condition
IA	CRT is indicated for patients who have LVEF ≤35%, sinus rhythm, LBBB with a QRS duration ≥150 ms, and NYHA class II, III, or ambulatory class IV symptoms on GDMT
IB	Level of evidence: B for NYHA class II
IIaA	CRT can be useful for patients who have LVEF ≤35%, sinus rhythm, a non-LBBB pattern with a QRS duration ≥150 ms, and NYHA class III or ambulatory class IV symptoms on GDMT
IIaB	CRT can be useful for patients who have LVEF ≤35%, sinus rhythm, LBBB with a QRS duration 120–149 ms, and NYHA class II, III, or ambulatory, IV symptoms on GDMT CRT can be useful in patients with atrial fibrillation and LVEF ≤35% on GDMT if: a) The patient requires ventricular pacing or otherwise meets CRT criteria and b) AV nodal ablation or pharmacologic rate control will allow near 100% ventricular pacing with CRT
IIaC	CRT can be useful for patients on GDMT who have LVEF ≤35% and are undergoing new or replacement device placement with anticipated requirement for significant (>40%) ventricular pacing
IIbB	CRT may be considered for patients who have LVEF ≤35%, sinus rhythm, a non-LBBB pattern with QRS duration 120–149 ms, and NYHA class III or ambulatory class IV on GDMT CRT may be considered for patients who have LVEF ≤35%, sinus rhythm, a non-LBBB pattern with a QRS duration ≥150 ms, and NYHA class II symptoms on GDMT
IIbC	CRT may be considered for patients who have LVEF ≤30%, ischemic etiology of HF, sinus rhythm, LBBB with a QRS duration of ≥150 ms, and NYHA class I symptoms on GDMT

Continued

Continued

Recommendation	Medical Condition
IIIB	CRT is not recommended for patients with NYHA class I or II symptoms and non-LBBB pattern with QRS duration <150 ms
IIIC	CRT is not indicated for patients whose comorbidities and/or frailty limit survival with good functional capacity to <1 year

CRT, cardiac resynchronization therapy; LVEF, left ventricular ejection fraction; LBBB, left bundle branch block; NYHA, New York Heart Association; GDMT, guideline directed medical therapy; AV, atrioventricular; HF, heart failure.

CONCLUSION

Heart failure patients often have an increased risk for SCD. Several landmark trials, including MADIT II, COMPANION, DEFINITE, SCD-HeFT, and MIRACLE ICD have provided ample evidence for the use of ICDs and CRT to protect heart failure patients from SCD. Strong recommendations exist for ICD placement in survivors of cardiac arrest, VF, unstable VT, and those with low LVEF post MI. Recommendations exist for other classes of patients as well. Strong recommendations regarding CRT have also been proposed, and CRT has been shown to improve quality of life, to increase functional status, and to reduce arrhythmias in several classes of patients. Patients with HCM represent a select group of high-risk patients that require appropriate risk-stratification and recommendation-based screening. Increasing numbers of HF patients and growing understanding of implantable electronic cardiac devices will mean a greater use of such devices over time. Therefore, knowledge of device indications and usage are important aspects of current and future care for patients with heart failure.

KEY POINTS

- Advanced heart failure patients can be at a risk for sudden cardiac death
- Implantable cardioverter defibrillator (ICD) can prevent such events
- Indications for ICD placement are based on landmark studies
- Hypertrophic cardiomyopathy is another indication for ICD placement
- Cardiac resynchronization therapy improved cardiac function in selected group of patients.

SUGGESTED READINGS

1. Antonio N, Teixeira R, Coelho L, Lourenço C, Monteiro P, Ventura M, et al. Identification of 'super-responders' to cardiac resynchronization therapy: the importance of symptom duration and left ventricular geometry. Europace. 2009;11(3):343-9.
2. Bardy GH, Lee KL, Mark DB, Poole JE, Packer DL, Boineau R, et al. Amiodarone or an implantable cardioverter-defibrillator for congestive heart failure. N Engl J Med. 2005;352:225-37.
3. Bristow MR, Saxon LA, Boehmer J, Krueger S, Kass DA, De Marco T, et al. Cardiac-resynchronization therapy with or without an implantable defibrillator in advanced chronic heart failure. N Engl J Med. 2004;350(21):2140-50.
4. Bristow MR, Saxon LA, Boehmer J, Krueger S, Kass DA, De Marco T, et al. Cardiac-resynchronization therapy with or without an implantable defibrillator in advanced chronic heart failure. N Engl J Med. 2004;350:2140-50.
5. Cleland JG, Daubert JC, Erdmann E, Freemantle N, Gras D, Kappenberger L, et al. The effect of cardiac resynchronization on morbidity and mortality in heart failure. N Engl J Med. 2005;352(15):1539-49.
6. Curtis AB, Worley SJ, Adamson PB, Chung ES, Niazi I, Sherfesee L, et al. Biventricular pacing for atrioventricular block and systolic dysfunction. N Engl J Med. 2013;368:1585-93.
7. Kadish A, Dyer A, Daubert JP, Quigg R, Estes NA, Anderson KP, et al. Prophylactic defibrillator implantation in patients with nonischemic dilated cardiomyopathy. N Engl J Med. 2004;350:2151-8.
8. Kutyifa V, Pouleur AC, Knappe D, Al-Ahmad A, Gibinski M, Wang PJ, et al. Dyssynchrony and the risk of ventricular arrhythmias. JACC Cardiovasc Imaging. 2013;6(4):432-44.
9. Kutyifa V1, Klein HU, Wang PJ, McNitt S, Polonsky B, Zima E, et al. Clinical significance of ventricular tachyarrhythmias in patients treated with CRT-D. Heart Rhythm. 201;10(7):943-50.
10. Maron BJ, Spirito P, Shen WK, Haas TS, Formisano F, Link MS, et al. Implantable cardioverter-defibrillators and prevention of sudden cardiac death in hypertrophic cardiomyopathy. JAMA. 2007;298:405-12.
11. Maron BJ. Hypertrophic cardiomyopathy: a systemic review. JAMA. 2002;287(10):1308-20.
12. Moss AJ, Zareba W, Hall WJ, Klein H, Wilber DJ, Cannom DS, et al. Prophylactic implantation of a defibrillator in patients with myocardial infarction and reduced ejection fraction. N Engl J Med. 2002;346:877-83.
13. Richardson P, McKenna W, Bristow M, Maisch B, Mautner B, O'Connell J, et al. Report of the 1995 World Health Organization/International Society and Federation of Cardiology Task Force on the Definition and Classification of cardiomyopathies. Circulation. 1996;93(5):841-2.
14. Sherrid MV, Chaudry FA, Swistel DG. Obstructive hypertrophic cardiomyopathy: echocardiography, pathophysiology, and the continuing evolution of surgery for obstruction. Ann Thorac Surg. 2003;75(2):620-32.
15. Young JB, Abraham WT, Smith AL, Leon AR, Lieberman R, Wilkoff B, et al. Combined cardiac resynchronization and implantable cardioversion defibrillation in advanced chronic heart failure: the MIRACLE ICD Trial. JAMA. 2003;289(20):2685-94.

20
CHAPTER

Clinical Decision-making in the Outpatient Setting: the Use of Galectin-3

Rogier van der Velde, Wouter C Meijers, Rudolf A de Boer

INTRODUCTION

Biomarkers can be used to diagnose heart failure (HF), but may also serve as predictors of prognosis. Improved risk prediction may help to better inform patients, but also helps to give patients a "personalized" treatment. In HF, risk prediction remains a challenge. In the last decade, several biomarkers have become available and showed their independent predictive value. Galectin-3 is one of those novel biomarkers, that was discovered as one of the most upregulated genes associated with the transition from compensated towards decompensated HF. An early increase in galectin-3 gene expression identifies individuals that are prone to develop HF. Therefore, galectin-3 may be used as a marker of "early stage" HF, and may steer treatment towards a more aggressive approach.

Galectin-3 is a β-galactosidase binding lectin derived from macrophages. It stimulates fibroblast proliferation, deposition of collagen with subsequent cardiac dysfunction and it is believed that galectin-3 reflects extracellular matrix turnover. Moreover, galectin-3 is required for the fibrotic response after stimulation with aldosterone. If galectin-3 is not expressed, there is no inflammatory and fibrotic response.

Unlike natriuretic peptides, galectin-3 is a fairly stable marker—galectin-3 plasma levels do not change much over time. But when galectin-3 levels do change, only a slight change of 15% can already predict an improved or worsened prognosis. This narrow range of biological variability is also independent from cardiac pressures: mechanical unloading of the heart with a mechanical circulatory support device is not reflected by a change in plasma galectin-3 levels. This implies that the prognostic value of galectin-3 can be measured at any time during the disease process and will not differ much when comparing a decompensated and recompensated state.

DIAGNOSTIC VALUE IN HEART FAILURE

In order to diagnose HF, galectin-3 is of limited value. In the N-terminal Pro-brain nitriuretic peptide (NT-proBNP) Investigation of Dyspnea in the Emergency Department (PRIDE) study, 599 acutely dyspnoeic patients were studied, from which 209 had acute HF as their final diagnosis. Receiver-operating characteristic analysis was performed to evaluate the utility of galectin-3, apelin, or NT-proBNP for the diagnosis of HF. This analysis showed an area under the curve (AUC) of 0.94 for NT-proBNP, an AUC of 0.72 for galectin-3 and 0.52 for apelin. These results indicate that NT-proBNP is by far the best biomarker to diagnose HF. Furthermore, galectin-3 levels are not elevated in all patients with HF. Approximately, 40–60% of HF patients present with high levels of galectin-3 (cutpoint 17.8 ng/mL) and can be identified as patients with a subtype of "fibrotic" HF.

PROGNOSTIC VALUE IN HEART FAILURE

After Myocardial Infarction

Fibrosis and cardiac remodeling are detrimental processes that occur after acute myocardial infarction. Since galectin-3 is involved in these pathways, it was hypothesized that galectin-3 is important in the development of HF. In patients after ST-elevated myocardial infarction (STEMI), galectin-3 was found to be significantly correlated with infarct size. Patients with galectin-3 levels above 10.9 ng/mL (median galectin-3 level), had a significant lower left ventricular ejection fraction (LVEF) after 4 months ($57.9 \pm 8.3\%$ vs $65.1 \pm 5.8\%$, $p = 0.022$). This implies that galectin-3 levels can be used to estimate infarct size and LVEF after myocardial infarction, but this has to be confirmed in larger studies.

Mortality in Acute Heart Failure

The PRIDE study, as briefly described above also evaluated, the prognostic value of galectin-3 in acute HF. Galectin-3 was superior over NT-proBNP in identifying high risk patients for short-term mortality and 30-day rehospitalization. The combination of both markers was found to be the best predictor for this composite endpoint. Galectin-3 was also an independent predictor for 60-day mortality only. These findings were confirmed by the results from the Co-ordinating Study Evaluating Outcomes of Advising and Counseling in Heart Failure (COACH). This study, comprising 592 patients that were hospitalized for HF with a follow-up period of 18 months, showed that galectin-3 was an independent predictor of the composite endpoint: all-cause mortality and HF hospitalization. Another interesting finding was that galectin-3, particularly, had strong predictive value in patients with HF with preserved ejection fraction (HFpEF), compared to patient with HF with reduced ejection fraction (HFrEF).

Mortality in Chronic Heart Failure

The prognostic value of galectin-3 in chronic HF patients was first studied in the Deventer–Alkmaar heart failure (DEAL-HF) study, in which patients were followed during 6.5 years. In these 232 patients with severe, chronic HF, galectin-3 was a significant predictor of mortality, also after adjusting for age, sex, NT-proBNP, and estimated glomerular filtration rates (eGFR). Again, the combination of elevated galectin-3 and NT-proBNP yielded the highest prognostic value (Fig. 1). These results were confirmed by several other studies in patients with chronic HF. However, the Controlled Rosuvastatin Multinational Trial in Heart Failure (CORONA) trial (n = 1462) showed that galectin-3 was a univariable predictor for mortality, but this effect was diminished after adjustment for NT-proBNP. In another large clinical trial Heart Failure: A Controlled Trial Investigating Outcomes of Exercise Training (HF-ACTION) (n = 895), galectin-3 was found to be a significant predictor of outcome, but after adjustment for eGFR, this predictive value was lost. It should be noted that these results were for the combined endpoint of mortality and HF hospitalization.

Rehospitalization in Heart Failure

Galectin-3 is a predictor for mortality in acute HF and in chronic HF, but can also be used as a predictor for rehospitalization. In a pooled analysis of three studies in patients with acute HF [COACH, PRIDE, and University of Maryland Pro-BNP for Diagnosis and Prognosis in Patients Presenting With Dyspnea (UMD) H-23258 (n = 902)], elevated levels of galectin-3 were found to be associated with short-

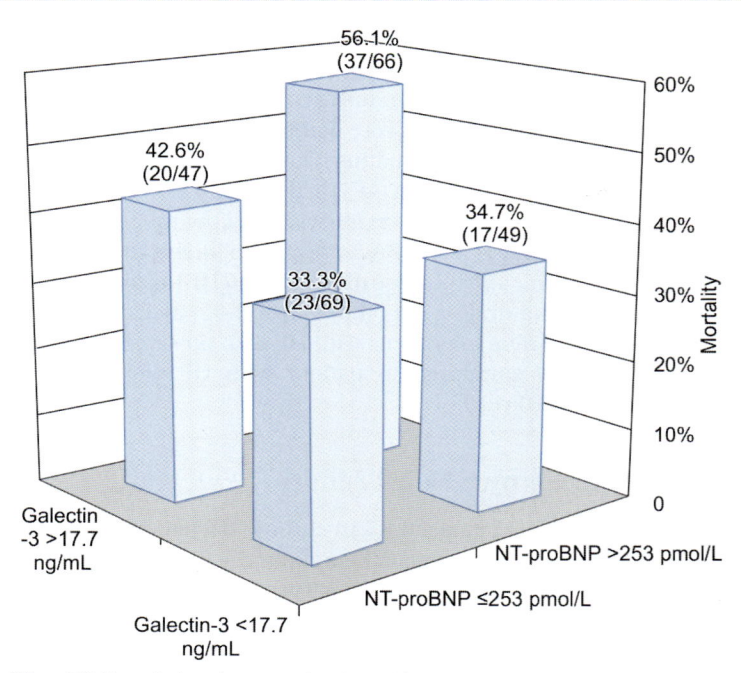

NT-proBNP, N-terminal pro-b-type natriuretic peptide.

FIG. 1: Mortality is presented in four categories of galectin-3, N-terminal pro-b-type natriuretic peptide (NT-proBNP)-probing (and their combination) in patients with severe, chronic heart failure. Increased levels of galectin-3 were associated with higher mortality and after adjustment for age, renal dysfunction, and NT-proBNP, remained an independent prognostic marker

term rehospitalization. Patients with galectin-3 levels above the Food and Drug Administration-approved cutpoint (17.8 ng/mL) had a three times higher risk for short-term rehospitalization (30, 60, 90, and 120 days). Galectin-3 remained an independent predictor for rehospitalization after adjustment for age, gender, eGFR, New York Heart Association class, LVEF, and NT-proBNP. Addition of galectin-3 to the risk model reclassified the risk of postdischarge rehospitalization at each time point (continuous net reclassification improvement at 30 days: 42.6%).

SERIAL MEASUREMENTS OF GALECTIN-3

Baseline galectin-3 levels provide prognostic value, but repeated measurements also bear prognostic consequences. In a substudy of the CORONA trial (n = 1329) and COACH study (n = 324), galectin-3 levels were measured at multiple time points. Rising galectin-3 levels over time (3–6 months) were associated with a significant higher rate of HF hospitalization and mortality compared with stable or decreasing galectin-3 levels. This was shown for categorical change (using 17.8 ng/mL cutpoint) as well as for percentage change (15% change cutpoint). This predictive value was independent of age, sex, diabetes mellitus, LVEF, renal function, medication, and NT-proBNP. The predictive value of repeated galectin-3 measurements was confirmed in the Valsartan Heart Failure Trial (Val-HeFT) and ProBNP Outpatient Tailored Chronic Heart Failure Therapy (PROTECT).

POTENTIAL USE IN CLINICAL DECISION-MAKING

Several studies have investigated the interaction between evidence-based HF drugs and galectin-3. A substudy of the Val-HeFT trial investigated the effect of valsartan on HF outcome, stratified to galectin-3 levels. The use of valsartan resulted in a significant reduction of 44% in hospitalizations for HF in patients with galectin-3 levels below the median (16.2 ng/mL). This was independent of all baseline variables including NT-proBNP. In patients with high galectin-3 levels, there was no effect of valsartan.

In a substudy of the CORONA trial, investigators studied the effect of statins in HF patients. Previously was found that statins only exerted effect in patients with low values of NT-proBNP. This substudy concluded that only patients with relatively low galectin-3 levels (<19 ng/mL) benefited from statin therapy. These results might be difficult to interpret, since it is thought that statins influence anti-inflammatory effects of the cytokine network, a pathway in which galectin-3 also plays a role. These results suggest that statins affect different pathways in inflammation.

Cardiac resynchronization therapy (CRT) can improve symptoms or even LVEF. It is believed that the success rate of CRT depends on the amount of fibrosis. Whether galectin-3, as a marker of fibrosis, can predict the response to CRT remains uncertain. A substudy of the Cardiac Resynchronization-Heart Failure (CARE-HF) (n = 260) concluded that galectin-3 does not predict response to CRT. The larger Multicenter Automatic Defibrillator Implantation Trial with Cardiac Resynchronization Therapy (MADIT-CRT) trial (n = 654) showed that CRT-defibrillator therapy was beneficial in patients with low and high galectin-3, but the absolute benefit of CRT was bigger in patients with high galectin-3 levels: patients with galectin-3 levels in the highest quartile had 65% reduction in risk of the primary endpoint, compared to 25% reduction in risk in the lowest quartile of galectin-3. These results suggest that galectin-3 levels may be used to prioritize patients that are eligible for CRT treatment.

Galectin-3 to Guide Therapy

Preclinical research has shown that aldosterone induced fibrosis is galectin-3 dependent. Mineralocorticoid receptor antagonists (MRAs) block the aldosterone receptor and, therefore, may affect galectin-3 pathways. Interestingly, both MRAs as well as galectin-3 antagonists blocked aldosterone induced fibrosis. Therefore, it is hypothesized that patients with high galectin-3 levels, and hence more fibrosis, will respond in a different manner to MRA treatment.

This hypothesis was first tested in a substudy of HF-ACTION. Spironolactone did not show a beneficial effect in patients with high galectin-3 levels, however, spironolactone failed to show any effect at all on mortality, compared to no MRA treatment. A second analysis in the COACH trial, involving 534 patients with acute HF, showed a reduction in 30-day event rate in patients that were discharged on spironolactone and this survival benefit was more prominent in patients with high galectin-3 levels. These results suggest that high galectin-3 levels can be used to identify high risk patients that are more likely to benefit from initiation or continuation of spironolactone therapy.

A PROPOSED ALGORITHM

The value of galectin-3 is based upon the fact that is it not dependent on "loading status", and reflects a different pathway than natriuretic peptides, which are highly dependent on fluid status. Galectin-3 can be used to discriminate high and low risk HF patients and is one of the best independent predictors in patients with acute HF, especially, for predicting short-term prognosis. There are conflicting results whether galectin-3 is also the best predictor for long-term prognosis and, therefore, NT-proBNP may also be used as a predictor for outcome. Several studies conclude that the combination of elevated levels of galectin-3 and NT-proBNP is the best prognostic predictor.

In the proposed algorithm (Algorithm 1), it is advised to treat low risk patients according to standard care. Post hoc analyses suggest the continuation of angiotensin receptor blockers and statins as a treatment for HF patients with low galectin-3 levels. Patients in

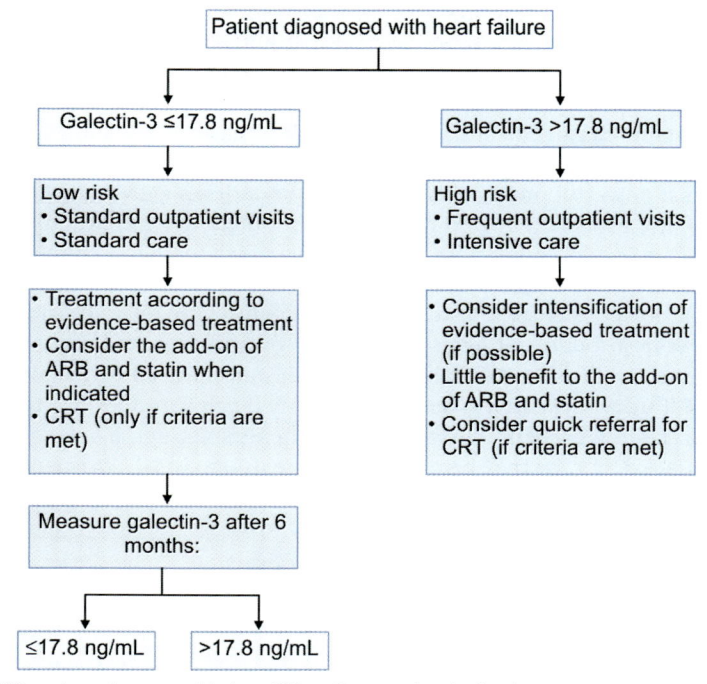

Clinical Decision-making in the Outpatient Setting: the Use of Galectin-3

```
                Patient diagnosed with heart failure
                        /                    \
            Galectin-3 ≤17.8 ng/mL      Galectin-3 >17.8 ng/mL
                    |                           |
            Low risk                      High risk
            • Standard outpatient visits  • Frequent outpatient visits
            • Standard care               • Intensive care
                    |                           |
            • Treatment according to      • Consider intensification of
              evidence-based treatment      evidence-based treatment
            • Consider the add-on of        (if possible)
              ARB and statin when         • Little benefit to the add-on
              indicated                     of ARB and statin
            • CRT (only if criteria are   • Consider quick referral for
              met)                          CRT (if criteria are met)
                    |
            Measure galectin-3 after 6
                    months:
                  /        \
            ≤17.8 ng/mL   >17.8 ng/mL
```

ARB, angiotensin receptor blockers; CRT, cardiac resynchronization therapy.

ALGORITHM 1: A proposed algorithm for the use of galectin-3 in clinical decision making. Galectin-3 measurements should complement established predictors like estimated glomerular filtration rates and N-terminal pro-brain natriuretic peptide

the high risk group have the worst prognosis and should be closely monitored, with frequent visits to the outpatient department and they should be treated with the optimal antifibrotic drug regimen, including MRAs and angiotensin converting enzyme inhibitors. It is suggested that the absolute benefit of CRT is more beneficial in patients with high galectin-3 levels; therefore, galectin-3 can be used to prioritize patients who are eligible for CRT.

Of note, this is a proposed algorithm, based on several peer-reviewed papers, but should not serve as a guideline for general practice, since no prospective studies have been performed yet. Caution should be exercised in the interpretation of galectin-3 levels in patients with low eGFR, since kidney function is responsible for a large part of the variability of galectin-3. Though prospective data are lacking that support the standard use of galectin-3 yet, the precise role of galectin-3 will emerge in the coming years.

CONCLUSION

In conclusion, galectin-3 is a protein that has established function in the development of myocardial fibrosis. Galectin-3 enters the systemic circulation and as such it may be measured as a biomarker. The last decade, it has been established that galectin-3 is one of the most powerful prognostic biomarkers in patients with acute heart failure, especially regarding short-term outcomes. Importantly, it can be of additional value on top of the stretch marker NT-proBNP, which appears logical because these two markers reflect different (patho-)physiology. Plasma levels of galectin-3 are relatively stable over time, but nevertheless, differences over time are of prognostic value in HF patients. Galectin-3 should not be used to diagnose HF. Current research is aimed to identify if galectin-3 levels might be used to install or withhold specific treatments, and if galectin-3 targeted therapy may be of use in the treatment of HF. Prospective studies are needed to validate proposed algorithms.

KEY POINTS

- Galectin-3 is involved in fibrosis and identifies heart failure (HF)-prone hearts
- Plasma levels are stable over time and are independent of "fluid status"
- Galectin-3 is one of the best short-term prognostic biomarkers in patients with acute heart failure and is particularly of value in patients with heart failure with preserved ejection fraction
- Galectin-3 can be used to select patients with high risk of short-term rehospitalization
- Galectin-3 identifies patients who are less sensitive for evidence-based cardiovascular medication, like angiotensin receptor blockers and statins.

SUGGESTED READINGS

1. Anand IS, Rector TS, Kuskowski M, Adourian A, Muntendam P, Cohn JN. Baseline and serial measurements of galectin-3 in patients with heart failure: relationship to prognosis and effect of treatment with valsartan in the Val-HeFT. Eur J Heart Fail. 2013;15(5):511-8.
2. Calvier L, Miana M, Reboul P, Cachofeiro V, Martinez-Martinez E, de Boer RA, et al. Galectin-3 mediates aldosterone-induced vascular fibrosis. Arterioscler Thromb Vasc Biol. 2013;33(1):67-75.
3. de Boer RA, Lok DJ, Jaarsma T, van der Meer P, Voors AA, Hillege HL, et al. Predictive value of plasma galectin-3 levels in heart failure with reduced and preserved ejection fraction. Ann Med. 2011;43(1):60-8.

4. Fiuzat M, Schulte PJ, Felker M, Ahmad T, Neely M, Adams KF, et al. Relationship between galectin-3 levels and mineralocorticoid receptor antagonist use in heart failure: analysis from HF-ACTION. J Card Fail. 2014;20(1):38-44.
5. Gullestad L, Ueland T, Kjekshus J, Nymo SH, Hulthe J, Muntendam P, et al. Galectin-3 predicts response to statin therapy in the Controlled Rosuvastatin Multinational Trial in Heart Failure (CORONA). Eur Heart J. 2012;33(18):2290-6.
6. Lok DJ, Van Der Meer P, de la Porte PW, Lipsic E, Van Wijngaarden J, Hillege HL, et al. Prognostic value of galectin-3, a novel marker of fibrosis, in patients with chronic heart failure: data from the DEAL-HF study. Clin Res Cardiol. 2010;99(5):323-8.
7. Maisel A, Xue Y, van Veldhuisen DJ, Voors AA, Jaarsma T, Pang PS, et al. Effect of spironolactone on 30-day death and heart failure rehospitalization (from the COACH Study). Am J Cardiol. 2014;114(5):737-42.
8. Mayr A, Klug G, Mair J, Streil K, Harrasser B, Feistritzer HJ, et al. Galectin-3: relation to infarct scar and left ventricular function after myocardial infarction. Int J Cardiol. 2013;163(3):335-7.
9. Meijers WC, Januzzi JL, deFilippi C, Adourian AS, Shah SJ, van Veldhuisen DJ, et al. Elevated plasma galectin-3 is associated with near-term rehospitalization in heart failure: a pooled analysis of 3 clinical trials. Am Heart J. 2014;167(6):853-60.e4.
10. Milting H, Ellinghaus P, Seewald M, Cakar H, Bohms B, Kassner A, et al. Plasma biomarkers of myocardial fibrosis and remodeling in terminal heart failure patients supported by mechanical circulatory support devices. J Heart Lung Transplant. 2008;27(6):589-96.
11. Sharma UC, Pokharel S, van Brakel TJ, et al. Galectin-3 marks activated macrophages in failure-prone hypertrophied hearts and contributes to cardiac dysfunction. Circulation. 2004;110(19):3121-8.
12. Stolen CM, Adourian A, Meyer TE, Stein KM, Solomon SD. Plasma galectin-3 and heart failure outcomes in MADIT-CRT (multicenter automatic defibrillator implantation trial with cardiac resynchronization therapy). J Card Fail. 2014; 20(11):793-9.
13. van der Velde AR, Gullestad L, Ueland T, Aukrust P, Guo Y, Adourian A, et al. Prognostic value of changes in galectin-3 levels over time in patients with heart failure: data from CORONA and COACH. Circ Heart Fail. 2013;6(2):219-26.
14. van Kimmenade RR, Januzzi JL Jr, Ellinor PT, Sharma UC, Bakker JA, Low AF, et al. Utility of amino-terminal pro-brain natriuretic peptide, galectin-3, and apelin for the evaluation of patients with acute heart failure. J Am Coll Cardiol. 2006;48(6):1217-24.

CHAPTER 21

ST2: How to Really Do It Right?

Jason M Duran, Lori B Daniels

INTRODUCTION

ST2 is a receptor for interleukin-33 (IL-33) and is expressed by cardiomyocytes and fibroblasts in response to mechanical stress. In animal models of pressure overload, IL-33 has been shown to protect against left ventricular hypertrophy and fibrosis. Two isoforms of the ST2 receptor are expressed through alternative splicing: membrane bound (ST2L) and soluble (sST2, hereafter denoted as ST2). In heart failure (HF), the soluble variant of ST2 is overexpressed and acts as a decoy receptor that binds IL-33 and prevents its antihypertrophic and antifibrotic activity. No prospective, randomized, and controlled clinical trials have examined the utility of ST2 as a clinical biomarker, but there is a growing body of retrospective and observational evidence suggesting its use as a prognostic indicator with implications for monitoring patients with HF and for driving therapy decisions. In this chapter, data provided by 18 of the many clinical studies have been provided, to outline a proposed algorithm of how ST2 may be used in the clinical setting.

ST2 MEASUREMENT IN THE INPATIENT SETTING: ST ELEVATION MYOCARDIAL INFARCTION AND NON-ST ELEVATION MYOCARDIAL INFARCTION

ST2 levels peak about 12 hours after ST elevation myocardial infarction (STEMI). Several retrospective analyses have demonstrated that higher levels of ST2 are associated with increased risk of new HF and death by 30 days after STEMI. The Metabolic

Efficiency with Ranolazine for Less Ischemia in Non-ST Elevation Acute Coronary Syndromes-thrombolysis in myocardial infarction (MERLIN-TIMI 36) trial examined patients with non-ST elevation myocardial infarction (NSTEMI), and demonstrated that ST2 levels greater than 35 ng/mL were associated with increased risk of HF and death at 30 days and at 1 year post-myocardial infarction (post-MI).

In addition to these prognostic uses of post-MI ST2 levels, a *post hoc* analysis of the Eplerenone Post-Acute Myocardial Infarction Heart Failure Efficacy and Survival Study (EPHESUS) trial of acute MI patients with left ventricular dysfunction demonstrated that aldosterone inhibition with eplerenone prevented adverse left ventricular remodeling (i.e., increased left ventricular end-systolic and end-diastolic volumes) only among patients with ST2 above the median. Of the patients included in this trial, 90% had STEMI and 10% had NSTEMI. Thus, when treating a patient with acute STEMI or NSTEMI and a left ventricular ejection fraction less than 40% who is already on optimal medical therapy including a β-blocker and an angiotensin converting enzyme inhibitor (ACEI) or angiotensin receptor blocker (ARB), ST2 levels might be useful for titrating therapy and determining which patients should be further treated with aldosterone blockade. One possible algorithm for use of ST2 in this setting is as follows:

1. After medical optimization, check an ST2 level
2. If ST2 is 35 ng/mL or less, continue current management. If ST2 levels are over 35 ng/mL and the patient's potassium levels and renal function are acceptable (potassium <5.0 mEq/L, serum creatinine <2.5 mg/dL for men, or <2.0 mg/dL for women, or estimated glomerular filtration rate >30 mL/min/1.73 m^2), start aldosterone inhibition e.g., spironolactone 25 mg PO daily
3. Continue to monitor serial ST2 levels (as an outpatient), and increase spironolactone, β-blocker, and/or ACEI/ARB dose if levels do not continue to decline less than or equal to 35 ng/mL or by at least 25% (Algorithm 1).

ST2 MEASUREMENT IN THE INPATIENT SETTING: ACUTE DECOMPENSATED HEART FAILURE

Retrospective evidence suggests that ST2 measurements can be beneficial for the treatment and risk stratification of patients admitted for acute decompensated heart failure (ADHF). Elevated ST2 levels in patients presenting to the emergency department with ADHF have been associated with higher mortality at 30 days and 1 year. Serial measurements of ST2 during the hospital course

Algorithms in Heart Failure

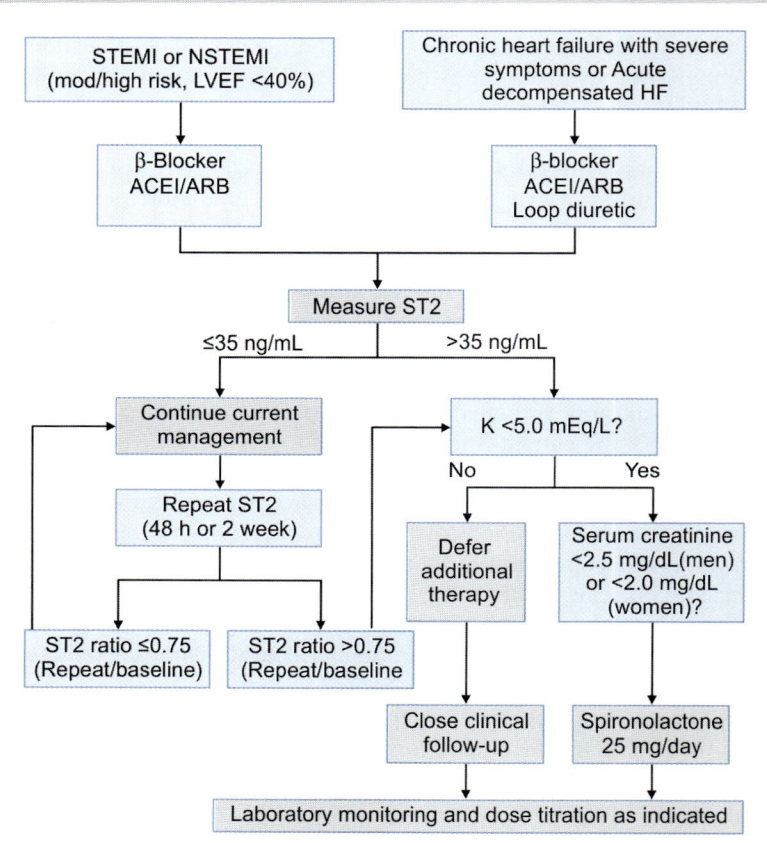

```
STEMI or NSTEMI              Chronic heart failure with severe
(mod/high risk, LVEF <40%)   symptoms or Acute
                             decompensated HF
         │                            │
         ▼                            ▼
    β-Blocker                    β-blocker
    ACEI/ARB                     ACEI/ARB
                                 Loop diuretic
         │                            │
         └─────────┬──────────────────┘
                   ▼
              Measure ST2
         ≤35 ng/mL │ >35 ng/mL
         ┌─────────┴─────────┐
         ▼                   ▼
   Continue current      K <5.0 mEq/L?
    management         No │        │ Yes
         │        ┌───────┘        └───────┐
         ▼        ▼                        ▼
    Repeat ST2   Defer            Serum creatinine
   (48 h or 2 week)  additional   <2.5 mg/dL (men)
                 therapy          or <2.0 mg/dL
                                  (women)?
   ┌─────┴─────┐         │                │
   ▼           ▼         ▼                ▼
ST2 ratio ≤0.75  ST2 ratio >0.75  Close clinical   Spironolactone
(Repeat/baseline) (Repeat/baseline) follow-up       25 mg/day

       Laboratory monitoring and dose titration as indicated
```

STEMI, ST elevation myocardial infarction; NSTEMI, non-ST elevation myocardial infarction; HF, heart failure; LVEF, left ventricular ejection fraction; ACEI, angiotensin converting enzyme inhibitor; ARB, angiotensin receptor blocker.

ALGORITHM 1: Proposed sample algorithm for how to use ST2 in the setting of myocardial infarction or heart failure

can also be beneficial for risk stratification. One study showed that patients whose ST2 levels failed to decrease by more than 25% in the first 48 hours after admission had higher mortality at 1 year. Similarly, a study at the VA San Diego Healthcare System showed that patients whose ST levels did not decrease by at least 15% had a higher 90-day mortality. As a result of these studies, the 2013 clinical practice guideline update from the American College of Cardiology or American Heart Association (ACC or AHA) now gives ST2 measurement a Class IIb recommendation for ADHF (level of evidence A) and for chronic heart failure (level of evidence B) (Table 1).

TABLE 1: Retrospective evidence for ST2 measurement ST elevation myocardial infarction, non-ST elevation myocardial infarction, and heart failure

	Trial	Findings
NSTEMI STEMI	TIMI 14 and 23	• ST2 peaks 12 h post-MI • Higher ST2 levels are associated with greater risk of new HF or death at 30 days post-MI
	CLARITY-TIMI	• Higher ST2 levels are associated with greater risk of HF and cardiovascular death at 30 days post-MI
	Dhillon, 2013	• Higher predischarge ST2 level associated with higher 30-day mortality
	EPHESUS	• 90% of patients had STEMI, 10% had NSTEMI • Higher ST2 levels were associated with increased left ventricular ESV and EDV at 24 weeks • This remodeling was attenuated in those randomized to eplerenone
	MERLIN-TIMI 36	• ST2 levels >35 ng/mL are associated with increased risk of HF or cardiovascular death at both 30 days and 1 year post-MI
ADHF	Socrates, 2010 Januzzi, 2007 Rehman, 2008	• Higher ST2 levels are associated with increased mortality at 30 days and 1 year in ED patients presenting with dyspnea • ST2 levels were complementary to natriuretic peptides
	Breidthardt, 2013	• ST2 "early responders" (whose ST2 levels decreased by 25% or more after 48 h) had lower 1 year mortality
	Boisot, 2008	• ADHF patients whose ST2 levels did not drop by at least 15% before discharge had a higher rate of death at 90 days

Continued

Continued

	Trial	Findings
Chronic heart failure	Broch, 2012 Ky, 2011 Bayes-Genis, 2012	• Higher ST2 levels were associated with a worse prognosis in ambulatory patients with HF
	Daniels, 2010	• ST levels predicted increased mortality at 1 year in outpatients referred for echocardiogram for any reason
	HF-ACTION	• Elevated baseline ST2 levels were associated with death or hospitalization, cardiovascular death or heart failure hospitalization, and all-cause mortality in ambulatory HF patients with reduced LVEF
	Wu, 2013	• ST2 has a lower long-term intra-individual variation than the NP's, so an increase in ST2 level on serial measurement may be a more accurate measure of a patient's risk of adverse events compared to NP's
	Bayes-Genis, 2010	• High ST2 Ratio >0.75 (2 weeks/baseline) associated with higher risk of death, HF admission, or cardiac transplantation at 1 year
	Weinberg, 2003	• Change in ST2 level at 2 weeks associated with risk of mortality or need for cardiac transplant, independent of NP's

HF, heart failure ; MI, myocardial infarction; STEMI, ST elevation myocardial infarction; NSTEMI, non-ST elevation myocardial infarction; ESV, end-systolic volume; EDV, end-diastolic volume; ED, emergency department; ADHF, acute decompensated HF; LVEF, left ventricular ejection fraction; NP, natriuretic peptide.

We propose that patients admitted with ADHF should have an initial ST2 level drawn, and patients with levels over 35 ng/mL, should be more closely monitored, especially if they also have an elevated natriuretic peptide or troponin level. Patients who do not show rapid clinical improvement may have a second ST2 level drawn after 48 hours or prior to discharge. If ST2 levels fail to drop by at least 25% on repeat measurement, pay particular attention to optimizing proven HF medications (β-blockers, ACEI or ARB, and loop diuretics) with inclusion of aldosterone antagonists if the patient's potassium level and renal function permit (Algorithm 1).

ST2 MEASUREMENT IN THE OUTPATIENT SETTING: CHRONIC HEART FAILURE

As in patients with ADHF, higher ST2 levels are associated with worse prognosis in patients with chronic HF. Furthermore, in outpatients referred for echocardiogram for any reason, higher ST2 levels predicted higher risk of death at 1 year. A separate study of ambulatory HF patients with reduced left ventricular ejection fraction demonstrated that elevated baseline ST2 levels (>35 ng/dL) were associated with higher risk of death or hospitalization, higher risk of cardiovascular death or HF hospitalization, and increased all-cause mortality. The strongest evidence for use of ST2 in chronic heart failure also involves serial monitoring, as several studies have previously demonstrated with natriuretic peptides. ST2 has a much lower long-term intra-individual variability than the natriuretic peptides, so increases in ST2 over time may be a more meaningful measure of progression of HF. Monitoring the progression of ST2 levels after recent decompensation can also help guide treatment. One study demonstrated that outpatients with decompensated HF who had an "ST2 ratio" (the ratio of ST2 levels at 2 weeks to the level at baseline) of greater than 0.75 had a higher risk of death, HF admission, or cardiac transplantation at 1 year, and the ST2 ratio was more predictive of outcome than baseline ST2 level alone. Another study of patients with severe nonischemic chronic heart failure showed that change in ST2 levels at 2 weeks was a better predictor of mortality or need for cardiac transplant compared to baseline ST2 level, and the association was independent of natriuretic peptide levels.

It is suggested that ST2 levels be checked in patients with chronic symptomatic HF after optimization with proven neurohormonal blockade medications (β-blocker, ACEI or ARB, and loop diuretics). As with STEMI/NSTEMI and ADHF, if ST2 is elevated at more than

35 ng/mL, and if potassium levels and renal function are permissive, start spironolactone 25 mg/dL. Continue to monitor serial serum ST2 and consider increasing spironolactone, β-blocker, or ACEI/ARB dose if levels do not begin to fall. In patients whose initial ST2 levels are less than or equal to 35 ng/mL, continue current medical management and recheck ST2 in 2 weeks. If ST2 ratio (2 week/baseline) is less than 0.75, continue current management. However, if ST2 ratio is greater than 0.75, and potassium levels and renal function permit, consider starting spironolactone 25 mg daily or uptitrating the β-blocker or ACEI/ARB (Algorithm 1).

CONCLUSION

The body of evidence supports the use of ST2 as a biomarker for prognosis in both the inpatient and outpatient settings. ST2 levels should optimally be measured early in STEMI and high risk NSTEMI patients to help guide therapy. ST2 levels may also be checked early after admission in ADHF as well as prior to discharge, and again about 2 weeks postdischarge. Patients whose ST2 level remains elevated may benefit from addition of aldosterone antagonists to their standard medical therapy, or from uptitration of their other neurohormonal blockade medications, and they would also likely benefit from closer clinical follow-up. Prospective studies testing these proposed algorithms for actionable uses of ST2 in acute MI and/or HF would be of great interest.

KEY POINTS

- ST2 is the receptor for interleukin-33 (IL-33), an anti-inflammatory cytokine that prevents cardiac remodeling and fibrosis
- ST2 is secreted as its soluble alternative splice variant during myocardial stress, and this soluble isoform acts as a decoy receptor for IL-33, thus exacerbating remodeling and fibrosis
- Elevated ST2 levels post-myocardial infarction (post-MI) are associated with higher risk of developing new heart failure and death
- Elevated ST2 levels are associated with development of adverse left ventricular remodeling, and elevated ST2 levels post-MI or in acute decompensated heart failure may help guide the initiation of aldosterone antagonist therapy
- Serial ST2 levels can be used to risk stratify patients with ST elevation myocardial infarction (STEMI) or non-STEMI (NSTEMI) or acute decompensated heart failure.

SUGGESTED READINGS

1. Bayes-Genis A, de Antonio M, Galan A, Sanz H, Urrutia A, Cabanes R, et al. Combined use of high-sensitivity ST2 and NTproBNP to improve the prediction of death in heart failure. Eur J Heart Fail. 2012;14:32-8.
2. Bayes-Genis A, Pascual-Figal D, Januzzi JL, Maisel A, Casas T, Valdes Chavarri M, et al. Soluble ST2 monitoring provides additional risk stratification for outpatients with decompensated heart failure. Rev Esp Cardiol. 2010;63:1171-8.
3. Berger R, Moertl D, Peter S, Ahmadi R, Huelsmann M, Yamuti S, et al. N-terminal pro-B-type natriuretic peptide-guided, intensive patient management in addition to multidisciplinary care in chronic heart failure a 3-arm, prospective, randomized pilot study. J Am Coll Cardiol. 2010;55:645-53.
4. Boisot S, Beede J, Isakson S, Chiu A, Clopton P, Januzzi J, et al. Serial sampling of ST2 predicts 90-day mortality following destabilized heart failure. J Card Fail. 2008;14:732-8.
5. Breidthardt T, Balmelli C, Twerenbold R, Mosimann T, Espinola J, Haaf P, et al. Heart failure therapy-induced early ST2 changes may offer long-term therapy guidance. J Card Fail. 2013;19:821-8.
6. Broch K, Ueland T, Nymo SH, Kjekshus J, Hulthe J, Muntendam P, et al. Soluble ST2 is associated with adverse outcome in patients with heart failure of ischaemic aetiology. Eur J Heart Fail. 2012;14:268-77.
7. Daniels LB, Clopton P, Iqbal N, Tran K, Maisel AS. Association of ST2 levels with cardiac structure and function and mortality in outpatients. Am Heart J. 2010;160:721-8.
8. Dhillon OS, Narayan HK, Khan SQ, Kelly D, Quinn PA, Squire IB, et al. Pre-discharge risk stratification in unselected STEMI: is there a role for ST2 or its natural ligand IL-33 when compared with contemporary risk markers? Int J Cardiol. 2013;167:2182-8.
9. Felker GM, Fiuzat M, Thompson V, Shaw LK, Neely ML, Adams KF, et al. Soluble ST2 in ambulatory patients with heart failure: Association with functional capacity and long-term outcomes. Circ Heart Fail. 2013;6:1172-9.
10. Januzzi JL Jr, Rehman SU, Mohammed AA, Bhardwaj A, Barajas L, Barajas J, et al. Use of amino-terminal pro-B-type natriuretic peptide to guide outpatient therapy of patients with chronic left ventricular systolic dysfunction. J Am Coll Cardiol. 2011;58:1881-9.
11. Januzzi JL Jr., Peacock WF, Maisel AS, Chae CU, Jesse RL, Baggish AL, et al. Measurement of the interleukin family member ST2 in patients with acute dyspnea: results from the PRIDE (Pro-Brain Natriuretic Peptide Investigation of Dyspnea in the Emergency Department) study. J Am Coll Cardiol. 2007;50:607-13.
12. Jourdain P, Jondeau G, Funck F, Gueffet P, Le Helloco A, Donal E, Aupetit JF, Aumont MC, Galinier M, Eicher JC, Cohen-Solal A and Juilliere Y. Plasma brain natriuretic peptide-guided therapy to improve outcome in heart failure: the STARS-BNP Multicenter Study. J Am Coll Cardiol. 2007;49:1733-9.
13. Kieser A, Goodnight J, Kolch W, Mischak H, Mushinski JF. Identification of the primary growth response gene, ST2/T1, as a gene whose expression is differentially regulated by different protein kinase C isozymes. FEBS Lett. 1995;372:189-93.
14. Kohli P, Bonaca MP, Kakkar R, Kudinova AY, Scirica BM, Sabatine MS, et al. Role of ST2 in non-ST-elevation acute coronary syndrome in the MERLIN-TIMI 36 trial. Clin Chem. 2012;58:257-66.
15. Ky B, French B, McCloskey K, Rame JE, McIntosh E, Shahi P, et al. High-sensitivity ST2 for prediction of adverse outcomes in chronic heart failure. Circ Heart Fail. 2011;4:180-7.
16. Pascual-Figal DA, Manzano-Fernandez S, Boronat M, Casas T, Garrido IP, Bonaque JC, et al. Soluble ST2, high-sensitivity troponin T- and N-terminal pro-B-type natriuretic peptide: complementary role for risk stratification in acutely decompensated heart failure. Eur J Heart Fail. 2011;13:718-25.

17. Rehman SU, Mueller T, Januzzi JL Jr. Characteristics of the novel interleukin family biomarker ST2 in patients with acute heart failure. J Am Coll Cardiol. 2008;52:1458-65.
18. Sabatine MS, Morrow DA, Higgins LJ, MacGillivray C, Guo W, Bode C, et al. Complementary roles for biomarkers of biomechanical strain ST2 and N-terminal prohormone B-type natriuretic peptide in patients with ST-elevation myocardial infarction. Circulation. 2008;117:1936-44.
19. Sanada S, Hakuno D, Higgins LJ, Schreiter ER, McKenzie AN, Lee RT. IL-33 and ST2 comprise a critical biomechanically induced and cardioprotective signaling system. J Clin Invest. 2007;117:1538-49.
20. Schmitz J, Owyang A, Oldham E, Song Y, Murphy E, McClanahan TK, et al. IL-33, an interleukin-1-like cytokine that signals via the IL-1 receptor-related protein ST2 and induces T helper type 2-associated cytokines. Immunity. 2005;23:479-90.
21. Shimpo M, Morrow DA, Weinberg EO, Sabatine MS, Murphy SA, Antman EM, et al. Serum levels of the interleukin-1 receptor family member ST2 predict mortality and clinical outcome in acute myocardial infarction. Circulation. 2004;109:2186-90.
22. Socrates T, deFilippi C, Reichlin T, Twerenbold R, Breidhardt T, Noveanu M, et al. Interleukin family member ST2 and mortality in acute dyspnoea. J Intern Med. 2010;268:493-500.
23. Tominaga S. A putative protein of a growth specific cDNA from BALB/c-3T3 cells is highly similar to the extracellular portion of mouse interleukin 1 receptor. FEBS Lett. 1989;258:301-4.
24. Troughton RW, Frampton CM, Yandle TG, Espiner EA, Nicholls MG, Richards AM. Treatment of heart failure guided by plasma aminoterminal brain natriuretic peptide (N-BNP) concentrations. Lancet. 2000;355:1126-30.
25. Weinberg EO, Shimpo M, Hurwitz S, Tominaga S, Rouleau JL, Lee RT. Identification of serum soluble ST2 receptor as a novel heart failure biomarker. Circulation. 2003;107:721-6.
26. Weir RA, Miller AM, Murphy GE, Clements S, Steedman T, Connell JM, et al. Serum soluble ST2: a potential novel mediator in left ventricular and infarct remodeling after acute myocardial infarction. J Am Coll Cardiol. 2010;55:243-50.
27. Wu AH, Wians F, Jaffe A. Biological variation of galectin-3 and soluble ST2 for chronic heart failure: implication on interpretation of test results. Am Heart J. 2013;165:995-9.
28. Yanagisawa K, Tsukamoto T, Takagi T, Tominaga S. Murine ST2 gene is a member of the primary response gene family induced by growth factors. FEBS Lett. 1992;302:51-3.
29. Yancy CW, Jessup M, Bozkurt B, Butler J, Casey DE Jr., Drazner MH, et al. 2013 ACCF/AHA guideline for the management of heart failure: a report of the American College of Cardiology Foundation/American Heart Association Task Force on Practice Guidelines. J Am Coll Cardiol. 2013;62:e147-239.

CHAPTER 22

Use of Cardiac Troponin to Assist in the Management of Patients with Congestive Heart Failure: A Practical Guide

Affan B Irfan, Wayne Miller, Allan S Jaffe

INTRODUCTION

The cardiac troponins (cTn) regulatory complex is comprised of three proteins; calcium binding (cTnC), tropomyosin-binding (cTnT), and inhibitory (cTnI) which regulate the calcium-mediated contractile interactions of actin and myosin. The cardiac isoforms of cTnT and cTnI are encoded by unique genes and thus are highly cardiac specific. The bulk of cTn protein is predominantly found structurally bound to other proteins intracellularly, with a small percentage more loosely bound (6–8% for cTnT and 3.5% for cTnI). There is controversy about whether cTn release requires death of cardiomyocytes from apoptosis, necrosis and/or autophagia. However, regardless of the mechanisms, ongoing cardiac injury appears to be a critical pathophysiological component in the progression of heart failure (HF). From a clinical perspective, it is impossible to distinguish one mechanism from another, and it is unclear if they have any differential impact on prognosis. Cardiac injury may be more overtly apparent in acute settings and more subtle, but just as important, in chronic HF where progressive loss of cardiomyocytes over time results in the progression of HF.

PRINCIPLES FOR USING CARDIAC TROPONIN

In order to achieve the clinical performance clinicians want, one must appreciate how to optimally utilize cTn determinations (Algorithm 1). Some quick rules for use include:

Algorithms in Heart Failure

```
┌─────────────────────────────────────────────────────────┐
│ Be cognizant of the specific cardiac troponin assay     │
│ being used (99th percentile — gender specific,          │
│ sensitivity, coefficient variation)                     │
└─────────────────────────────────────────────────────────┘
                          ↓
┌─────────────────────────────────────────────────────────┐
│ Understand when to expect both normal and abnormal      │
│ troponin levels and identify changing patterns among    │
│ the target population                                   │
└─────────────────────────────────────────────────────────┘
                          ↓
┌─────────────────────────────────────────────────────────┐
│ Measure and interpret baseline and serial troponin      │
│ levels in the clinical setting                          │
└─────────────────────────────────────────────────────────┘
```

ALGORITHM 1: Clinical use of troponin testing

- The appropriate cutoff value for an abnormal cTn value is the 99th percent of an upper reference limit (URL). In many institutions, this is not what is reported as an abnormal value, however, checking with your lab concerning this value is a key
- Almost all high sensitivity assays will require the use of gender specific cutoff values
- Having good precision at low levels allows for changing values to be more easily identifiable. However, modest imprecision (between 10 and 20%) which is less than ideal does not cause false positive assessments and, as such, assays with less than ideal precision are usable
- It is important to have some sense of the relative sensitivity of the assay used in any given institution. Many assays developed years ago are still being used and there are many new very sensitive assays
- False positive and false negative results are uncommon but can occur. One should ask the laboratory to repeat values that do not fit with the clinical presentation of the patient
- An understanding of the range of values normally expected with any given clinical situation will help clinicians determine if consideration of other processes as well as the primary one can be helpful. For example, with chronic heart failure, the cTn elevations that occur tend to be modest
- The criteria for a changing pattern of values are unique to each assay and to the timing of the evaluations. At present, we endorse the use of the guidelines recommended by the European Society of Cardiology (ESC).

POSSIBLE MECHANISMS FOR ELEVATED CARDIAC TROPONIN

Cardiac troponin is released from cardiomyocyte apoptosis, necrosis, and/or autophagia; i.e., all processes that lead to

Nonischemic

- Inflammatory cytokines
  - TNF-α
  - Interleukins
- Oxidative stress
- Neurohomonal activation
  - Renin
  - Angiotensin II
  - Norepinephrine
  - Vasopressin
  - Endothelin

Ischemic

- Epicardial CAD or endothelial dysfunction
- Chronic hypoxia
- Subendocardial ischemia
  - Increased wall stress, left ventricular hypertrophy and dilatation
  - Other supply-demand mismatch (e.g., anemia, hypotension)

```
         Reversible injury
        /      |      \
Apoptosis → Proteolysis ← Necrosis
              ↑
Aging and → Cardiac troponin and degradation
renal dysfunction    products release
```

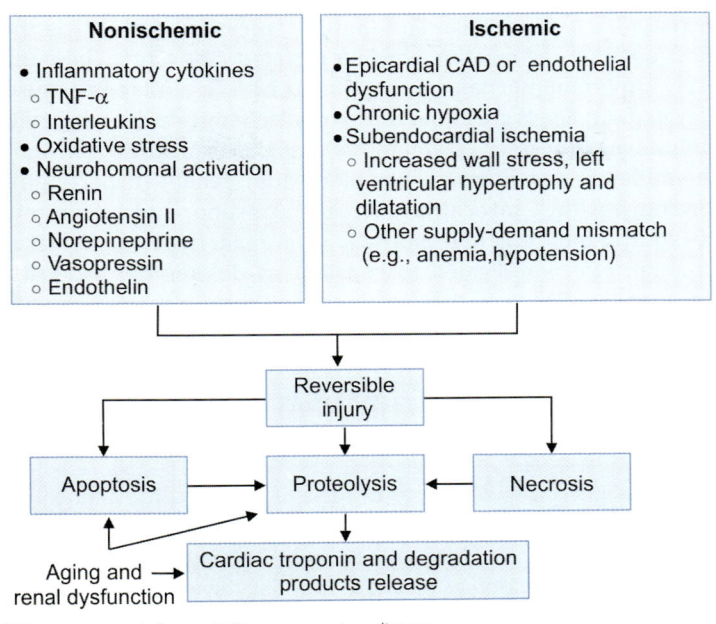

TNF, tumor necrosis factor; CAD, coronary artery disease.

ALGORITHM 2: Release of cardiac troponin from reversible injury, necrotic and apoptotic myocardial cell death through ischemic and nonischemic etiologies in heart failure

myocyte death. A wide variety of causes can lead to cTn release through several different putative mechanisms in chronic and decompensated heart failure (HF) (Algorithm 2). Acute ischemic heart disease is a common cause of both acute and chronic heart failure. Data from the EuroHeart Failure Survey suggest that acute ischemic heart disease may be present in up to 20% of patients with acute heart failure (AHF). Type I myocardial infarction (MI) is spontaneous infarction that appears to occur due to acute plaque rupture or erosion. Type II MI encompasses other forms of ischemic cardiac injury such as those due to hemodynamic compromise, for example due to tachycardia, hypotension or hypertension in patients with fixed coronary artery disease, events related predominantly to coronary endothelial dysfunction, and/or vasospasm. In most studies, cTn elevations are similar between patients with ischemic and nonischemic etiologies of HF emphasizing the importance of other mechanisms in the HF circumstance. Acute preload induced stretch leads to the release of cTn from apoptotic cells and an increased left ventricular end-diastolic pressure (LVEDP) is the most common association with an elevated cTn value. These are likely important mechanisms in patients with HF and renal failure. Elevated cTn levels are found due to nonischemic cardiomyopathy; infiltrative processes (sarcoidosis), toxic exposures (alcohol, chemotherapeutic drugs, carbon monoxide), genetic (hypertrophic cardiomyopathy), myocarditis, stress (takotsubo) and peripartum cardiomyopathy, and in response to ventricular hypertrophy. Thus, although one is obligated to consider as differential diagnoses, elevations of cTn, even those with a rising pattern in patients with HF, do not in and of themselves mandate a diagnosis of acute MI.

BACKGROUND FOR THE INPATIENT USE OF CARDIAC TROPONIN

There has been a wide range (6–80%) of reported prevalences of elevated cTn levels in the hospital setting. With high sensitivity cardiac troponin (hs-cTn) assays, up to 90% of patients hospitalized for HF without evidence of acute coronary syndrome are likely to have hs-cTn elevations. These differences in prevalence are dependent on the selection of study patients [i.e., etiology of HF, New York Heart Association class, ejection fraction, etc.] and also on the sensitivity of the immunoassays and the cutoff values used to define elevations. Patients with elevated cTn values have an adverse prognosis.

The largest data in acute decompensated HF emanated from the Acute Decompensated Heart Failure National Registry (ADHERE) study. Cardiac troponins I and T were measured and considered elevated in 3,253 patients (5.3%) and 1,035 patients (13.1%), respectively. The adjusted odds ratio for death in patients with an elevated cTn was 2.55 (95% confidence interval, 2.24–2.89) (Fig. 1). Another report from the ADHERE investigators showed that elevations of cTn I or T and brain natriuretic peptide were positively synergistic with mortality risk. These analyses included a variety of assays and cutoff values and likely underestimate the extent of the prognostic importance of cTn values.

Serial measurements of cTn during hospitalization further assist in evaluating the severity of myocardial injury, the impact of therapy, and provide additional prognostic information in these patients. It has been suggested that targeting cTn levels would help in optimization of therapy and better salvage the myocardium at risk, but the data supporting such an approach is lacking at present.

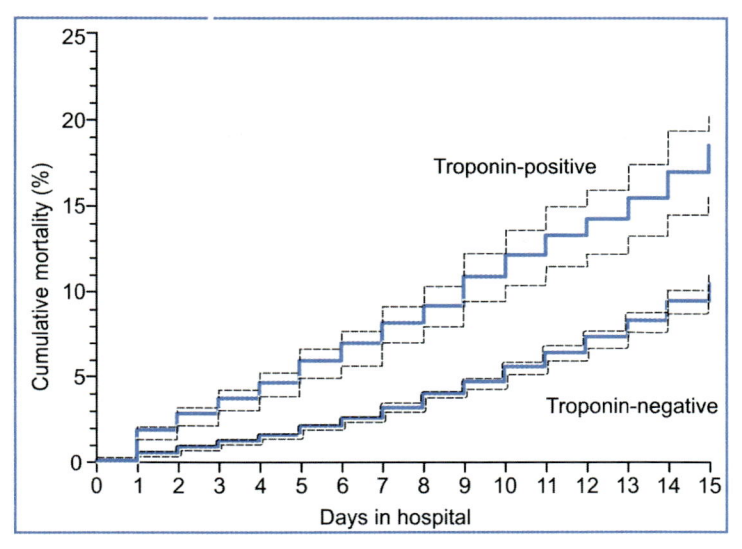

FIG. 1: Mortality according to number of days in the hospital and troponin status at presentation. By the log-rank test, p <0.001. Dashed lines show 95% confidence intervals

RECOMMENDATIONS FOR THE USE OF CARDIAC TROPONIN IN HOSPITALIZED PATIENTS

- Serial measurements of cTn are necessary whenever there is suspicion of acute ischemic heart disease
- The diagnosis of an acute ischemic event should not be made solely on the basis of cTn. Cardiac troponin values must be interpreted in proper clinical context
- A nonischemic etiology such as an increased LVEDP should be considered as a possible cause for elevated cTn values (Algorithm 3)
- It is reasonable to serially measure cTn in all patients admitted with AHF. A rising pattern and persistently elevated values are an adverse prognostic finding. However, the optimal change criteria to use or what exactly should be done to remediate this adverse prognosis has yet to be defined
- Like natriuretic peptides, hs-cTn measurements should be considered as continuous variables across a spectrum of risk and not simply detectable or undetectable
- Patients with adverse prognosis, including those identified with elevated cTn, should be considered for changes in acute therapy and outpatient surveillance (Algorithm 4).

Algorithms in Heart Failure

Vitals	Hypo-/hypertension, hypoxia, tachy-/bradyarrhythmias
Volume status	Hypervolemia (from heart failure or renal dysfunction)
Underlying causes	Sepsis, anemia, PE, stroke, aortic dissection, ARDS
Other primary causes	Cardiomyopathy (stress, drugs, perimyocarditis, trauma, etc.)

Note: There may be more than one cardiomyocyte injury process occurring at the same time.
PE, pulmonary embolism; ARDS, acute respiratory distress syndrome.

ALGORITHM 3: Common nonacute coronary syndrome etiologies and workup for troponin release in acute heart failure patients

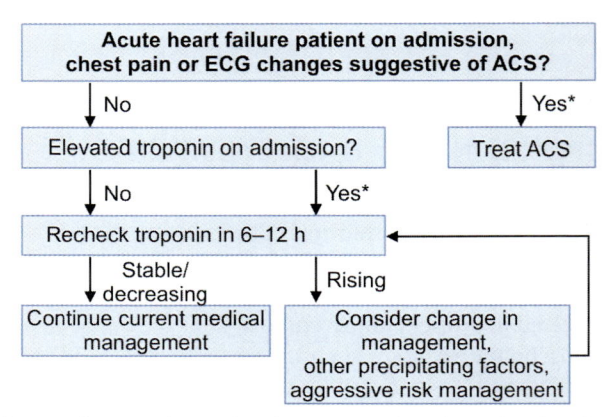

Acute heart failure patient on admission, chest pain or ECG changes suggestive of ACS?
- Yes* → Treat ACS
- No → Elevated troponin on admission?
  - Yes* → Recheck troponin in 6–12 h
  - No → Recheck troponin in 6–12 h
    - Stable/decreasing → Continue current medical management
    - Rising → Consider change in management, other precipitating factors, aggressive risk management → (recheck loop)

*Consider nonischemic etiologies of cardiac troponin release (as in algorithm 3) and treat accordingly.
ECG, electrocardiogram; ACS, acute coronary syndrome.

ALGORITHM 4: Clinical use of troponin testing in acute heart failure patients

Background for the Outpatient use of Cardiac Troponin

Elevated cTn levels also have been found in stable HF patients and seem to carry a significant independent short-term and long-term

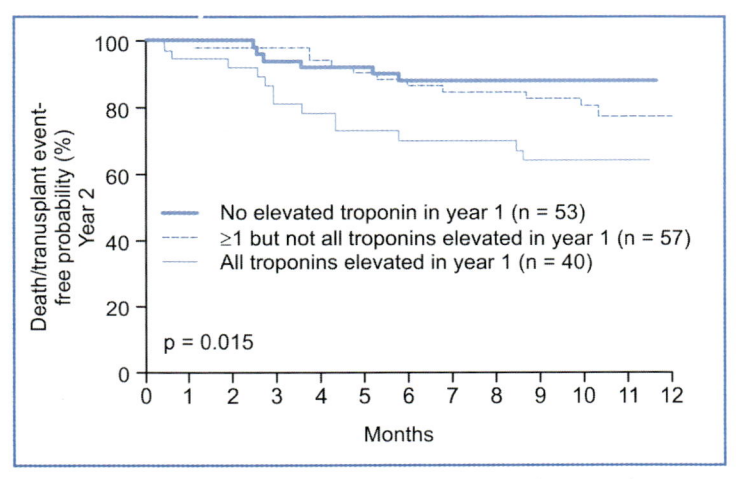

FIG. 2: Kaplan-Meier analysis of the risk of death or cardiac transplantation in year 2 based on cardiac troponin T patterns from year 2 of clinical follow-up

high mortality risk. With high sensitive assays, the prevalence of elevated cTn values that are detectable has been reported to be 50–90% compared to only 10–50% with standard assays. Similar to patients with acute decompensated HF, higher concentrations of hs-cTn within the normal range (below the 99th percent URL) carry prognostic value in stable patients. Even deciles of risk can be determined.

Serial cTn monitoring in stable patients allows early identification of patients at risk of disease progression and mortality. In a 200 patient cohort study, Miller and colleagues have shown that even modest changes in cTn but not natriuretic peptides are important predictors of prognosis. Also, persistent elevations of serial troponin in ambulatory HF patients were associated with increased risk of future events (Fig. 2). The data suggest that cTn might be a good way to monitor patients and or to use to direct therapy. Recently, analyses from two large randomized clinical trials of 5,284 patients with chronic heart failure have seemed to confirm the speculation that changes over time (3–4 months) in the circulating levels of hs-cTn T are associated with the severity and progression of HF and have a robust prognostic value (median follow-up time was >24 months). It is likely that hs-cTn assays will further facilitate this approach.

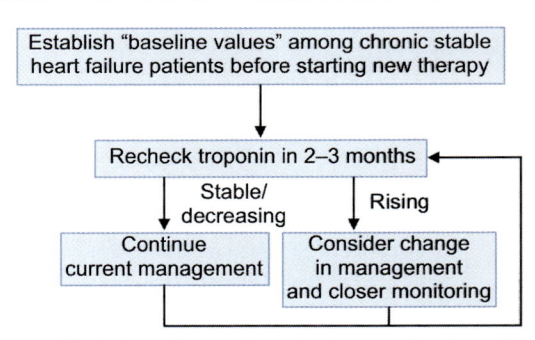

```
┌─────────────────────────────────────────────┐
│ Establish "baseline values" among chronic stable │
│ heart failure patients before starting new therapy │
└─────────────────────────────────────────────┘
                        │
                        ▼
        ┌─────────────────────────────┐◄─────┐
        │ Recheck troponin in 2–3 months │      │
        └─────────────────────────────┘      │
           Stable/              Rising        │
         decreasing                           │
           │                    │             │
           ▼                    ▼             │
    ┌──────────────┐    ┌──────────────────┐ │
    │   Continue   │    │  Consider change │ │
    │current management│ │  in management   │─┘
    └──────────────┘    │and closer monitoring│
                        └──────────────────┘
```

ALGORITHM 5: Clinical use of troponin testing in outpatient heart failure patients and those on cardiotoxic drug. This area of work looks promising and more studies are needed before criteria for baseline values, and change in pattern over length of time could be determined

Recommendations for the use of Cardiac Troponin in Outpatients

- Elevated cTn values with contemporary assays are associated with increased risk. Thus, such measurements are worth considering in chronic heart failure patients to help assess prognosis
- Specific therapeutic interventions in response to elevated cTn levels in these patients have not yet been defined
- Like, natriuretic peptides, identifying a "baseline value" for cTn could help to distinguish chronic elevations from acute cardiac injury
- It is reasonable but unproven to measure cTn before and after starting medical therapy for HF management (including device therapy) to guide therapy
- Routine cTn measurements should be obtained in patients on medications known to cause cardiotoxicity (e.g., chemotherapeutic drugs) to provide early identification of patients at risk and to guide therapeutic interventions (Algorithm 5).

SPECIAL SITUATIONS

Even in patients with HF with preserved left ventricular ejection fraction, elevations in cTn are prevalent and strongly associated with abnormal left ventricular relaxation, increased left ventricular mass and poor long-term and short-term outcomes.

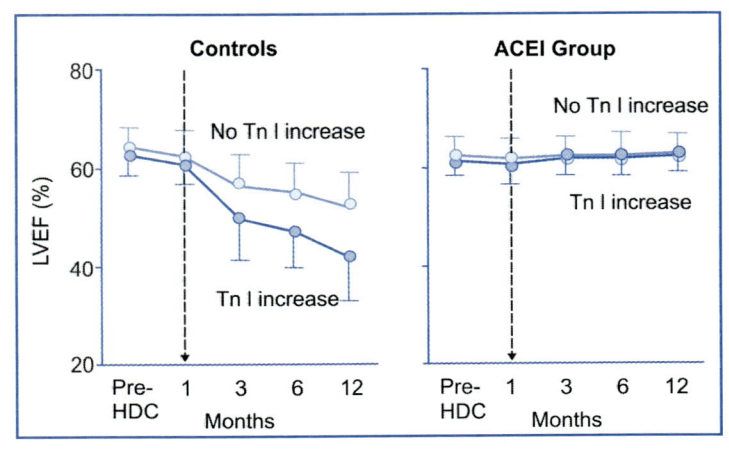

FIG. 3: Patients without elevations of cardiac troponin I did not manifest a marked reductions in ejection fractions over time. Those with elevations in the control group did however. This decrease was ablated with the use of an angiotensin converting enzyme inhibitor

Tn I, troponin I; ACEI, angiotensin converting enzyme inhibitor; LVEF, left ventricular ejection fraction; HDC, high dose chemotherapy.

Cardiac troponin has been used in experimental and clinical studies to evaluate cardiac and noncardiac medications (e.g., chemotherapeutic agents) which are suspected to cause cardiotoxicity and HF. Among patients on such treatment, angiotensin converting enzyme inhibitors have been found not only to reduce cTn values but also the propensity to the development of HF (Fig. 3).

Aarones et al. has shown the ability of hs-cTn T to predict the response to cardiac resynchronization therapy with the lowering of values being associated with a better response. Despite such convincing data with serial monitoring of cTn, we are still far from using serial cTns in daily practice for this purpose.

Studies in community populations and amongst subgroups of patients (e.g., those with chronic kidney disease) have shown strong independent associations between values of hs-cTn T and HF prevalence. Furthermore, several studies have observed that in selected patients (e.g., the elderly) elevated hs-cTn T levels at baseline are independent predictors of HF. Recent data indicate that the exercise may lower hs-cTn T values.

Because there are different 99% values for men and women with hs-cTn assays and different pathophysiologies with more heart failure with a preserved ejection fraction in women, it is likely that women will require different cutoff values. To date, no studies specifically studying this issue in patients with HF have been reported but the data in other areas is robust.

CONCLUSION

Using cTn in patients with HF is extremely attractive based on the available clinical information at present. Additional studies are necessary to refine this ability and to develop more evidence based diagnosis and treatment algorithms necessary to make this a reality.

KEY POINTS

- Besides acute ischemia (such as in type I and type II myocardial infarction), there are multiple other mechanisms both, acute and chronic, leading to myocardial injury and cardiac troponin (cTn) release in heart failure (HF) patients. Thus, clinical judgment is essential in evaluating these elevations. Literature shows a wide range of "troponin elevations" among inpatient and outpatient HF patients due to the differences in selection of study patients, the different sensitivities of the immunoassays and cutoff values used to define elevations
- "Normal" expected values can now be determined with the advent of "high sensitive" troponin assays, making them attractive for use, once approved in the United States among inpatients and outpatients with HF
- Elevated cTn values are robust short-term and long-term mortality risk and other adverse outcome prognosticator among acute and chronic heart failure patients.
- Serial measurements of cTn among inpatient and outpatient patients may have a role in screening and predicting therapy outcome. However, future studies are needed to make it a reality
- Cardiac troponin provides information additional and synergistic to natriuretic peptides.

SUGGESTED READINGS

1. Aarones M, Gullestad L, Aakhus S, Ueland T, Skaardal R, Aass H, et al. Prognostic value of cardiac troponin T in patients with moderate to severe heart failure scheduled for cardiac resynchronization therapy. Am Heart J. 2011;161(6):1031-7.
2. Cardinale D, Colombo A, Sandri MT, Lamantia G, Colombo N, Civelli M, et al. Prevention of high-dose chemotherapy-induced cardiotoxicity in high-risk patients by angiotensin-converting enzyme inhibition. Circulation. 2006;114(23):2474-81.

3. deFilippi CR, de Lemos JA, Christenson RH, Gottdiener JS, Kop WJ, Zhan M, et al. Association of serial measures of cardiac troponin T using a sensitive assay with incident heart failure and cardiovascular mortality in older adults. JAMA. 2010;304(22):2494-502.
4. Fonarow GC, Peacock WF, Horwich TB, Phillips CO, Givertz MM, Lopatin M, et al. Usefulness of B-type natriuretic peptide and cardiac troponin levels to predict in-hospital mortality from ADHERE. Am J Cardiol. 2008;101(2):231-7.
5. Gheorghiade M, Gattis Stough W, Adams KF Jr., Jaffe AS, Hasselblad V, O'Connor CM. The Pilot Randomized Study of Nesiritide Versus Dobutamine in Heart Failure (PRESERVD-HF). Am J Cardiol. 2005;96(6A): 18G-25G.
6. Jaffe AS, Apple FS. High-sensitivity cardiac troponin assays: Isn't it time for equality? Clin Chem. 2014;60:7-9.
7. Januzzi JL Jr, Filippatos G, Nieminen M, Gheorghiade M. Troponin elevation in patients with heart failure: on behalf of the third Universal Definition of Myocardial Infarction Global Task Force: Heart Failure Section. Eur Heart J. 2012;33(18):2265-71.
8. Latini R, Masson S, Anand IS, Missov E, Carlson M, Vago T, et al. Prognostic value of very low plasma concentrations of troponin T in patients with stable chronic heart failure. Circulation. 2007;116(11):1242-9.
9. Masson S, Anand I, Favero C, Barlera S, Vago T, Bertocchi F, et al. Serial measurement of cardiac troponin T using a highly sensitive assay in patients with chronic heart failure: data from 2 large randomized clinical trials. Circulation. 2012;125(2):280-8.
10. Miller WL, Hartman KA, Burritt MF, Grill DE, Jaffe AS: Profiles of serial changes in cardiac troponin T concentrations and outcome in ambulatory patients with chronic heart failure. J Am Coll Cardiol. 2009;54(18):1715-21.
11. Peacock WF 4th, De Marco T, Fonarow GC, Diercks D, Wynne J, Apple FS, et al. Cardiac troponin and outcome in acute heart failure. N Engl J Med. 2008;358(20):2117-26.
12. Perna ER, Aspromonte N, Cimbaro Canella JP, Di Tano G, Macin SM, Feola M, et al. Minor myocardial damage is a prevalent condition in patients with acute heart failure syndromes and preserved systolic function with long-term prognostic implications: a report from the CIAST-HF (Collaborative Italo-Argentinean Study on cardiac Troponin T in Heart Failure) study. J Card Fail. 2012;18(11):822-30.
13. Thygesen K, Mair J, Katus H, Plebani M, Venge P, Collinson P, et al. Recommendations for the use of cardiac troponin measurement in acute cardiac care. Eur Heart J. 2010;31(18):2197-204.
14. Xue Y, Clopton P, Peacock WF, Maisel AS. Serial changes in high-sensitive troponin I predict outcome in patients with decompensated heart failure. Eur J Heart Fail. 2011;13(1):37-42.

SECTION 4

Special Issues in Heart Failure

23
CHAPTER

Heart Failure in the Nursing Home Setting

Corrine Y Jurgens

INTRODUCTION

Nursing home residents diagnosed with heart failure (HF) pose several unique challenges for healthcare providers. Accurate diagnosis in the context of comorbid illness, cognitive dysfunction, and an atypical HF symptom profile contribute to the complexity of identifying HF in this older population. Comorbidity complicates accurate attribution of symptoms to HF or less threatening illnesses because of overlapping symptom profiles. Other management challenges in the nursing home setting include lack of routine monitoring of HF status and reliance on direct care personnel to report changes in condition to licensed providers. A diagnosis of HF requires vigilant monitoring and management similar to other chronic illnesses (e.g., diabetes, hypertension). The purpose of this chapter is to provide step-by-step guidance on initiating a HF management protocol in the nursing home setting.

STEP-BY-STEP GUIDANCE ON INITIATING A HEART FAILURE MANAGEMENT PROTOCOL IN THE NURSING HOME

Step 1: Identification of Nursing Home Residents with Heart Failure and Devices

Identification of residents diagnosed with HF (e.g., armband, medical record alerts) is important so all staff know which residents have HF. Identification helps to ensure implementation of vigilant

Algorithms in Heart Failure

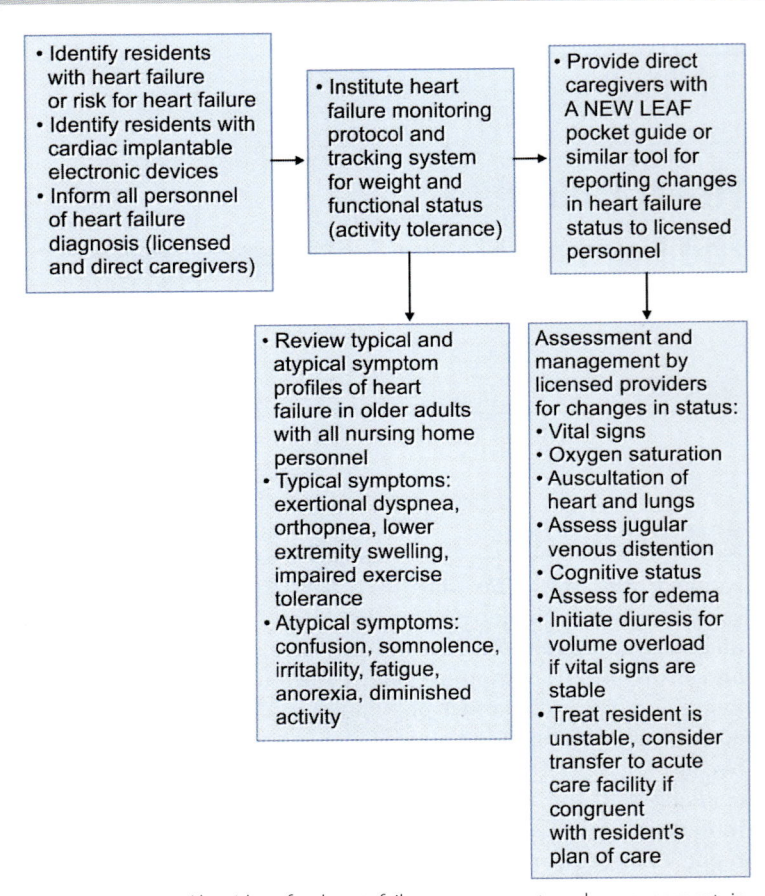

Box 1:
- Identify residents with heart failure or risk for heart failure
- Identify residents with cardiac implantable electronic devices
- Inform all personnel of heart failure diagnosis (licensed and direct caregivers)

Box 2:
- Institute heart failure monitoring protocol and tracking system for weight and functional status (activity tolerance)

Box 3:
- Provide direct caregivers with A NEW LEAF pocket guide or similar tool for reporting changes in heart failure status to licensed personnel

Box 4:
- Review typical and atypical symptom profiles of heart failure in older adults with all nursing home personnel
- Typical symptoms: exertional dyspnea, orthopnea, lower extremity swelling, impaired exercise tolerance
- Atypical symptoms: confusion, somnolence, irritability, fatigue, anorexia, diminished activity

Box 5:
Assessment and management by licensed providers for changes in status:
- Vital signs
- Oxygen saturation
- Auscultation of heart and lungs
- Assess jugular venous distention
- Cognitive status
- Assess for edema
- Initiate diuresis for volume overload if vital signs are stable
- Treat resident is unstable, consider transfer to acute care facility if congruent with resident's plan of care

ALGORITHM 1: Algorithm for heart failure assessment and management in nursing homes

monitoring and treatment of acute decompensation as appropriate (Algorithm 1). Residents with devices such as implantable cardioverter-defibrillators (ICDs) and pacemakers also should be clearly identified in the event when device deactivation is necessary. The cardiologist managing the device and schedule of follow-up care should be documented in the medical record.

Step 2: Monitoring Nursing Home Residents with Heart Failure

Frequency of monitoring varies based on the clinical status of the resident (Box 1). Residents with stable HF can be monitored weekly.

Heart Failure in the Nursing Home Setting

Those with recent hospitalizations and other risk factors should be assessed daily. Pocket cards, posters, and notations in the medical record serve as reminders as to who requires daily versus weekly monitoring. The pocket card with the acronym "A NEW LEAF" can be used as a screening-tool designed for direct caregivers for detection of changes in HF status (Box 2).

Factors reported to increase risk for hospitalization within 6 months among patients with HF with reduced ejection fraction include age above 70 years, history of diabetes, stroke, arrhythmia, abnormal serum sodium, blood urea nitrogen greater than 43 mg/dL, and absence of β-blocker therapy. Although increasing weight and symptoms of HF occur relatively late in the trajectory of acute decompensation, documentation of daily weights and tracking of signs and symptoms using a HF assessment protocol is essential. In addition, adherence to HF guidelines with respect to medications supports symptom management and avoidance of hospitalization. A low sodium diet or fluid restriction may be required for some residents.

Box 1: Frequency of monitoring

High risk: monitor daily
- Hospitalized in last 6 months for heart failure
- Primary diagnosis of heart failure
- Active secondary diagnosis of heart failure
- NYHA class III or IV
- Hypertensive BP >150/90 mmHg

Low risk: monitor weekly
- More than 6 months since last heart failure hospitalization
- NYHA class I or II

NYHA, New York Heart Association; BP, blood pressure.

Box 2: "A NEW LEAF": a heart failure screening tool for direct caregivers[3]

- **A**: Acute agitation or anxiety
- **N**: Nighttime shortness of breath or increase in nighttime urination
- **E**: Edema in lower extremities
- **W**: Weight gain (2–4 pounds per week)
- **L**: Lightheadedness
- **E**: Extreme shortness of breath lying down
- **A**: Abdominal symptoms (nausea, pain, decreased appetite, distention)
- **F**: Fatigue

Direct caregivers will come to know and recognize subtle differences in residents under their care. It is critically important to appreciate and act on their reports of residents' changes in behavior, cognition or functional status. Examination of HF status over time, comparing functional status and symptoms with activity from day-to-day, and reporting these changes to licensed nursing home personnel and medical staff is essential for averting hospitalization.

Monitoring Signs and Symptoms of Heart Failure

Detecting a change in HF status is particularly difficult. Signs and symptoms of HF are outlined in box 3. Early symptoms of impending decompensation of HF such as fatigue or activity intolerance are nonspecific and easily missed. Cognitive dysfunction, common among nursing home residents, limits patients' ability to report symptoms. Importantly, symptoms of HF may be atypical based on sedentary lifestyles and compensatory changes in the pulmonary vasculature in older adults (Box 4). As a result, hallmark symptoms of HF such as dyspnea on exertion, orthopnea, and nocturnal dyspnea may not be evident. Furthermore, absence of symptoms at rest does not necessarily indicate clinical stability. Behavioral changes may be of more value in detecting a change in status in this population. Acute changes in mental status should prompt an evaluation of cardiac status in residents with a history or risk factors for HF.

A standard weight protocol to avert errors in daily weights is important for tracking HF status. For example, variations in blankets, shoes, use of different scales, and wheelchairs can result in errors in accuracy of weight.

Box 3: Signs and symptoms of heart failure

- Dyspnea on exertion
- Fatigue
- Orthopnea
- Lower extremity swelling
- Impaired exercise tolerance
- Weight gain
- Jugular venous distention
- Increasing abdominal girth

> **Box 4: Atypical signs and symptoms of heart failure in older adults**
> - Confusion
> - Somnolence
> - Irritability
> - Fatigue
> - Loss of appetite
> - Lower body mass index
> - Nocturnal dyspnea

Step 3: Nonpharmacological Management

Balancing dietary preferences in the context of quality of life and HF management is often an issue in nursing homes. Lowering the sodium content in food is difficult. Not all facilities offer low sodium diets, family members bring in high sodium content food, and residents potentially decrease their food intake with a lower sodium diet. Furthermore, resident weight loss can be a confounding condition for patients with HF. Although weight loss related to treatment of volume overload is appropriate for patients with HF, weight gain is often considered a sign of quality care in long-term care facilities. For residents without a diagnosis of HF, weight loss is a marker of inadequate nutrition. Interdisciplinary collaboration and HF dietary education for all personnel are essential components in the management of HF in nursing homes. A physician, nurse practitioner or physician assistant champion, weekly interdisciplinary rounds, and monitoring the implementation of the HF disease management program are keys to success.

Step 4: Co-ordination of Care

Successful HF management requires coordination of care among interdisciplinary healthcare providers, residents, and family members. As HF is a chronic and progressive illness, its management typically entails periodic transitions in delivery of care. Minimizing unnecessary transitions to acute care facilities is generally preferred as hospitalization is associated increased risk of iatrogenic complications and increased healthcare costs. Meticulous communication of the medical history leading to hospitalization is essential in the event transition to another facility is warranted. With careful planning and training, particularly

Step 5: Maintaining Quality of Life

Quality of life over longevity is preferred by some patients with HF. Accordingly, guideline therapy must be individualized to maximize quality of life, minimize symptom burden, and avoid both negative side effects and drug-to-drug interactions. Cardiac medications outlined in the Beers criteria as potentially inappropriate in older adults include several antiarrhythmic drugs and higher doses of spironolactone and digoxin. Consideration of the patient's and family goals, functional and cognitive status is paramount when determining the plan of care including medications.

Device Management

In the event of inappropriate ICD shocks or emergent need to disable the device, ICDs can be deactivated by placing a donut magnet placed over the device. Access to a magnet with accompanying policies for use is needed in nursing homes for timely deactivation of devices to avoid unnecessary shocks while waiting for reprogramming.

Step 6: Transition to End-of-life Care

Although prognostication is difficult, several factors may indicate increased risk for mortality in 6 months or less (Box 5). For HF patients with significant cardiac dysfunction, current National Heart Failure guidelines recommend end-of-life care, such as hospice, as an option for stage D HF. Specifically, recommendations are that clinicians conduct careful discussions of prognosis, goals of care, and options available for end-of-life when all conventional strategies used in evidence based HF care have been implemented and no further therapies are deemed appropriate. Options include continuing HF therapies from earlier stages that stabilize the patient provide symptom relief or improve quality of life. Every HF patient should receive optimal, guideline directed care. Safety, privacy, open and flexible visiting hours, family support, and access to both palliative care teams and other professionals are criteria of quality end-of-life care in nonhome settings.

> **Box 5: Prognostic factors for median survival of 6 months or less***
> - Increased age
> - Poor left ventricular ejection fraction
> - Elevated serum B-type natriuretic peptide
> - Elevated cardiac troponin I
> - Elevated C-reactive protein
> - Multiple hospitalizations
> - Decreased functional status
> - Malnutrition
> - Systolic hypotension
> - Renal, vascular, or other comorbid diseases
>
> *Presence of three or more factors indicates risk of decreased median survival

Step 7: Clinical Management at End-of-life

Recommendations on HF management at end-of-life in the nursing home setting include aggressive symptom management, patient and family discussions, education, psychosocial and spiritual care, and possible interventions. Palliation of symptoms becomes a primary focus in end-of-life care and regular assessment, ideally by patient rating is preferred. The most common symptoms are dyspnea, pain, depression, fatigue, and edema. These symptoms are related to HF or to comorbidities or common geriatric syndromes. Options for symptom management are outlined in algorithm 2. Fatigue can be managed using stimulants as well as exploring secondary causes including anemia, depression, and sleep disordered breathing. All treatments ordered earlier in the HF trajectory including ICDs should be reevaluated in light of the goals of care. Only essential pharmacological agents should be used. Therapies that are burdensome or not symptom focused may need to be discontinued or titrated down. Therapies that manage neurohormonal (e.g., angiotensin converting enzyme inhibitors; angiotensin receptor blockers) or sympathetic disorders should be continued as long as the patient tolerates them. Open and caring discussions between clinicians and patients or families are a key element of quality palliative care. Psychosocial and spiritual support is part of best practice palliative care. Consultative services can be used by nursing home personnel without current resources to provide this interprofessional level of care.

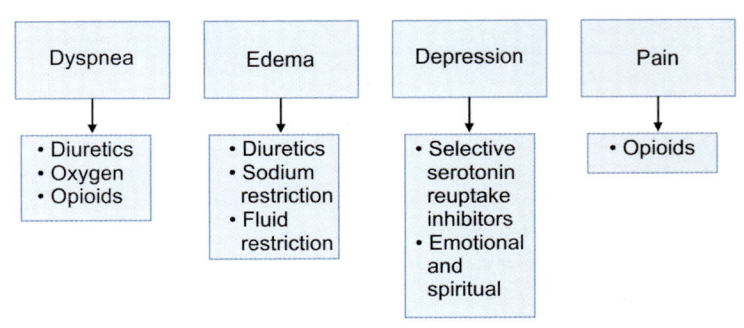

```
┌──────────┐   ┌──────────┐   ┌──────────┐   ┌──────────┐
│ Dyspnea  │   │  Edema   │   │Depression│   │   Pain   │
└────┬─────┘   └────┬─────┘   └────┬─────┘   └────┬─────┘
     ↓              ↓              ↓              ↓
• Diuretics    • Diuretics    • Selective     • Opioids
• Oxygen       • Sodium         serotonin
• Opioids        restriction    reuptake
               • Fluid          inhibitors
                 restriction  • Emotional
                                and
                                spiritual
```

ALGORITHM 2: Symptom management options at end-of-life

CONCLUSION

Nursing home residents diagnosed with HF often are older and frail with multiple comorbid illnesses including cognitive dysfunction that complicates detection of a change in HF status. Accordingly, regularly monitoring for subtle changes in activity tolerance and cognition may support early intervention and avert a hospital admission. Assessing symptoms with activity and tracking symptoms over time is particularly important in determining a resident's HF status.

KEY POINTS

- ❑ Routine assessment and tracking of heart failure status (signs and symptoms) is needed to avert hospitalization among nursing home residents diagnosed with heart failure
- ❑ Older aged residents diagnosed with heart failure may have atypical symptoms that overlap with other comorbid illnesses
- ❑ Behavioral changes may be a better indicator of impending decompensation of heart failure
- ❑ Lack of heart failure symptoms at rest does not indicate a stable clinical status. Symptoms should be assessed with activity when possible
- ❑ Heart failure management should be based on heart failure guidelines from diagnosis to end-of-life to control symptoms and support quality of life.

SUGGESTED READINGS

1. Abraham A, Kutner JS, Beaty B. Suffering at the end of life in the setting of low physical symptom distress. J Palliat Med. 2006;9:658-65.
2. Adler ED, Goldfinger JZ, Kalman J, Park ME, Meier DE. Palliative care in the treatment of advanced heart failure. Circulation. 2009;120:2597-606.
3. Ahmed A, Allman RM, Aronow WS, DeLong JF. Diagnosis of heart failure in older adults: predictive value of dyspnea at rest. Arch Gerontol Geriatr. 2004;38:297-307.
4. Allen LA, Hernandez AF, Peterson ED, Curtis LH, Dai D, Masoudi FA, et al. Discharge to a skilled nursing facility and subsequent clinical outcomes among older patients hospitalized for heart failure. Circ Heart Fail. 2011;4:293-300.
5. Borlaug BA, Paulus WJ. Heart failure with preserved ejection fraction: Pathophysiology, diagnosis, and treatment. Eur Heart J. 2011;32:670-9.
6. Boxer RS, Dolansky MA, Frantz MA, Prosser R, Hitch JA, Pina IL. The Bridge project: Improving heart failure care in skilled nursing facilities. J Am Med Dir Assoc. 2012;13:83.e1-7.
7. Dolansky MA, Hitch JA, Pina IL, Boxer RS. Improving heart failure management in skilled nursing facilities: Lessons learned. Clin Nur Res. 2013:22:432-47.
8. Goodlin SJ, Hauptman PJ, Arnold R, Grady K, Hershberger RE, Kutner J, et al. Consensus statement: Palliative and supportive care in advanced heart failure. J Card Fail. 2004;10(3):200-9.
9. Goodlin SJ, Hauptman PJ, Arnold R, Grady K, Hershberger RE, Kutner J, et al. Consensus statement: Palliative and supportive care in advanced heart failure. J Card Fail. 2004;10: 200-9.
10. Goodlin SJ. Palliative care for end-stage heart failure. Curr Heart Fail Rep. 2005;2:155-60.
11. Goodlin SJ. Palliative care in congestive heart failure. J Am Coll Cardiol. 2009;54:386-96.
12. Harrington CC. Assessing heart failure in long-term care facilities. J Gerontol Nurs. 2008;34:9-14.
13. Jurgens, CY, Goodlin S, Dolansky M, Ahmed A, Fonarow GC, Boxer R, ... the Heart Failure Society of, A. (2015). Heart failure management in skilled nursing facilities: a scientific statement from the American Heart Association and the Heart Failure Society of America. Circ Heart Fail. 8(3), 655-687. doi: 10.1161/HHF.0000000000000005
14. Lampert R, Hayes DL, Annas GJ, Farley MA, Goldstein NE, Hamilton RM, et al. HRS expert consensus statement on the management of cardiovascular implantable electronic devices (CIEDs) in patients nearing end of life or requesting withdrawal of therapy. Heart Rhythm. 2010;7:1008-26.
15. Lorenz KA, Lynn J, Dy SM, Shugarman LR, Wilkinson A, Mularski RA, et al. Evidence for improving palliative care at the end of life: a systematic review. Ann Intern Med. 2008;148:147-59.
16. Oudejans I, Mosterd A, Bloemen JA, Valk MJ, van Velzen E, Wielders JP, et al. Clinical evaluation of geriatric outpatients with suspected heart failure: Value of symptoms, signs, and additional tests. Euro J Heart Fail. 2011;13:518-27.
17. Ouslander JG, Lamb G, Tappen R, Herndon L, Diaz S, Roos BA, et al. Interventions to reduce hospitalizations from nursing homes: evaluation of the INTERACT II collaborative quality improvement project. J Am Geriatr Soc. 2011;59:745-53.
18. Rich MW, Kitzman DW. Heart failure in octogenarians: A fundamentally different disease. Am J Geriatr Cardiol. 2000;(Supp)9:97-104.
19. Rich MW. Heart failure in older adults. Med Clin North Am. 2006;90:863-85, xi.

20. Stanek EJ, Oates MB, McGhan WF, Denofrio D, Loh E. Preferences for treatment outcomes in patients with heart failure: Symptoms versus survival. J Card Fail. 2000;6:225-32.
21. Tresch DD. Clinical manifestations, diagnostic assessment, and etiology of heart failure in elderly patients. Clin Geriatr Med. 2000;16:445-56.
22. Yancy CW, Jessup M, Bozkurt B, Butler J, Casey DE Jr, Drazner MH, et al. 2013 ACCF/AHA guideline for the management of heart failure: a report of the American College of Cardiology Foundation/American Heart Association Task Force on practice guidelines. Circulation. 2013;128:e240-327.

CHAPTER 24

Heart Failure from the Nursing Perspective

Nancy M Albert

INTRODUCTION

This chapter provides algorithms, tables, and 1 box) of nursing management of patients with heart failure. Heart failure is a complex condition, with a complex treatment plan that involves polypharmacy, self-care adherence and internal cardiac devices. All-cause mortality has not been reduced sufficiently when previous eras of management are compared with the current era of cardiac medications and cardiac-device therapies and may be related to interactions and relationships between healthcare providers, patients and families; especially related to heart failure self-care. Patients' physical, psychological, emotional, social, economic, spiritual, and cultural factors may affect care discussions and decisions related to medication, cardiac devices, and other treatment decisions. Care delivery, evaluation, and general monitoring routes (home, telemonitoring, office, combined, or other assessment and communication methods) are influenced by healthcare providers, patient needs and system constraints.

Nursing management may be augmented or fragmented based on healthcare provider decisions; communication and coordination between multiple care providers and specialty-care services, and patients' willingness to adhere to follow-up medical and nursing care expectations. Other factors that influence nursing management of patients with heart failure are nurses' knowledge about heart failure and management, training, licensure, and

Algorithms in Heart Failure

certifications (for example, prescriptive authority and ability to write orders for consultative services and hospital admission), and nurse span of control, which may involve system-based or individual supervisor-based beliefs, policies, procedures and key job responsibilities of the scope of nursing management.

Thus, algorithms, tables and the box below (Algorithms 1, 2; Table 1–6; Box 1) provide a global perspective of nursing assessment and considerations in management, and do not consider services that may have minimal research evidence or are highly specific to individual-care needs or specific cardiomyopathies (for example, amyloidosis, arrhythmogenic right ventricular dysplasia, hypertrophic or takotsubo cardiomyopathies).

GENERAL NURSING ASSESSMENT OF HEART FAILURE

General nursing assessment of heart-failure status includes: (a) general subjective assessment; (b) general objective assessment, and (c) objective assessment related to diagnostic tests.

Nurses are responsible for coordination in patients' care and are often called upon to facilitate development and operation of programs that assure optimal care transitions, patient safety, and patient stability. The following algorithms, tables, and box provide an overview of nurse considerations and research opportunities related to assessing patients for care transitions, stability, and safety.

General Subjective Assessment

Markers of Hypervolemia

Presence of new or worsening:
- Dyspnea, orthopnea, or paroxysmal nocturnal dyspnea
- Edema, ascites, anasarca, or acute pulmonary edema
- Cough or rales
- Sudden, unexpected weight gain of four or more pounds above ideal (dry) weight
- Nocturia
- S3 gallop, neck-vein distension, elevated jugular venous pressure (>10 cm H_2O pressure), or positive hepatojugular reflux test
- Anxiety related to inability to breathe easily
- Sleep-disordered breathing (central sleep apnea).

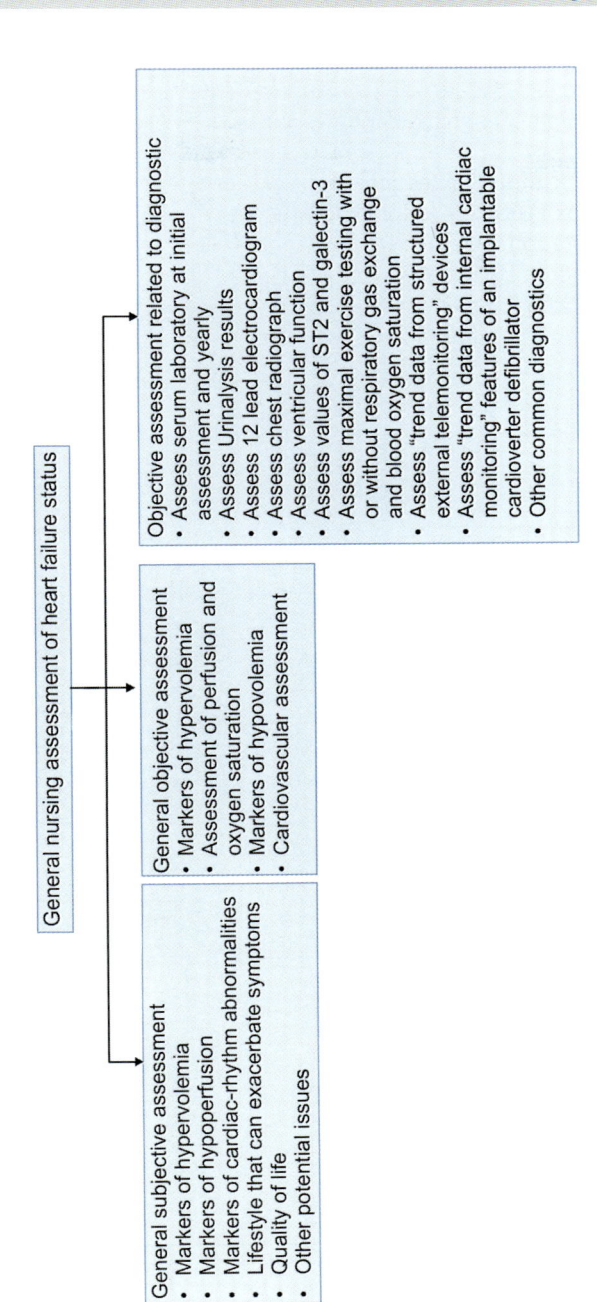

Heart Failure from the Nursing Perspective

General nursing assessment of heart failure status

General subjective assessment
- Markers of hypervolemia
- Markers of hypoperfusion
- Markers of cardiac-rhythm abnormalities
- Lifestyle that can exacerbate symptoms
- Quality of life
- Other potential issues

General objective assessment
- Markers of hypervolemia
- Assessment of perfusion and oxygen saturation
- Markers of hypovolemia
- Cardiovascular assessment

Objective assessment related to diagnostic
- Assess serum laboratory at initial assessment and yearly
- Assess Urinalysis results
- Assess 12 lead electrocardiogram
- Assess chest radiograph
- Assess ventricular function
- Assess values of ST2 and galectin-3
- Assess maximal exercise testing with or without respiratory gas exchange and blood oxygen saturation
- Assess "trend data from structured external telemonitoring" devices
- Assess "trend data from internal cardiac monitoring" features of an implantable cardioverter defibrillator
- Other common diagnostics

ALGORITHM 1: General nursing assessment of heart failure status

Algorithms in Heart Failure

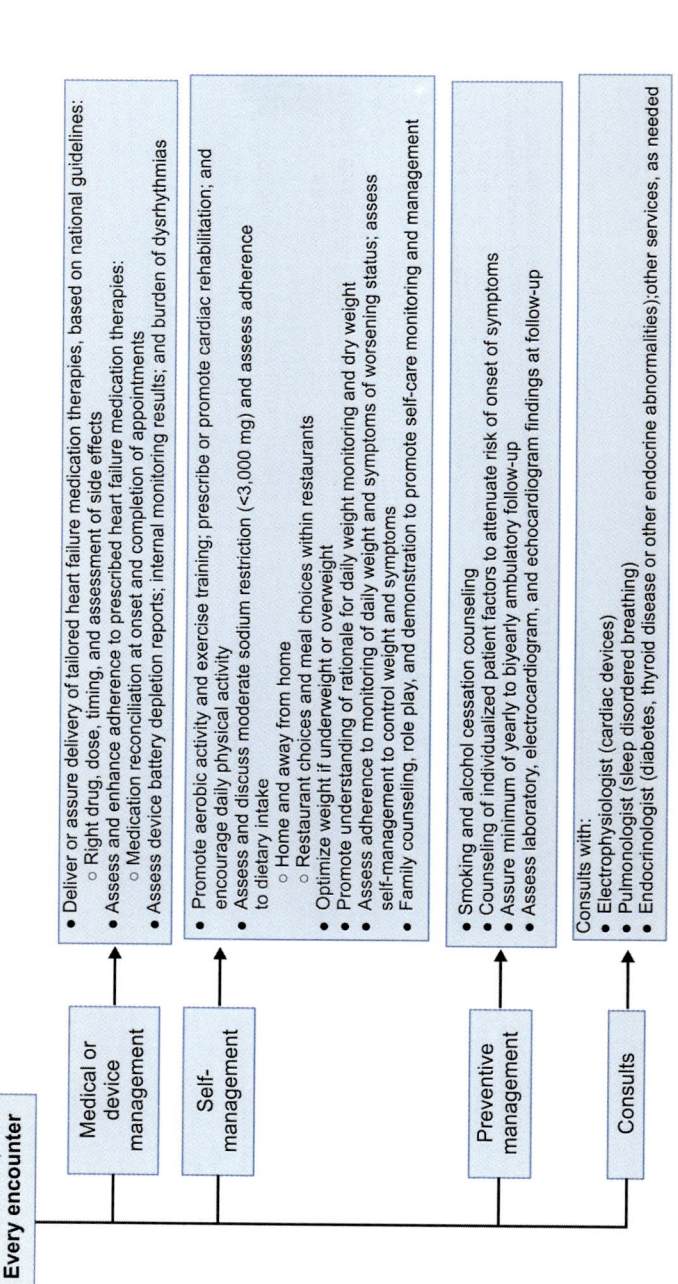

Every encounter

Medical or device management
- Deliver or assure delivery of tailored heart failure medication therapies, based on national guidelines:
  - Right drug, dose, timing, and assessment of side effects
- Assess and enhance adherence to prescribed heart failure medication therapies:
  - Medication reconciliation at onset and completion of appointments
- Assess device battery depletion reports; internal monitoring results; and burden of dysrhythmias

Self-management
- Promote aerobic activity and exercise training; prescribe or promote cardiac rehabilitation; and encourage daily physical activity
- Assess and discuss moderate sodium restriction (<3,000 mg) and assess adherence to dietary intake
  - Home and away from home
  - Restaurant choices and meal choices within restaurants
- Optimize weight if underweight or overweight
- Promote understanding of rationale for daily weight monitoring and dry weight
- Assess adherence to monitoring of daily weight and symptoms of worsening status; assess self-management to control weight and symptoms
- Family counseling, role play, and demonstration to promote self-care monitoring and management

Preventive management
- Smoking and alcohol cessation counseling
- Counseling of individualized patient factors to attenuate risk of onset of symptoms
- Assure minimum of yearly to biyearly ambulatory follow-up
- Assess laboratory, electrocardiogram, and echocardiogram findings at follow-up

Consults
Consults with:
- Electrophysiologist (cardiac devices)
- Pulmonologist (sleep disordered breathing)
- Endocrinologist (diabetes, thyroid disease or other endocrine abnormalities); other services, as needed

ALGORITHM 2: Nursing management of asymptomatic heart failure

Heart Failure from the Nursing Perspective

TABLE 1: Nursing overview of medication considerations in heart failure and reduced ejection fraction

Vasodilators	Beta-blockers	Mineralocorticoid receptor antagonists	Diuretics	Other drugs
• Assess kidney function for insufficiency before assuming that a decrease in ACE-i, ARNI, ARB, or H/N is needed for transient asymptomatic hypotension or lightheadedness • During initiation and up-titration, hold decreasing ACE-i, ARNI or ARB dose due to transient, mild increase in SCr or BUN, especially when associated with aggressive diuretic therapy • Assess for inappropriate use of the combo of ACE-i, ARB, renin inhibitor and ARNI or any of the above and MRA therapy	• Promotes improved left ventricular systolic and diastolic function, reverses remodeling, controls heart rate, prevents malignant arrhythmias, and lowers cardiac afterload and preload • If not receiving amiodarone and has asymptomatic bradycardia with heart rate >50 bpm, therapy may not require down-titration • Assess usage of evidence-based therapies (carvedilol, metoprolol succinate or bisoprolol)	• Appropriate to use in mild, moderate, and severe symptomatic HF if potassium and kidney function criteria are met • Use early post-MI if reduced ejection fraction and diabetes or HF symptoms • Obtain basic metabolic profile (for serum potassium and creatinine) frequently, when drug therapy initiated or dose up-titrated	• Bioavailability of oral loop diuretics and pharmacologic half-life differ by drug • Add nitrate therapy (preload reduction) to improve dyspnea and signs of fluid overload when diuretic therapy (in addition to other core HF therapies) fails to resolve fluid overload • In diuretic resistance, add a thiazide or thiazide-like agent	**Digoxin:** • Decrease dose, if renal insufficiency • Decrease dose, if receiving amiodarone therapy • Therapeutic serum digoxin concentration: 0.5–0.9 ng/mL • May decrease all-cause 30-day rehospitalization • Do not use in atrial fibrillation • Do not use post-MI

Continued

Continued

Vasodilators	Beta-blockers	Mineralocorticoid receptor antagonists	Diuretics	Other drugs
• If combo of once-daily ACE-i or ARB + β-blocker lead to dizziness or lightheadedness, stagger ACE-i/ARB to dinner time and keep twice-daily β-blocker with breakfast and bed time. If 2 twice-daily agents are used, for example ARNI and β-blocker, stagger so that β-blocker is taken with meals and ARNI is taken at alternate times • When SCr >2 mg/dL at baseline, despite an acute increase in SCr after ACE-i initiation, chronic use will decrease SCr in most patients • Maintain during ADHF • Use to reduce mortality and hospitalization for HF	• Up-titrate to target or highest tolerated dose • If BP decreases with use, switch twice-daily dosing from breakfast and dinner to breakfast and bedtime • Maintain during ADHF • Use to reduce mortality and hospitalization for HF	• Withhold use if serum potassium >5.5 mEq/L or creatinine >2.5 mg/dL (men) and 2.0 mg/dL (women) • May reduce hospitalization for HF	• Increased risk of hyponatremia with chlorthalidone (compared to HCTZ)	**Anticoagulants in AF:** • Unless contraindicated, VTE prophylaxis should include anticoagulants rather than anti-platelets (especially if <80 years old) **Statins:** • In RCT, no benefit on morbidity and mortality in chronic HF • In AF, may improve clinical outcomes **Sinus node funny channel inhibitor (ivabradine):** • In RCT, patients with symptomatic HF who could not tolerate β-blocker or were on target dose of therapy and had heart rate >70 bpm had lower rehospitalization rates over time when ivabradine was added to therapy.

ACE-i, angiotensin converting enzyme inhibitor; ADHF, acute decompensated heart failure; ARB, angiotensin receptor blocker; ARNI, angiotensin receptor neprilysin inhibitor; BP, blood pressure; BUN, blood urea nitrogen; HCTZ, hydrochlorothiazide; HF, heart failure; H/N, hydralazine/nitrate combination; MI, myocardial infarction; MRA, mineralocorticoid receptor antagonists; RCT, randomized controlled trials; SCr, serum creatinine; VTE venous thromboembolism; AF, atrial fibrillation; MI, mycardial infarction.

Heart Failure from the Nursing Perspective

TABLE 2: Nursing overview of medication considerations in heart failure and preserved ejection fraction*

Vasodilators	Beta-blockers	Mineralocorticoid receptor antagonists	Diuretics	Other drugs

ACE-i and ARB:
• Decreases BP and improve ventricular relaxation, but do not improve clinical outcomes (mortality or HF hospitalization) when outcomes reviewed over time (both short-term and long-term)
   ○ Conflicting evidence
• Over 12-year follow-up, ACE-i improved overall mortality and major cardiovascular events
• The ARB, candesartan reduced hospital admissions in one RCT study
   ○ Conflicting evidence
• Maintain during ADHF
• When SCr > 2 mg/dL at baseline, despite an acute increase in SCr after ACE-i initiation, chronic use will decrease SCr in most patients
• Use to treat comorbidities associated with HFPEF: hypertension and CAD, post-MI
	• In two randomized trials, β-blockers were not associated with all-cause mortality or HF hospitalization (but were underpowered); however, survival benefit was found in studies with mean age <75 years
	• In multiple observational studies, β-blockers decreased all-cause mortality, but not HF hospitalization
	• Beta blockers decreased mortality in post-MI patients with HFPEF
	   ○ Conflicting evidence
		• Spironolactone does not reduce the incidence of the composite of death from cardiovascular causes, aborted cardiac arrest, or hospitalization for HF management
		• Spironolactone increased serum creatinine levels, doubled the rate of hyperkalemia and reduced hypokalemia in HFPEF
			• Use for symptom relief
			• Bioavailability of oral loop diuretics and pharmacologic half-life differ by drug
			• Add nitrate therapy (preload reduction) to improve dyspnea and signs of fluid overload when diuretic therapy fails to resolve fluid overload
			• In diuretic resistance, add a thiazide or thiazide-like agent
				Digoxin:
				• Increased the risk of 30-day all-cause hospital admission, but not during longer follow-up
				• No benefit in patients in normal sinus rhythm
				• Do not use in atrial fibrillation
				• Do not use post-MI
				Anticoagulants in AF:
				• Unless contraindicated, VTE prophylaxis should include anticoagulants rather than antiplatelets (especially if < 80 years old)

Continued

Continued

Vasodilators	Beta-blockers	Mineralocorticoid receptor antagonists	Diuretics	Other drugs

Calcium channel blockers:
• Verapamil increased exercise capacity, increased ventricular filling rate, and improved subjective HF scores compared to placebo; but did not improve survival
• In older patients (mean age, 80 years) amlodipine and non-amlodipine calcium channel blockers had no associations with composite or individual endpoints of mortality or HF hospitalization
• Over 12-year follow-up, calcium channel blockers improved overall mortality and major cardiovascular events
  ○ Conflicting evidence
	• Improves early (E) to late (A) mitral valve flow velocity and quality of life; benefits greater in patients with high heart rate at baseline
	• Promotes improved left ventricular diastolic function, controls heart rate, prevents malignant arrhythmias, and lowers cardiac afterload and preload
	• Maintain during ADHF
		• In older patients (mean age, 80 years), aldosterone antagonists had no association with clinical outcomes	• Increased risk of hyponatremia with chlorthalidone (compared to HCTZ)	**Statins:**
				• May be associated with reduced mortality; in one report, statin users had a 40% lower risk of mortality
				  ○ Need more evidence

*Drug therapies goal is risk-factor modification.

ACE-i, angiotensin converting enzyme inhibitor; ADHF, acute decompensated heart failure; ARB, angiotensin receptor blocker; BP, blood pressure; HCTZ, hydrochlorothiazide; HF, heart failure; MI, myocardial infarction; RCT, randomized controlled trials; SCr, serum creatinine; VTE, venous thromboembolism; CAD, coronary artery disease; HFPEF, heart failure and preserved ejection fraction; AF, atrial fibrillation

TABLE 3: Registered nurse capabilities in heart failure management—no advanced practice training

General nurse capabilities (examples in parentheses are not inclusive)	Ambulatory and general hospital care	Critical- or heart failure specialty-care
A. Can perform (☑) or is capable of performing after education or training (~); Generally not trained to perform: (-)		
Provide objective assessment of excessive intravascular and interstitial volume overload (edema, lung crackles, dyspnea)	☑	☑
Provide objective assessment of excessive intravascular volume depletion (orthostatic symptoms from excessive diuretic use, diarrhea, fever, sweating)	- / ~	☑
Provide assessment of patients' current knowledge of HF and barriers to readiness to change; given time to complete	- / ~	~ / ☑
Deliver in-depth patient education on HF medications; given time to complete	- / ~ / ☑	~ / ☑
Deliver in-depth patient education on self-care expectations (diet, fluid management, activity or exercise, and signs or symptoms of worsening HF); given time to complete	- / ~ / ☑	~ / ☑
Assess and provide patient education about factors that increase risk for worsening condition (obesity, smoking, alcohol or substance abuse)	~ / ☑	☑
Determine current NYHA-functional status and stage of HF	~ / ☑	~ / ☑
Determine atrial fibrillation contribution to current subjective or objective health status	~ / ☑	☑
Use serum laboratory changes, current medications and subjective or objective health status to determine dilutional hyponatremia, worsening renal or liver function, and myocardial instability requiring emergency care, hospitalization or readiness for hospice or palliative care	- / ~	~ / ☑
Use echocardiogram, subjective or objective health status and other measures to determine need for surgical-care approaches (coronary artery bypass surgery, or valve procedures)	- / ~	~ / ☑

Continued

Continued

Algorithms in Heart Failure

General nurse capabilities (examples in parentheses are not inclusive)	Ambulatory and general hospital care	Critical- or heart failure specialty-care
Assess psychosocial, cultural and economic-care needs and patient preferences, given time to complete	☑	☑
Screen patients for advanced therapies or need for change in setting (home to hospital; hospital floor to critical care)	∼	☑
Assess patients for non-HF conditions that could worsen HF or require use of therapies that could cause progressive worsening of condition (anemia, thyroid disease, chronic lung diseases, peripheral vascular diseases, sleep disorders, gout, cardiac dysrhythmias, hypertension, hypotension, degenerative joint disease)	∼	☑
Evaluate effectiveness of current HF medication therapies and need for up-or down-titration	∼	☑
Evaluate effectiveness of current nonpharmacological HF therapies and need for revision or consultation of other healthcare personnel	∼	☑
Request internal or external interdisciplinary care consultation to advance clinical therapies	∼ / ☑	∼ / ☑
Communicate with healthcare providers and caregivers to advance clinical therapies	☑	☑
Participate in developing, implementing and assessing effectiveness of quality or process improvement activities at a local level	∼ / ☑	∼ / ☑
Review HF literature for highest strength and quality of research evidence on clinical and nonclinical management topics important to managing patients clinically	– / ∼ / ☑	– / ∼ / ☑
Translate best practice, research-based evidence in clinical setting	– / ∼ / ☑	– / ∼ / ☑
Participate in gap analysis of issues with healthcare provider performance	– / ∼ / ☑	– / ∼ / ☑
Participate in gap analysis of issues with clinical-care delivery and/or outcomes of clinical care (rehospitalization, mortality, quality of life)	– / ∼ / ☑	– / ∼ / ☑

Continued

Continued

General nurse capabilities (examples in parentheses are not inclusive)	Ambulatory and general hospital care	Critical- or heart failure specialty-care
Communicate with physician and other non-nurse healthcare providers to minimize gaps in care and promote evidence-based practices	-/~/✓	-/~/✓
B. May be (~) or may not be (-) capable of performing without consistent application or regular competency assessments		
Provide fine objective assessment of fluid status (S3 heart sound, JVD-P, new or worsening murmur, PND, sleep apnea; hepatojugular reflex; serum laboratory changes)	-	~
Provide fine objective assessment of left ventricular dysfunction (laterally displaced point of maximal impulse; pulsus alternans; chest pain or palpitations in left lateral position; echocardiogram findings-LVEDP/V)	-	~
Understand hemodynamics beyond high or low blood pressure, oxygen saturation or respirations; and tachycardiac heart rate or bradycardiac heart rate	-	~
Understand physical examination findings that differentiate systolic from diastolic dysfunction (S3 and S4 heart sounds, peripheral edema, JVD-P, and cardiomegaly); and those that are similar (rales)	~	~
Provide subjective assessment of new or worsening status, given time to complete	~	~
Determine a patients' "dry" weight (weight without excess fluid) and assess for optimization of weight	-	-/~
Assess cognitive, psychological, literacy, health literacy and preferred method of learning, given time to complete and standardized tools	-/~	~
Assess use of prescription (thiazolidinediones, dronedarone) and over-the-counter substances (NSAIDs, ephedrine, effervescent antacids) that should be avoided or are contraindicated	-/~	~
Assess readiness for a cardiac device (cardiac resynchronization or implantable cordioverter-defibrillator) based on QRS width, presence of q waves and/or left BBB	-/~	~

BBB, bundle branch block; HF, heart failure; LVEDP/V, left ventricular end diastolic pressure/volume; NSAIDs, non-steroidal anti-inflammatory drugs; NYHA, New York Heart Association; JVD-P, jugular venous distention-pressure; PND, paroxysmal nocturnal dyspnea.

Algorithms in Heart Failure

TABLE 4: Capabilities of advanced-practice nurses with training and experience in heart-failure management

Can perform (☑) or is capable of performing after education/training (~)	Patient care focused	Population focused
Provide gross objective assessment of excessive intravascular and interstitial volume overload (edema, lung crackles, dyspnea)	☑	☑
Provide gross objective assessment of excessive intravascular volume depletion (orthostatic symptoms from excessive diuretic use, diarrhea, fever, sweating)	☑	☑
Provide fine objective assessment of fluid status (S3, JVD-P, new or worsening murmur, PND, sleep apnea; hepatojugular reflex; serum laboratory changes)	☑	☑
Provide fine objective assessment of left ventricular dysfunction (laterally displaced point of maximal impulse; pulsus alternans; chest pain or palpitations in left lateral position; echocardiogram findings-LVEDP/V)	~ / ☑	☑
Understand hemodynamics beyond high or low blood pressure, oxygen saturation or respirations; and tachycardic heart rate or bradycardic heart rate	☑	☑
Understand physical examination findings that differentiate and are similar for systolic and diastolic dysfunction (S3 and S4 heart sounds, peripheral edema, JVD-P, and cardiomegaly)	☑	☑
Provide subjective assessment of new or worsening status, given time to complete	☑	☑
Provide assessment of patients' current knowledge of heart failure and barriers to readiness to change; given time to complete	☑	☑
Deliver in-depth patient education on HF medications; given time to complete	~ / ☑	~ / ☑
Deliver in-depth patient education on self-care expectations related to diet, fluid management, activity or exercise, and signs or symptoms of worsening HF; given time to complete	~ / ☑	~ / ☑

Continued

Continued

Can perform (☑) or is capable of performing after education/training (~)	Patient care focused	Population focused
Assess and provide patient education about factors that increase risk for worsening condition (obesity, smoking, alcohol or substance abuse)	☑	☑
Determine patients' "dry" weight (weight without excess fluid) and optimize weight	~ / ☑	~ / ☑
Determine current NYHA-functional status and stage of HF	☑	☑
Determine atrial fibrillation contribution to current subjective or objective health status	☑	☑
Use serum laboratory changes + current medications and subjective or objective health status to determine dilutional hyponatremia, worsening renal or liver function, and myocardial instability requiring emergency care, hospitalization or readiness for hospice or palliative care	~ / ☑	~ / ☑
Use echocardiogram, subjective or objective health status and other measures to determine need for surgical-care approaches (coronary artery bypass surgery, or valve procedures)	☑	☑
Assess psychosocial, cultural and economic-care needs and patient preferences, given time to complete	☑	☑
Assess cognitive, psychological, literacy, health literacy and preferred method of learning, given time to complete and standardized tools	☑	☑
Assess use of prescription (thiazolidinediones, dronedarone) and over-the-counter substances (NSAIDs, ephedrine, effervescent antacids) that should be avoided or are contraindicated	☑	~ / ☑
Assess readiness for a cardiac device (cardiac resynchronization or implantable cardioverter-defibrillator) based on QRS width, presence of q waves and/or left bundle branch block	☑	~ / ☑
Screen patients for advanced therapies or need for change in setting (home to hospital; hospital floor to critical care)	☑	☑

Continued

Continued

Can perform (☑) or is capable of performing after education/training (~)	Patient care focused	Population focused
Assess patients for non-HF conditions that could worsen HF or require use of therapies that could cause progressive worsening of condition (anemia, thyroid disease, chronic lung diseases, peripheral vascular diseases, sleep disorders, gout, cardiac dysrhythmias, hypertension, hypotension, degenerative joint disease)	☑	☑
Evaluate effectiveness of current medication therapies and need for up-titration or down-titration	☑	☑
Evaluate effectiveness of current nonpharmacological therapies and need for revision or consultation of other healthcare personnel	☑	☑
Participate in developing, implementing and assessing effectiveness of quality or process improvement activities at a local level	☑	☑
Participate in gap analysis of issues with health-care provider performance	~ / ☑	~ / ☑
Participate in gap analysis of issues with clinical care delivery and/or outcomes of clinical care (rehospitalization, mortality, quality of life)	~ / ☑	~ / ☑
Request internal or external interdisciplinary care consultation to advance clinical therapies	☑	☑
Communicate with physician and other nonnurse health-care providers to advance clinical therapies	☑	☑
Communicate with physician and other nonnurse health-care providers to minimize gaps in care and promote evidence-based practices	☑	~ / ☑
Review HF literature for highest strength and quality of research evidence on clinical and nonclinical management topics important to managing patients clinically	☑	☑
Translate best practice, research-based evidence in clinical setting	☑	☑

HF, heart failure; LVEDP/V, left ventricular end diastolic pressure/volume; NSAIDs, non-steroidal anti-inflammatory drugs; NYHA, New York Heart Association; JVD-P, jugular venous distention-pressure; PND, paroxysmal nocturnal dyspnea.

TABLE 5: Nurse consideration at transitions point of care

Transition point	Nurse considerations: assess and manage, when applicable
Hospital to home (or assisted living center) to hospital	- Local social support and postdischarge community resources - Health literacy; language barriers - Frailty issues and risk for falls - Cognitive status - Depression and other emotions - Medication reconciliation at admission and predischarge - Polypharmacy and (a) need for all medications, (b) dosage, (c) timing of use and (d) interactions with other medications - Transportation to receive medications and attend follow-up care - Presence of written materials before discharge related to: self-care; signs and symptoms of worsening condition; follow-up appointment date, time; and provider contact information - Documentation of and delivery of the following to next care provider(s): Admitting diagnosis, ejection-fraction percentage, care delivered, medical-test reports, plan of care during hospitalization, treatments needed after discharge, signs and symptoms of heart failure at discharge, and functional status - Completion of in-hospital delivery of services - Presence of advance directives - Presence and effects of treatment(s) on comorbidities - Care coordinator (navigator) assigned to patient, or other system (i.e., checklist) that verifies completion of predischarge expectations that support healthcare provider and patient-provider communication, collaboration and services delivery

Continued

Continued

Transition point	Nurse considerations: assess and manage, when applicable
Home to ED services to home, to acute care hospital or SNF	- Same as hospital to home, and: - Transcription of all home medications - Medication reconciliation at admission and before next point of care - Continuation of home medications in ED, when appropriate - Documentation of all point-of-care laboratory, radiology, and other diagnostic-test results
Hospital to SNF to home or to acute care hospital	- Patient's: (a) level of moral distress; (b) ability to interpret heart failure signs, symptoms, and acuity; (c) desire for reactive or proactive care services; and (d) access to resources - Information flow among healthcare providers and between health-care providers and patients - Documentation of and transmission of the following to SNF provider(s): Admitting diagnosis, ejection fraction percentage, hospital care delivered, medical-test reports, plan of care post hospitalization, treatments needed after discharge, signs and symptoms of heart failure at discharge, and medication details, especially, tranquilizers, sleep aides, anticoagulants and other medications that could impact patient safety and quality of care; smoking and alcohol-intake status - Documentation of functional status at SNF admission and expectations during stay; especially, related to physical therapy - Advance directives status - Polypharmacy and (a) need for all medications, (b) dosage, (c) timing of use and (d) interactions with other medications - Physician involvement in care - SNF personnel knowledge and skills in assessing and managing patients with HF - Care coordinator (navigator) assigned to patient, or other system (i.e., checklist) that verifies completion of new admission and predischarge expectations related to healthcare provider and patient-provider communication, collaboration and service delivery

Continued

Continued

Transition point	Nurse considerations: assess and manage, when applicable
Hospital to palliative care or hospice care	- Advance-care planning - Social and financial supports - Anxiety and depression - Uncertainty (related to patient, family, and healthcare providers) - Family caregiver concerns, knowledge, and support - Medication regimens to retain and delete - Psychological support for patients and families - Symptom management plan of care - Prognostic tools used in determining individual patient status - Referrals required to optimize care and comfort - Triggers related to treatment and palliation - Methods for managing "congestion" - Health-care provider knowledge and support of heart failure treatments

SNF, skilled nursing facility; ED, emergency department.

TABLE 6: Nurse tips of safety and self-care behaviors at home

Patient safety and self-care promotion	Nurse considerations: assess and manage, when applicable

Falls prevention or minimization	• Provide optimal information to family and caregivers
	• Consider walking aids (cane, walker, etc.) and support when ambulating, especially, if dizzy or lightheaded
	• Instructed to stop activity and sit when dizzy or lightheaded
	• Assess fluid status and nutritional status; dehydration may cause dizziness that leads to falls
	• Consider assessing and intervening related to HF
	   ○ If urgency, frequency or nocturia, consider adult diapers, underpants liners or other interventions that would decrease fast motions that could lead to fall events
	   ○ If frail, has cognitive issues, delirium, or Alzheimer's disease, develop interventions, vetted and understood by the patient and all family members, for consistent application; i.e., assistance or support when walking
	   ○ If prescribed an anticoagulant or antiplatelet medication, assess home situation to prevent bumping and bruising (corners of the home, texture of walls), assess and discuss risk for falls (location, how, time of day, with what activity, etc.) with an adverse bleeding event

Tips on medication adherence	• Ensure patient and family understand medication prescription:
	   ○ Use teach back or other methods to assess understanding
	   ○ Elements to understand: why taking, name, medication type, dose, when to take, how to take, what to do if a dose is missed, common side-effects, drug interactions, and how to store
	• Keep a written list of all current medications with name, dose, and other characteristics above:
	   ○ Bring to each health-care provider appointment, no matter who is treating the patient
	• Incorporate medication taking into daily routines. If morning or night-time dose, keep by toothbrush in bathroom; if taking with meals, keep on person who is available when traveling:
	   ○ Use pill box or other storage solutions

Continued

Continued

Patient safety and self-care promotion	Nurse considerations: assess and manage, when applicable
	- Call health-care provider one week before medication runs out, to reorder - Leave notes or other reminders to take medications - Leave notes, check boxes, or other reminders after taking medication to prevent doubling up - Communicate medication schedule to family or friends

Tips on low-sodium diet adherence	- Consider what motivates you to follow the prescribed diet
	- Consider current eating habits and how to incorporate a low-sodium diet:
	  ○ Ease of purchasing the right foods
	  ○ How to control or offset hunger and cravings for high-sodium foods
	  ○ How to overcome challenges that lead to nonadherence
	  ○ Who you live with and their dietary needs
	- Make a list of when a low-sodium diet is hardest to follow (at restaurants and others homes) and communicate your needs to family and friends
	- Plan meals ahead and consider sodium content as well as vitamin and mineral content and general nutrition goals
	- Use a smaller plate and eat slowly, while sitting down so you are aware of consumption
	- Keep track of low-sodium foods consumed, so you can create diet staples
	- Read all labels for sodium content and serving size. At each meal, consider the sodium consumed by multiplying sodium content by serving size
	- Choose fresh foods whenever possible (foods generally on the perimeter of food stores)
	- Remove the salt shaker from the table

Continued

Continued

Patient safety and self-care promotion	Nurse considerations: assess and manage, when applicable

	- Avoid (or eat sparingly):
	   ○ Condiments, sauces, and gravies. If using, do not place on food. Set aside and dip fork tongs into the item before spearing food with fork
	   ○ Fried foods (breading is high in sodium); choose baked or broiled
	   ○ Pizza (sodium in crust, sauce, processed cheese, and toppings)
	   ○ Soups unless home made without salt or other seasonings that contain sodium
	   ○ Deli meats (sodium used to maintain shelf life [preservative])
	   ○ Breads (read all labels to find the brand with the lowest sodium content) and other foods with high-flour content (bagels, spaghetti, pretzels, etc.)
	   ○ Deli sandwiches
	   ○ Snack chips (potato chips, pretzels, corn chips, buttered, salted popcorn, and others)
	   ○ Boxed, canned, and bagged foods (generally, high in sodium content). Frozen foods can be high or low sodium- read labels
	 - Stay accountable to yourself by keeping a food diary of sodium content, every day
	 - Recognize that you are in-charge of making food choices
	 - If you snack, binge or have cravings (when tired, bored, studying, etc.: (a) set aside low-sodium foods to meet needs and (b) remove high sodium foods from the home
	 - If you become thirsty within 2 hours of eating a meal, the meal was probably high in sodium; assess foods eaten and avoid or moderate in the future
	 - Your taste buds will adjust to a low-sodium diet within 1 month, be patient

Continued

Continued

Patient safety and self-care promotion	Nurse considerations: assess and manage, when applicable

	- At restaurants:
	  - Avoid fast-food restaurants and those where most food is shipped in precooked or preprepared
	  - Ask waiter to tell the chef to cook without sodium and to limit seasonings with high-salt content
	  - Select menu items that are naturally low in sodium (salads, vegetables, whole baked potato, broiled and baked foods without sauces, butter, etc.)
	  - Ask for all sauces, salad dressing, gravies to come on the side. You control what you eat
	  - Avoid soups, bread in basket (before meal served), fried menu items (french fries) and those known to be high in sodium: cheese, bacon, deli meats
	  - Ask waiter for sodium level of food content (some restaurants have a chart of this information, along with fat content and total calories)
	  - Use butter sparingly

Tips on physical activity and exercise	- Assess current status and advance exercise slowly - Determine patient perspectives of barriers and benefits to physical activity and exercise - Determine if comorbid conditions interfere with independent physical activity and exercise - Explain benefits of regular physical activity and exercise - Explain usual expectations of exercise (dyspnea, increase in heart rate, and diaphoresis) to decrease patients' worry over their actions and normal physiologic responses - Overcome fears related to exercise and palpitations, elevated heart rate, chest pain, and implantable cordioverter-defibrillator firing - Use the "talk test" method of teaching patients about exercise limitations - Teach patients about the need for and simple methods of completing warm-up and cool-down exercises (5 min each) - Discuss the benefits of attending cardiac rehabilitation classes, especially, if uncertain about activity and exercise capabilities

Continued

Continued

Patient safety and self-care promotion	Nurse considerations: assess and manage, when applicable
Tips on communicating with health-care providers	<ul><li>Keep a log of questions and bring to appointments</li><li>Write down health-care provider responses</li><li>Request a written report of office visit information, including an updated medication list</li><li>Bring someone with you to an appointment who will ask questions and/or relay information after an appointment</li><li>Use "I" when asking questions and making statements</li><li>Be assertive in raising questions and letting your healthcare provider know when you do not understand</li><li>Ask for contact information (name, office phone number, and other communication systems) and keep with important health-care information</li><li>Be honest in communicating adherence to the treatment plan. Health-care providers make decisions based on your responses</li><li>Repeat what you thought you heard to your health-care provider and ask if that is correct</li><li>Ask for written materials that match instructions given</li></ul>

HF, heart failure.

Heart Failure from the Nursing Perspective

> **Box 1: Examples of contemporary nursing research opportunities**
>
> **Themes in nursing assessment of patients' needs**
>
> - Interplay of physiological and psychological state related to NYHA functional class and symptom burden
> - Timing of end-of-life care acceptance and cultural, spiritual, education, and psychosocial needs
> - Critical factors of self-care adherence that influence clinical outcomes that nurses need to accurately assess in ambulatory and hospital encounters
> - Nurses critical thinking based on current scientific information or guideline-directed medical therapies
> - Influence of cardiac and vascular assessment skills (cardiac physiology, dysrhythmia recognition, effects on end organ function) and (a) meeting population and family needs and (b) healthcare provider communication and collaboration
> - Nursing resources (time, knowledge, and others) and HF clinical outcomes
> - Factors that would increase nurses' knowledge, comfort and frequency of educating patients about self-care principles in multiple care settings
> - Setting of care (home, assisted living, skilled nursing home) and patterns and variances in patient assessment
> - Synthesis of available data and relevance to assessment patterns and variances
>
> **Themes in nursing interventions**
>
> - Interplay of physiological and psychological state related to NYHA functional class and symptom burden
> - Timing of end-of-life care acceptance and cultural, spiritual, education, and psychosocial needs of patients and family
> - Nurses critical thinking based on current scientific information or guideline directed medical therapies
> - Influence of cardiac and vascular assessment skills (cardiac physiology, dysrhythmia recognition, effects on end-organ function) and (a) meeting population and family needs and (b) healthcare provider communication and collaboration
> - Nursing resources used (time, knowledge, and processes and supplies used in role paly and demonstration) and clinical outcomes
> - Novel nurse-directed and implemented interventions that improve self-care adherence, including HF medication adherence
> - Novel nurse-directed and implemented interventions that improve adherence to follow-up visits, especially early discharge care

Continued

Continued

Themes in nursing interventions and outcomes

- Novel nurse-directed implemented interventions that improve clinical outcomes: short-term and long-term mortality and hospitalization
- Factors influencing desire to initially use and continually use telemonitoring devices, especially, newer smart phone applications and/or small, externally applied devices that provide knowledge, skills, and reinforcement of care expectations
- Use of telemonitoring devices, especially, newer smart phone applications and/or small, externally applied devices and (a) communication and collaboration with primary HF providers and (b) clinical outcomes
- Modes of patient education (in-person, pre-recorded apps, visual, handouts, kiosk, demonstration, etc. features) and efficiency and effectiveness of (a) patient and (b) family caregiver uptake
- Quality of life at end-of-life related to specific guideline recommended interventions
- Nursing interventions and age, gender, body size, cultural, emotional, environmental, spiritual, and economic related outcomes
- Differences in clinical outcomes of nursing directed interventions based on HF type: reduced or preserved ejection fraction
- Setting of care (home, assisted living, skilled nursing home) and (a) nurses' delivery of patient education, (b) patients' understanding of self-care expectations, medication management, and when to contact health care professionals
- Patient values; implicit beliefs and attitudes; relationships to medication and self-care adherence, and clinical outcomes
- Determinants in adherence to HF-guideline directed medical therapies based on non-HF factors (such as pain, health literacy, depression, anxiety, frailty, fall risk, etc.)
- Determinants of clinical outcomes based on non-HF factors (such as pain, health literacy, depression, anxiety, frailty, fall risk, etc.)
- Ideal level of low-sodium diet recommendations and (a) patient adherence and (b) clinical outcomes
- Ideal level of patient activity and exercise and (a) patient adherence and (b) clinical outcomes
- Ideal communication regarding weight and (a) patient adherence and (b) clinical outcomes
- Safest transitions from hospital to home

NYHA, New York Heart Association; HF, heart failure.

Markers of Hypoperfusion

Presence of new or worsening:
- General fatigue
- Decreased exercise tolerance
- Need for naps
- Mental obtundation or confusion
- Dizziness or lightheadedness; presyncope
- Nausea, anorexia, change in bowel habits
- Resting tachycardia (> 85 beats per minute)
- Decreased systolic blood pressure
- Increased intracardiac pressures
- Pulsus alternans
- Proportional pulse pressure less than 25% (subtract diastolic blood pressure from systolic blood pressure, then divide results by systolic blood pressure)
- Decreased ability to walk or carry out physical activity due to leg weakness
- Chest pain, or surrogates of cardiac pain
- Changes in urine output and diuretic effectiveness.

Markers of Cardiac Rhythm Abnormalities

Presence of new or worsening:
- Palpitations, especially when resting on left side
- Slow, rapid, or irregular heart rate associated with dizziness, lightheadedness, syncope, or near syncope

Lifestyle that can Exacerbate Symptoms

Presence of new or worsening:
- Alcohol use or substance abuse
- Tobacco use
- Fluid indiscretion with or without uncontrollable thirst
- High-sodium intake
- Inactivity or passive activity
- Failure to complete regular exercise
- Anxiety, depression, personality D, vital exhaustion, or poor stress management
- Medication nonadherence based on the plan of care
- Social isolation or lack of social support
- Economic constraints related to purchase of fresh foods, medications; and transportation to health-care providers
- Nonadherence to daily weight and signs or symptoms of heart-failure monitoring

- Nonadherence to notifying health-care providers of changes in health status
- Comorbid diagnoses and medication side-effects
- Medication management; i.e., taking all daily medications at the same time; causing hypotension; dizziness.

Quality of Life

Assess via formal tool (many require permission to use):
- Minnesota Living with Heart failure Questionnaire (20-item, Likert-type survey)
- Kansas City Cardiomyopathy Questionnaire (23-item Likert-type survey)
- Specific Activity Scale (five-item tool that objectively measures NYHA-functional class)
- Six-minute walk test (objective measure of distance in meters walked in 6 minutes).

Other Potential Issues

Assess for nonclinical factors that could lead to nonadherence to medical therapies and decompensation:
- Frailty
- Lack of social support
- Cognitive decline
- Health literacy
  - Inability to read medication labels
  - Inability to read food labels
- Uncertainty about which healthcare provider to notify for new or worsening symptoms

General Subjective Assessment

Markers of Hypervolemia

Assess:
- Presence of peripheral edema in legs, fingers, abdomen; ascites in abdomen; anasarca, scrotal or presacral-area edema
- Sitting and standing blood pressure to determine level of jugular venous distension
- Positive hepatojugular reflux test; presence and severity of organ distension (pulmonary congestion and hepatomegaly)
- Presence of elevated jugular venous pressure (most reliable sign of fluid overload)
- Short-term elevation in body weight

- New onset or worsening of S3 heart sound or systolic murmur
- Subjective assessment of new or worsening orthopnea, paroxysmal nocturnal dyspnea, nocturia, dyspnea with activity or at rest, exercise intolerance or sleep-disordered breathing (central sleep apnea) are most common

Assessment of Perfusion and Oxygen Saturation

- Blood pressure and orthostatic blood pressure changes
- Narrow pulse pressure may indicate hypoperfusion
- Audible S4 heart sound may indicate hypertension
- Audibly distant S2 heart sound, diminished pulse amplitude, narrowed pulse pressure, pulsus alternans, and/or laterally displaced apical beat may indicate poor cardiac function and poor perfusion
- Cool, mottled skin; cognitive dysfunction or altered mentation; and change in bowel habits may indicate poor perfusion
- Tachycardia and/or frequent premature ventricular beats could decrease perfusion
- Resting heart rate below 80 beats per minute on optimal heart-failure medical therapies is associated with improved survival
- Oxygen saturation greater than 92% reflects adequate cardiac output

Markers of Hypovolemia

- Flat neck veins
- Dry mucous membranes or mouth
- Clear lung fields
- Absence of edema.

Cardiovascular Assessment

- Assess for normal and abnormal or extra heart sounds in aortic, pulmonary, tricuspid, and mitral regions and apex if point of maximal impulse is not near the mitral region due to cardiac enlargement; murmurs
- Palpate apex for visible pulsations, thrills (if mitral stenosis, roll patient to left side to hear thrill), and heaves (at apex)
- Assess general color, temperature (cool extremities may indicate hypoperfusion), peripheral pulses, presence of peripheral vascular disease, ulceration, and edema (pitting versus non-pitting).

Pulmonary Assessment

- If using accessory muscles of respiration may be due to pulmonary edema, asthma, fulminant pneumonia, chronic pulmonary obstructive disease (COPD); pursed lip breathing may be due to emphysema; audible noises while breathing; ability to speak and breathe at same time
- Assess, if dyspnea plus wheezing (or whistling), present; may be due to asthma, COPD, or worsening heart failure
- Cheyne-Stokes breathing may be due to stroke, worsening heart failure, sedation, or uremia
- Cough may be due to worsening heart failure, pneumonia, angiotensin converting enzyme (ACE) inhibitor therapy, common cold or flu
- Muffled sounds may be due to pleural effusion; scratchy sound (similar to rubbing strands of hair together) may be due to rales (crackles); rales are rare in chronic heart failure
- Cyanosis in nail beds
- Obstructive sleep apnea may cause sleep disturbances
- Palpate abdomen in liver area for tricuspid regurgitation and hepatojugular reflux
- Inspect chest under left and right clavicle area for pacemaker, cardiac resynchronization therapy or implantable cordioverter-defibrillator devices.

Objective Assessment Related to Diagnostic Tests

Serum Laboratory

Assess at initial assessment and yearly for:
- Electrolyte balance: basic metabolic panel, calcium, magnesium; assess for abnormalities that cause:
  - Hypervolemia (decreased serum sodium)
  - Hypokalemia (prolonged administration of diuretics)
  - Hyperkalemia (reductions in glomerular filtration rate or inadequate delivery of sodium to the distal tubular sodium-potassium exchange sites of the kidney. This is more common when receiving potassium-sparing diuretics (spironolactone and eplerenone,) ACE-inhibitors or angiotensin II receptor blockers
  - Hypomagnesemia (prolonged administration of diuretics; accompanies potassium loss)
- Renal function: blood urea nitrogen, creatinine or glomerular filtration rate that provide evidence of poor renal blood flow

- Thyroid function: thyroid-stimulating hormone
- Complete blood count for infection or anemia
- Fasting blood glucose: high values increase the risk for heart failure
- Glycosylated hemoglobin (HbA1c) in patients with diabetes and heart failure: U-shaped relationship:
  - Best outcomes in the HbA1c category are levels of more than 7% to less than or equal to 9%.
  - Unlike patients with diabetes who do not have HF, mortality is higher when levels are less than 7%
  - When more than 9%, mortality increases
- Lipid profile:
  - Generally, lower total cholesterol and triglyceride levels were predictive of worse outcomes (all-cause mortality, cardiovascular mortality, or hospitalizations) after adjustment for baseline factors
  - Patients on statin therapy had reductions in mortality
- Liver function tests may reveal elevated liver-enzyme levels and liver dysfunction due to heart failure.

Urinalysis

Assess results for proteinuria.

Electrocardiogram

Assess for:
- Atrial or ventricular dysrhythmias or abnormalities
- New myocardial ischemia and/or injury; or new or prior myocardial infarction (nontransmural [Non ST elevated myocardial infarction; NSTEMI] or transmural [STEMI]), diffuse myocardial disease, and coronary artery disease that may provide a cause of heart failure
- Right or left bundle branch block (BBB); QRS width more than 150 ms, reflecting ventricular dyssynchrony. Left BBB could provide partial evidence of the need for cardiac resynchronization therapy
- Intraventricular or other conduction delays
- Left ventricular hypertrophy and axis deviations.

Chest Radiograph

Assess (posterior-anterior and lateral) to detect:
- Cardiac enlargement
- Pulmonary congestion

Algorithms in Heart Failure

- Other pulmonary disease when there is pulmonary distress requiring emergency care.

Ventricular Function

Assess:
- Brain natriuretic peptide or N-terminal pro-BNP:
  - When clinical diagnosis of heart failure is uncertain
  - When heart failure is known but it is uncertain if current symptoms reflect worsening heart failure or another medical condition
- ST2, an interleukin-1 receptor-like family of proteins; a marker of myocardial strain, associated with myocardial fibrosis, remodeling, and worse cardiovascular outcomes:
  - When decompensation etiology is uncertain and fibrosis is suspected
  - Values more than or equal to 35 ng/mL reflect worse prognosis; therefore, treat heart failure aggressively and reassess more frequently or determine palliative-care status
- Galectin-3, a galactosidase binding lectin secreted by macrophages or other inflammatory cells in interstitial spaces of the heart; a marker of myocardial strain, associated with myocardial fibrosis and cardiac remodeling and worse cardiac outcomes:
  - When decompensation etiology is uncertain and fibrosis is suspected
  - Values ≥17.8 ng/mL reflect worse prognosis; therefore, treat heart failure aggressively and reassess or determine palliative care status

Maximal Exercise Testing

Maximal exercise testing with or without respiratory gas exchange and/or blood oxygen saturation to assess:
- Cardiac and pulmonary function with activity and exercise
- Ability to walk without restrictions and for more than short distances (provides prognostic information)
- For a decrease in peak oxygen consumption that reflects severe disease requiring advanced therapies
- To determine if heart failure is the cause of exercise limitation
  Assess "trend data from structured external telemonitoring" devices:
- To assess ongoing status
- To assess decompensation

Two-dimensional Echocardiogram

Use coupled with Doppler-flow studies to:
- Determine whether abnormalities of myocardium, heart valves, or pericardium are present and which chambers are involved
- Evaluate the presence and severity of left ventricular dysfunction
- Determine subjective assessment of ejection fraction
- Reveal segmental wall motion abnormalities, chamber size, ventricular thrombus, and degree of cardiac dyssynchrony
- Reveal right ventricular size, right ventricular systolic performance, and right atrial size:
  - The single, most useful diagnostic tool in the evaluation of heart failure
  - Less expensive and more generally available than radionuclide ventriculography; it does not require preparation
  - Numerical data should include:
    - Estimate of ejection fraction
    - Ventricular dimensions and volumes
    - Wall thickness and chamber geometry
    - Regional wall motion
    - Left atrial dimensions and volume
    - Anatomic and flow abnormalities in all four valves
    - Secondary changes in valve function, with attention to mitral and tricuspid valve insufficiency.

Trend Data from Internal Cardiac Monitoring

Assess features of an implantable cardioverter defibrillator:
- Burden of atrial fibrillation (prevalence over 24-hour period)
- Ventricular heart rate while in atrial fibrillation
- Atrial and ventricular heart rate during the day and at night
- Activity level
- Intrathoracic impedance (reflects intrathoracic fluid volume)
- Heart rate variability
- Pulmonary artery systolic and diastolic pressures (and waveform configurations).

Other Common Diagnostics

- Screening for sleep-disordered breathing, hemochromatosis, human immunodeficiency virus, amyloidosis, rheumatologic diseases, or pheochromocytoma
- Magnetic resonance imaging or computed tomography provides chamber size, ventricular mass, ventricular function and ejection fraction.

CONCLUSION

Nursing care of clients with heart failure may be broad or very narrow in scope depending on work settings, work expectations and focus, knowledge of and clinical experiences in assessing, planning, delivering and evaluating heart failure therapies, licensure and credentialing to practice, and number and type of care partners assisting in meeting client (and family) needs and preferences. From a global perspective, nursing care must promote client health and safety (including safe client environments), and nurses must advocate for client health, be committed to practicing with compassion and respect, be accountable and demonstrate responsibility for nursing practice and ensure optimal communication and collaboration with multiple health professionals. In addition, nurses are responsible for advancing the profession through research and scholarly inquiry. Box 1 provides just a few ideas for nursing research in heart failure that could reduce health disparities, promote best practices in optimal care and health policy, enhance healthcare delivery, and establish novel care delivery methods and care outcomes that could improve the lives of heart failure clients.

Nurses are key stakeholders in managing heart failure. No matter their capabilities in assessing and delivering care to clients, they are responsible for protecting the health and well-being of vulnerable populations such as clients with heart failure who may have complex care needs due to multiple chronic medical conditions, frailty, cognitive impairment, or geographical or cultural isolation. It is imperative that nurses caring for clients with heart failure focus on providing heart failure education and using creative methods that improve adherence to self-care behaviors known improve quality of life and minimize morbidity and mortality. Finally, nurses are integral to assuring high quality care delivery and to improving communication and collaboration during transitions in care. Nurses must be actively involved in quality improvement initiatives and translation of new knowledge into clinical practice.

KEY POINTS

- Nurses providing general care to patients with heart failure are capable of collecting comprehensive data, deriving a nursing diagnosis from assessment data, identify outcomes of importance, plan and implement care that matches guideline-directed medical therapies recommendations, coordinate and evaluate care delivery that improves patients' overall and heart failure health

Continued

Continued

- Nurses with the appropriate knowledge and experience in cardiovascular and heart failure principles provide holistic care, health teaching, health promotion, and consultation that include families and other health-care providers and identifies barriers to effective care and communication
- Nurses synthesize the totality of available subjective and objective patient and healthcare provider data to identify patterns and variances in heart failure care delivery and patient adherence to increase stakeholder awareness of heart failure expectations, negotiate care responsibilities and promote optimal decision-making
- Advanced practice nurses use knowledge and skills in general care (described above) and also in prescriptive authority, referrals, and treatments, in accordance with state laws to attain optimal patient outcomes, based on guideline-directed medical therapies and patient preferences
- Nurses, at any level can be involved in structural, system or process changes that improve or advance the quality and scope of care, so that patients are assured of best practices.

SUGGESTED READINGS

1. Albert NM, Cohen B, Liu X, Best CH, Aspinwall L, Pratt L. Hospital nurses' comfort in and frequency of delivering heart failure self-care education. Eur J Cardiovasc Nurs. 2015;14(5):431-40.
2. Albert NM. A systematic review of transitional-care strategies to reduce rehospitalization in patients with heart failure. Heart Lung. 2016;45(2):100-13.
3. Albert NM, Paul S, Murray M. Complexities of care for patients and families living with advanced cardiovascular diseases: overview. J Cardiovasc Nurs. 2012;27:103-13.
4. Albert NM. Fluid management strategies in heart failure. Crit Care Nurse. 2012;32(2):20-32.
5. Bavishi C, Chatterjee S, Ather S, Patel D, Messerli FH. Beta-blockers in heart failure with preserved ejection fraction: a meta-analysis. Heart Fail Rev. 2015;20(2):193-201.
6. Currie K, Strachan PH, Spaling M, Harkness K, Barber D, Clark AM. The importance of interactions between patients and healthcare professionals for heart failure self-care: A systematic review of qualitative research into patient perspectives. Eur J Cardiovasc Nurs. 2015;14(6):525-35.
7. Goldberg RJ, Gurwitz JH, Saczynski JS, Hsu G, McManus DD, Magid DJ, et al. Comparison of medication practices in patients with heart failure and preserved versus those with reduced ejection fraction (from the Cardiovascular Research Network [CVRN]). Am J Cardiol. 2013;111:1324-9.
8. Heckman GA, Boscart VM, McKelvie RS. Management considerations in the care of elderly heart failure patients in long-term care facilities. Future Cardiol. 2014;10:563-77.

9. Liu G, Zheng XX, Xu YL, Ru J, Hui RT, Huang XH. Meta-analysis of the effect of statins on mortality in patients with preserved ejection fraction. Am J Cardiol. 2014;113:1198-204.
10. Loh JC, Creaser J, Rourke DA, Livingston N, Harrison TK, Vandenbogaart E, et al. Temporal trends in treatment and outcomes for advanced heart failure with reduced ejection fraction from 1993-2010: findings from a university referral center. Circ Heart Fail. 2013;6:411-9.
11. Patel K, Fonarow GC, Ahmed M, Morgan C, Kilgore M, Love TE, et al. Calcium channel blockers and outcomes in older patients with heart failure and preserved ejection fraction. Circ Heart Fail. 2014;7(6):945-52.
12. Pitt B, Pfeffer MA, Assmann SF, Boineau R, Anand IS, Claggett B, et al. Spironolactone for heart failure with preserved ejection fraction. N Engl J Med. 2014;370:1383-92.
13. Reed BN, Rodgers JE, Sueta CA. Polypharmacy in heart failure: drugs to use and avoid. Heart Fail Clin. 2014;10:577-90.
14. Reed JL, Pipe AL. The talk test: a useful tool for prescribing and monitoring exercise intensity. Curr Opin Cardiol. 2014;29:475-80.
15. Wu CK, Lee JK, Chiang FT, Lin LY, Lin JW, Hwang JJ, et al. Prognostic factors of heart failure with preserved ejection fraction: a 12-year prospective cohort follow-up study. Int J Cardiol. 2014;171:331-7.

SECTION 5

Advanced Heart Failure

CHAPTER 25

Left Ventricular Assist Device Versus Transplantation: How to Decide?

Patrick McCann, Eric Adler

INTRODUCTION

Advanced heart failure (HF) is a dynamic disease process with complex pathophysiology requiring synthesis of multiple data points including, but not limited to, volume status, comorbidities, exacerbating factors and prognosis. Estimates suggest end-stage HF (American Heart Association stage D HF) is associated with 50% annual mortality rate. Treatment of stage D HF is limited to three options: mechanical circulatory support (MCS); heart transplantation; and hospice. Previously, heart transplantation provided the only option for patients with stage D HF refractory to medical therapy. Limited donor heart variability extends waiting periods with extremely reduced functional capacity and many die (approximately 10%) while waiting (Algorigthm 1). Recent advances in technology and outcomes with ventricular assist devices (VADs) have markedly changed the approach to advanced HF management. This chapter provides an overview of the indications for advanced therapies with a focus on VAD and transplant.

INDICATIONS FOR MECHANICAL CIRCULATORY SUPPORT

The indications for VAD use have evolved with growing experience and longer duration of use. The rapid development of technology has allowed expansion of indications for MCS. Short-term circulatory support devices for left ventricular [left ventricular assist device (LVAD)] or right ventricular [right ventricular assist device

Algorithms in Heart Failure

Stage D heart failure
Refractory HF symptoms, recurrent hospitalization, cardiogenic shock ↓BP, end-organ damage, RV failure, cardiorenal HOCM, refractory angina, VT, cardiac tumor

Reversible cause? ischemia, optimal medical/device therapy?

Sick enough? VO_{2max}, InterMac 1–7 HFSS, SHFM

Consider transplant
SHFS 1 year survival <50–80%
HFSS medium/high risk
$VO_{2\,Max}$ <10

Gray zone
Retransplant
CHD

Defer
SHFS 1 year survival >80%
HFSS low risk
VO_{2max} >14

Transplant candidate?
Medical, surgical, psychosocial evaluation

Interval re-eval
Refer to advance HF center

Yes
Transplant
VAD BTT

No
Palliative consult
Home inotropes
Turn ICD off?
VAD DT

INTERMACS and time frame of need for advance therapy
- Critical cardiogenic shock: hours
- Progressive decline: days to week
- Stable but inotrope: weeks months
- Recurrent advanced HF: weeks to months
- Exertion intolerant: months Exertion limited
- Advanced NYHA class III

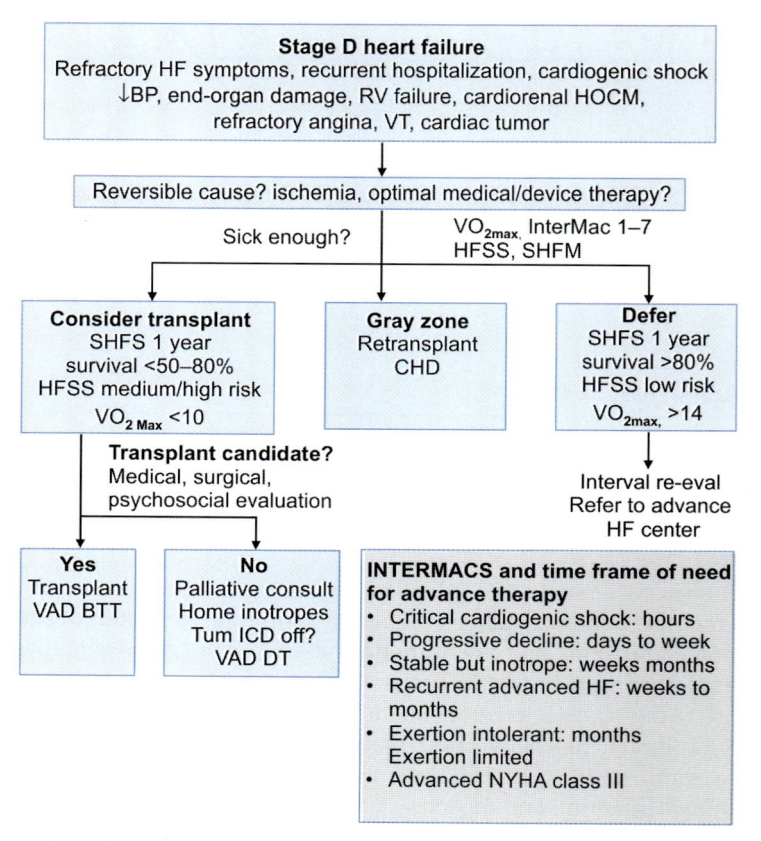

HF, heart failure; BP, blood pressure; RV, right ventricle; HOCM, hypertrophic obstructive cardiomyopathy; VT, ventricular tachycardia; HFSS, Heart Failure Survival Score; SHFM, Seattle Heart Failure Model; CHD, coronory heart disease; VAD, ventricular assist device; BTT, bridge to transplant; ICD, implantable cardioverter-defibrillator; DT, destination therapy; NYHA, New York Heart Association.

ALGORITHM 1: Sample treatment algorithm for stage D heart failure

(RVAD)] support are indicated for refractory cardiogenic shock. Examples include acute fulminant myocarditis and cardiac arrest during interventional cardiac procedures. The decision between an LVAD or RVAD or both primarily depends on right ventricular function and pulmonary artery resistance.

Durable circulatory support devices are typically indicated for patients with advanced HF [New York Heart Association (NYHA) class IV] who continue to worsen despite optimal medical therapy. Three groups have been identified that benefit from durable devices.

The first group consists of patients with severe HF who remain hemodynamically unstable despite maximal pharmacologic support and meet criteria for cardiac transplantation. These patients undergo LVAD implantation as a "bridge to transplant" (BTT). The second group encompasses patients with NYHA class IV who are not transplant candidates. These patients have an LVAD implanted for "destination therapy" (DT). The last group of patients usually present with cardiogenic shock in circumstances where candidacy for cardiac transplantation cannot be determined. These patients receive MCS as a "bridge to decision" (BTD).

BRIDGE TO TRANSPLANT

Currently, the most common indication for MCS is BTT in patients who deteriorate and develop refractory HF while awaiting heart transplant. Historically, 20–30% of patients who had a VAD implanted as a BTT did not survive to transplantation regardless of the device used or year of implantation owing to the severity of HF and complications associated with the device. However, this mortality has been reduced significantly with the advent of continuous flow devices. Recent changes to prioritize use of donors for 1A patients by the united network for organ sharing guidelines for organ sharing have also had a significant impact on the use of LVADs. This change in approach to transplantation and the reduction in mortality with newer generation VADs have contributed to a rapid increase in the use of LVADs.

Other than MCS, the only other option for unstable patients awaiting heart transplant is intravenous inotropes. Data from several studies have shown the outcome with VADs is significantly better than therapy with intravenous inotropes. Furthermore, the Investigation of Nontransplant-eligible Patients Who are Inotrope Dependent (INTrEPID) trial that declined LVAD implantation showed a 20% survival at 1 year. The success of LVADs compared to the low survival rates of intravenous inotropes has nearly eliminated inotrope therapy as an option for advanced HF. In patients with shorter expected waiting times for heart transplant being treated with inotropes delay in VAD transplant should be approached with extreme caution.

DESTINATION THERAPY

In contrast to patients that are transplant eligible, DT is reserved for patients who are deemed ineligible for heart transplant. The development of DT is a result of an aging population and limited donor availability. Two prospective trials have examined the outcome of MCS in patients that are not eligible for transplant. The first study was the Randomized Evaluation of Mechanical Assistance for the Treatment of Congestive Heart Failure (REMATCH) trial, which compared the outcome of first generation LVADs versus medical therapy in patients that were not eligible for transplant. The primary endpoint was death from any cause. The trial showed an absolute risk reduction of 27% at 1 year. However, the authors noted significant morbidity and mortality with the LVAD resulting in a 2-year survival rate of 23%.

More recently, the outcomes with MCS in DT patients were examined comparing the first generation pulsatile XVE device versus the second generation continuous flow HeartMate II device. The primary endpoint was a composite of survival at 2 years, free of disabling stroke or reoperation to replace the device. The survival estimate at 2 years in the continuous flow device was 55% compared to 24% with the pulsatile flow device. However, the risk of death from index hospitalization was 56% regardless of device, similar to results noted in the REMATCH trial. These data emphasize the importance of candidate selection in determining the outcomes with MCS.

BRIDGE TO DECISION

Mechanical circulatory support must be initiated in an appropriate and timely fashion to achieve the best outcomes. It is not uncommon for patients to present with cardiogenic shock, multisystem organ failure, and uncertain neurologic status. Such patients present a unique situation where implantation of durable MCS may be associated with poor outcomes and is not cost effective. These clinical circumstances may require nondurable MCS support as a BTD to provide support until the clinical situation allows for the implantation of a permanent device. A multidisciplinary approach and excellent communication between local hospitals and specialized MCS centers can make this an effective strategy.

It is important for medical teams to consider which patients will benefit from nondurable MCS and what modality of MCS device should be used. The ongoing evolution of these devices presents a challenging landscape to navigate when evaluating the appropriateness of a device for a particular patient. The current recommendation is to use the device that is familiar to the team and can best serve the needs of the patient. Quick and appropriate intervention with MCS can provide stabilization which may ultimately improve survival.

INDICATIONS FOR TRANSPLANT

Cardiac transplantation remains the treatment of choice for patients with end stage HF who are symptomatic despite optimal medical therapy. Unfortunately, this therapy is not available to the majority of people who need it secondary to a shortage of available donors. In the past 2 decades, approximately 2,200 heart transplants have been performed annually. As a result, screening for transplant involves an extensive evaluation to identify factors that may increase perioperative risk or decrease long-term survival.

Multiple indications for heart transplant exist and are outlined by Mancini and Lietz in selection of cardiac transplantation candidates. The following circumstances are indicated for cardiac transplant; cardiogenic shock requiring continuous intravenous inotrope therapy or MCS with an intra-aortic balloon pump device or MCS, persistent NYHA class IV congestive HF symptoms refractory to maximal medical therapy [left ventricular ejection fraction (LVEF) <20%; peak VO_2 <12 mL/kg/min], intractable or severe angina symptoms in patients with coronary artery disease not amenable to percutaneous or surgical revascularization, intractable life-threatening arrhythmias unresponsive to medical therapy, catheter ablation, and/or implantation of intracardiac defibrillator.

PATIENT SELECTION

The approach to implementing advanced therapies for HF is determined by the trajectory of HF progression, etiology of HF, and overall clinical status. Appropriate patient selection is essential to achieving excellent clinical outcomes. This principle extends to all therapies including MCS and heart transplant. Before evaluation for either therapy can proceed, a candid discussion between the HF team and the patient regarding prognosis and postoperative care or responsibilities is paramount as caregiver burden after advanced therapies is high. In addition to a review of advanced therapies, the benefits and risks of therapies, resuscitation and deactivation of devices should be explained to the patient and the patient's family.

Whether patients receive MCS or cardiac transplant is determined by a variety of medical and psychosocial factors. Psychosocial factors including barriers to care, informed consent, end-of-life care, and patient preferences should all be discussed prior to MCS or transplant. Informed consent should be discussed with both the patient and the patient's family. Both parties should be made aware of the all the risks and benefits, including lifestyle changes that are required for both MCS and heart transplant. Furthermore, end-of-life discussions, including palliative care, availability of hospice, and device deactivation need to be reviewed. Lastly, patient preferences must be identified before proceeding with evaluation for MCS or transplant. This may take time as patients consider their diagnosis, prognosis, and treatment options. Occasionally, an ethics consult may be helpful in decision-making for the patients and their family. Patients may also benefit from meeting others that have undergone LVAD and/or cardiac transplantation so they can ask them the questions about their lifestyle post-procedure.

As previously noted, medical factors play a significant role in screening patients for MCS or transplant. Univariate and multivariate analyses have examined the data to develop predictors of survival in HF. These analyses have also tried to compare predictors for subgroups of HF including systolic versus diastolic, acute versus chronic, and outpatient versus inpatient with HF.

CONCLUSION

Surgical therapy for stage D HF has undergone a radical transformation as a result of the rapid development and evolution of MCS. Selection of appropriate therapeutics has become a complicated multifactorial decision that is influenced by the etiology of the HF, the severity of disease and patient preferences. A multidisciplinary systematic approach is necessary to maximize the likelihood of a good outcome in this highly morbid patient population.

KEY POINTS

- Advanced heart failure is associated with significant mortality
- Treatment options consist of intravenous inotropes, mechanical circulatory support, and cardiac transplant
- Mechanical circulatory support is a viable option with excellent outcomes for patients that are ineligible to receive cardiac transplant.

SUGGESTED READINGS

1. Deng MC, Edwards LB, Hertz MI, Rowe AW, Keck BM, Kormos R, et al. Mechanical circulatory support device database of the International Society for Heart and Lung Transplantation: third annual report. J Heart Lung Transplant. 2005;24:1182-7.
2. Haft JW, Pagani FD, Romano MA, Leventhal CL, Dyke DB, Matthews JC. Short- and long-term survival of patients transferred to a tertiary care center on temporary extracorporeal circulatory support. Ann Thorac Surg. 2009;88:711-7.
3. Lloyd-Jones D, Adams RJ, Brown TM, Carnethon M, Dai S, De Simone G, et al. Heart disease and stroke statistics—2010 update: a report from the American Heart Association. Circulation. 2010;121:e46-e215.
4. Mancini D, Lietz K. Selection of cardiac transplantation candidates in 2010. Circulation. 2010;122:173-83.
5. Mulligan MS, Shearon TH, Weill D, Pagani FD, Moore J, Murray S. Heart and lung transplantation in the United States, 1997-2006. Am J Transplant. 2008;8:977-87.
6. Peura JL, Colvin-Adams M, Francis GS, Grady KL, Hoffman TM, Jessup M, et al. Recommendations for the use of mechanical circulatory support: device strategies and patient selection: a scientific statement from the American Heart Association. Circulation. 2012;126:2648-67.
7. Rogers JG, Butler J, Lansmann SL, Gass A, Portner PM, Pasque MK, et al. Chronic mechanical circulatory support for inotrope-dependent heart failure patients who are not transplant candidates: results of the INTrEPID trial. J Am Coll Cardiol. 2007;50:741-7.
8. Rose EA, Geljins AC, Moskowitz AJ, Heitjan DF, Stevenson LW, Dembitsky W, et al. Long-term use of a left ventricular assist device for end-stage heart failure. N Engl J Med. 2001;345:1435-43.
9. Slaughter MS, Rogers JG, Milano CA, Russell SD, Conte JV, Feldman D, et al. Advanced heart failure treated with continuous-flow left ventricular assist device. N Engl J Med. 2009;361:2241-51.
10. Stevenson LW, Miller LW, Desvigne-Nickens P, Ascheim DD, Parides MK, Renlund DG, et al. Left ventricular assist device as destination for patients undergoing intravenous inotropic therapy: a subset analysis from REMATCH (Randomized Evaluation of Mechanical Assistance in Treatment of Chronic Heart Failure). Circulation. 2004;110:975-81.

26
CHAPTER

Approach to Left Ventricular Assist Devices and Follow-up in Advanced Congestive Heart Failure

Anthony J Choi, Keshav R Nayak, Brian E Jaski

INTRODUCTION

The role of mechanical support for patients with advanced heart failure has expanded with bridge to destination and bridge to transplant indications for left ventricular assist devices (LVAD). Referral of patients requires an understanding of the role of LVAD in the overall care of the advanced heart failure. Patient selection for LVADs including identification of markers of mortality for patients who undergo HeartMate II implantation should be considered. As the use of such devices becomes widespread, initial presentation of LVAD patients may not be solely limited to centers with mechanical support and acute initial management of emergencies associated with LVADs should be widely disseminated. This section provides an overview of key management decisions in patients with LVADs.

CONTINUOUS FLOW MECHANICAL SUPPORT IN ADVANCED HEART FAILURE

Patient Selection

Treatment of congestive heart failure (CHF) should always begin with goal directed medical therapy (GDMT). Coronary revascularization should be considered in parallel with efforts to achieve GDMT. Cardiac resynchronization therapy should also be considered in patients with a QRS greater than 150 ms, and ejection

Approach to Left Ventricular Assist Devices and Follow-up...

```
Heart failure symptoms (INTERMACS profile 2, 3, and 4)
                        ↓
              Optimal medical therapy
                        ↓
       Consider revascularizaton if ischemic etiology
            ↓                                    ↓
      QRS >150 ms                           QRS <150 ms
   ┌──────────────────┐                ┌──────────────────┐
   │ Consider CRT if NSR, LBBB │       │ Consider ICD if after 3 │
   │ LVEF <35% and NYHA class II │     │ months of optimal │
   │ (class I B) or III/ambulatory │   │ medical therapy │
   │ IV (class I A) │                  └──────────────────┘
   └──────────────────┘
   Reassess response after 3 months ──┐
                                      ↓
              1–2 year mortality >50%
                        ↓
   Assess for candidacy based on clinical and psychosocial evaluation
                        ↓
              Consideration for MCS
```

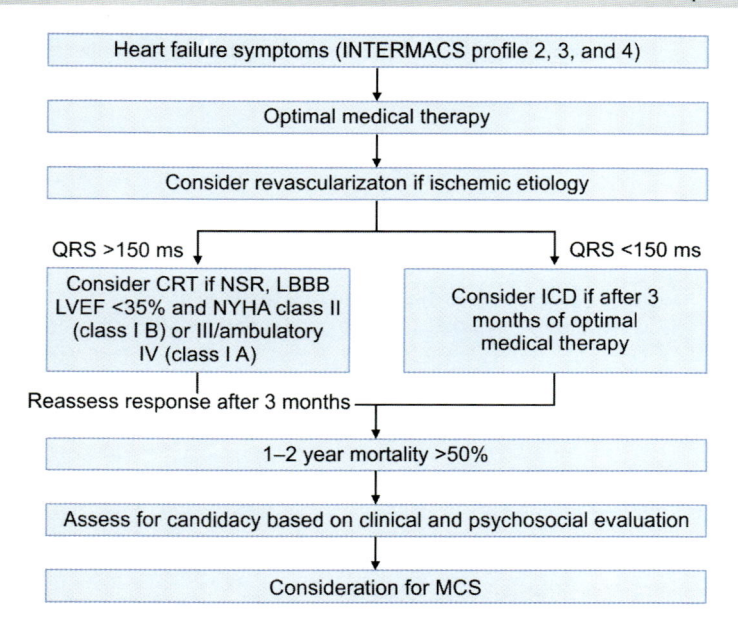

INTERMACS, Interagency Registry for Mechanically Assisted Circulatory Support; CRT, cardiac resynchronization therapy; NSR, normal sinus rhythm; LBBB, left bundle branch block; LVEF, left ventricular ejection fraction; NYHA, New York Heart Association; ICD, implantable cardioverter-defibrillator; MCS, mechanical circulatory support.

ALGORITHM 1: Systolic failure management overview

fraction less than 35% with New York Heart Association class II to ambulatory IV symptoms (Algorithm 1).

Should the patient remain in refractory CHF despite GDMT, revascularization, and cardiac resynchronization, the role of further mechanical care to include left ventricular assist devices (LVAD) should be carefully considered. Should LVAD be pursued, a multidisciplinary evaluation of the patient, family, and home support should be carried out in an attentive and methodical manner. Implantation should not be considered for patients with comorbidities that would preclude a good outcome despite LVAD support. Lastly, psychosocial concerns such as poor family or caregiver involvement, unresolved psychological or psychiatric issues, and compliance issues should be carefully weighed before consideration of an LVAD (Algorithm 2).

To aid in the medical screening of the LVAD patient, the Interagency Registry for Mechanically Assisted Circulatory Support defined patient profiles to help standardize the severity of the

Algorithms in Heart Failure

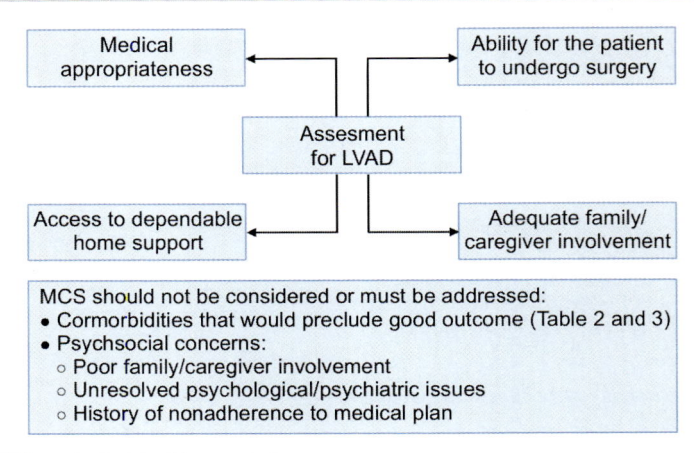

```
    Medical              Ability for the patient
 appropriateness  ←→    to undergo surgery
        ↕                       ↕
              Assessment
               for LVAD
        ↕                       ↕
 Access to dependable    Adequate family/
    home support    ←→  caregiver involvement
```

MCS should not be considered or must be addressed:
- Cormorbidities that would preclude good outcome (Table 2 and 3)
- Psychsocial concerns:
  - Poor family/caregiver involvement
  - Unresolved psychological/psychiatric issues
  - History of nonadherence to medical plan

MCS, mechanical circulatory support.

ALGORITHM 2: Pre-assesment for mechanical circulatory support

TABLE 1: Interagency Registry for Mechanically Assisted Circulatory Support patient profiles and timing of left ventricular assist device support

Profiles	Description	Time to left ventricular assist device
1	Crashing and burning: critical cardiogenic shock	Within hours
2	Progressive decline: inotrope dependence with continuing deterioration	Within a few days
3	Stable but inotrope dependent	Within a few weeks
4	Recurrent advanced heart failure: with recurrent rather than refractory decompensation	Within weeks to months
5	Exertion intolerant: comfortable at rest, but exercise intolerant	Variable
6	Exertion limited: patient who is able to do some mild activity, but fatigue within a few minutes	Variable
7	Advanced NYHA II: reasonably stable, able to tolerate reasonable level of comfortable activity. Decompensation history that is not recent	Not a candidate

NYHA, New York Heart Association.

candidate profile (Table 1). To identify patients who may successfully undergo implant or to identify comorbidities, elegant risk models were developed from the HeartMate XVE left ventricular assist device (LVAD) destination therapy registry to estimate one year mortality derived from a cumulative weighted risk score (Tables 2 and 3).

In patients who screen as appropriate for LVAD therapy, preoperative optimization directly impacts timing and success of LVAD implantation. The general workup for patients to undergo LVAD implantation as well as preoperative metabolic goals are shown in table 4. Ideally, right ventricular function should be optimized by addressing pulmonary hypertension and circulatory volume status in the preoperative period. Intraoperative hypoxia or pulmonary insult can result in right ventricular dysfunction. Additionally, preoperative assessment of cardiac valvular testing, bleeding risk, and nutrition can help reduce intraoperative and postoperative complications (Algorithm 3). Preoperative laboratory, dental, and imaging investigations are required for the preoperative risk assessment, management, and optimization of patients to undergo LVAD implantation. Depending on the socioeconomic or

TABLE 2: Risk factors for 90 day from the HeartMate II Risk Score

Variable	Coefficient
Age (in years) ×	0.0274
Albumin (g/dL) ×	0.723
Creatinine (mg/dL) ×	0.740
INR ×	1.136
Center LVAD volume (1 point if <15) ×	0.807
HRMS score =	Σ(variable × coefficient)

HRMS, HeartMate Risk Score.

TABLE 3: Risk category and survival (based on derivation and validation cohorts)

HRMS	Risk category	90 Day survival	1 year survival	2 year survival
<1.58	Low risk	94±1%	83±2%	74±3%
1.58–2.48	Medium risk	86±2%	72±2%	61±3%
>2.48	High risk	73±3%	58±3%	49±4%

HRMS, HeartMate Risk Score.

Algorithms in Heart Failure

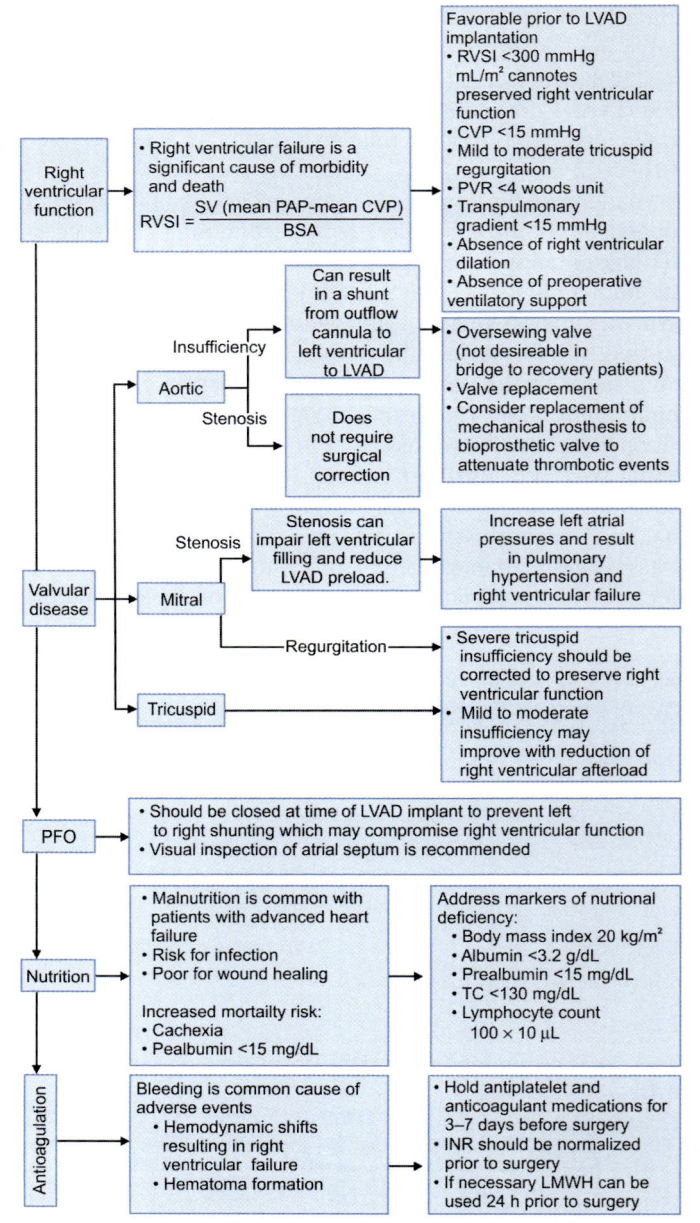

Right ventricular function
- Right ventricular failure is a significant cause of morbidity and death

$$RVSI = \frac{SV\ (mean\ PAP - mean\ CVP)}{BSA}$$

Favorable prior to LVAD implantation
- RVSI <300 mmHg mL/m² cannotes preserved right ventricular function
- CVP <15 mmHg
- Mild to moderate tricuspid regurgitation
- PVR <4 woods unit
- Transpulmonary gradient <15 mmHg
- Absence of right ventricular dilation
- Absence of preoperative ventilatory support

Valvular disease

Aortic — Insufficiency: Can result in a shunt from outflow cannula to left ventricular to LVAD
- Oversewing valve (not desireable in bridge to recovery patients)
- Valve replacement
- Consider replacement of mechanical prosthesis to bioprosthetic valve to attenuate thrombotic events

Aortic — Stenosis: Does not require surgical correction

Mitral — Stenosis: Stenosis can impair left ventricular filling and reduce LVAD preload. → Increase left atrial pressures and result in pulmonary hypertension and right ventricular failure

Mitral — Regurgitation

Tricuspid:
- Severe tricuspid insufficiency should be corrected to preserve right ventricular function
- Mild to moderate insufficiency may improve with reduction of right ventricular afterload

PFO
- Should be closed at time of LVAD implant to prevent left to right shunting which may compromise right ventricular function
- Visual inspection of atrial septum is recommended

Nutrition
- Malnutrition is common with patients with advanced heart failure
- Risk for infection
- Poor for wound healing

Increased mortaility risk:
- Cachexia
- Pealbumin <15 mg/dL

Address markers of nutrional deficiency:
- Body mass index 20 kg/m²
- Albumin <3.2 g/dL
- Prealbumin <15 mg/dL
- TC <130 mg/dL
- Lymphocyte count 100 × 10 µL

Antioagulation

Bleeding is common cause of adverse events
- Hemodynamic shifts resulting in right ventricular failure
- Hematoma formation

- Hold antiplatelet and anticoagulant medications for 3–7 days before surgery
- INR should be normalized prior to surgery
- If necessary LMWH can be used 24 h prior to surgery

RVSI, right ventricular systolic index; SV, stroke volume; PAP, pulmonary artery pressure; CVP, central venous pressure; BSA, body surface area; LVAD, left ventricular assist device; PVR, pulmonary vascular resistance; PFO, patent foramen ovale; INR, international normalized ratio; LMWH, low-molecular-weight heparin; TC, total cholesterol.

ALGORITHM 3: Preoperative optimization

TABLE 4: Preoperative assessment for patients undergoing left ventricular assist devices

Laboratory tests	Studies	Other
• CBC with differential and platelet count • Complete chemistry panel • Uric acid • Thyroid profile • Lactate dehydrogenase • PT/PTT, INR • Plasma renin activity • Pregnancy test in women • Iron, transferrin, ferritin • Glycosylated hemoglobin • HIT antibody if clinically suspected. Should be followed by a serotonin release assay if HIT antibodies are positive • Urinalysis, culture, and sensitivity	• Chest x-ray (AP and lateral) • Carotid Doppler if history of CAD or >5 years old • Chest or abdominal CT if prior surgery • ABI if history of claudication or diabetes • Abdominal ultrasound for AAA if >60 years old or if PAD • EGD or colonoscopy in the last 2 years • Echocardiography • Right heart catheterization	• Dental evaluation with Panorex image

CBC, complete blood count; PT, prothrombin time; PTT, partial thromboplastin time; INR, international normalized ratio; HIT, heparin-induced thrombocytopenia; AP, anteroposterior; CAD, coronary artery disease; CT, computed tomography; ABI, ankle-brachial index; AAA, abdominal aortic aneurysm; PAD, peripheral arterial disease; EGD, esophagogastroduodenoscopy.

locality where the patient resides, screening for indolent infectious diseases such as tuberculosis and coccidiomycosis should also be considered (Table 4).

Ongoing Management

As the indications for continuous flow LVADs expand and long-term management of patients with LVADs improve, medical encounters outside of specialized centers will naturally increase. As such, a basic understanding of key principles of management will be useful in the approach to the LVAD patient. Four key areas of considerations in these patients are evaluation and management of blood pressure, right ventricular function, anticoagulation, and identifying LVAD infection (Box 1 and Algorithm 4).

Box 1: Key areas of the ongoing management of left ventricular assist devices

Blood pressure
- Frequently little pulse pressure and diminished Korotkoff sounds
- Doppler should be used for unformity although blood pressure can be estimated by automated blood pressure cuff
- Goal MAP 70–90 mmHg
- Hypertension results in increased afterload which can deteriorate the device cannula valve
- Increased blood pressure decreases left ventricular to aortic gradient resulting in reduced output from device

Right ventricular function
- Key predictor of morbidity and mortality in LVAD patients
- Early postoperative volume shifts can affect right ventricular function and geometry
- Leftward sepal shift from right ventricular volume overload can obstruct the outflow canula
- Reduction of right ventricular preload translates to left ventricular preload reduction
- Right ventricular evaluation with varying LVAD speeds is recommended

Anticoagulation
- Immediate post operative patients should not be given anticoagulation unless other indication (i.e., atrial or ventricular thrombus). In this period, risk of bleeding out weighs thrombotic risk
- Continuous flow LVADs require chronic oral anticoagulation with warfarin
- Goal range for warfarin oral anticoagulation is INR 1.8–2.4
- Aspirin 81 mg daily should be given

Infection
- Frequent cause of readmission at any time after implant (10–26%)
- LVAD infection associated with 30% reduced sruvival
- Three categories of infection: drive line infection, pump pocket infection, and pump endocarditis

MAP, mean arterial pressure; LVAD, left ventricular assist devices; INR, international normalized ratio.

TROUBLESHOOTING AND MONITORING STABLE DEVICE FUNCTION

Proper LVAD function can be monitored by parameters provided by the LVAD to include pump speed, power, pulsatility index and estimated flow. These parameters along with surveillance echocardiography provide excellent indicators of device function. Physicians caring for LVAD patients should be familiar with the following LVAD conditions and their acute management (Algorithm 5).

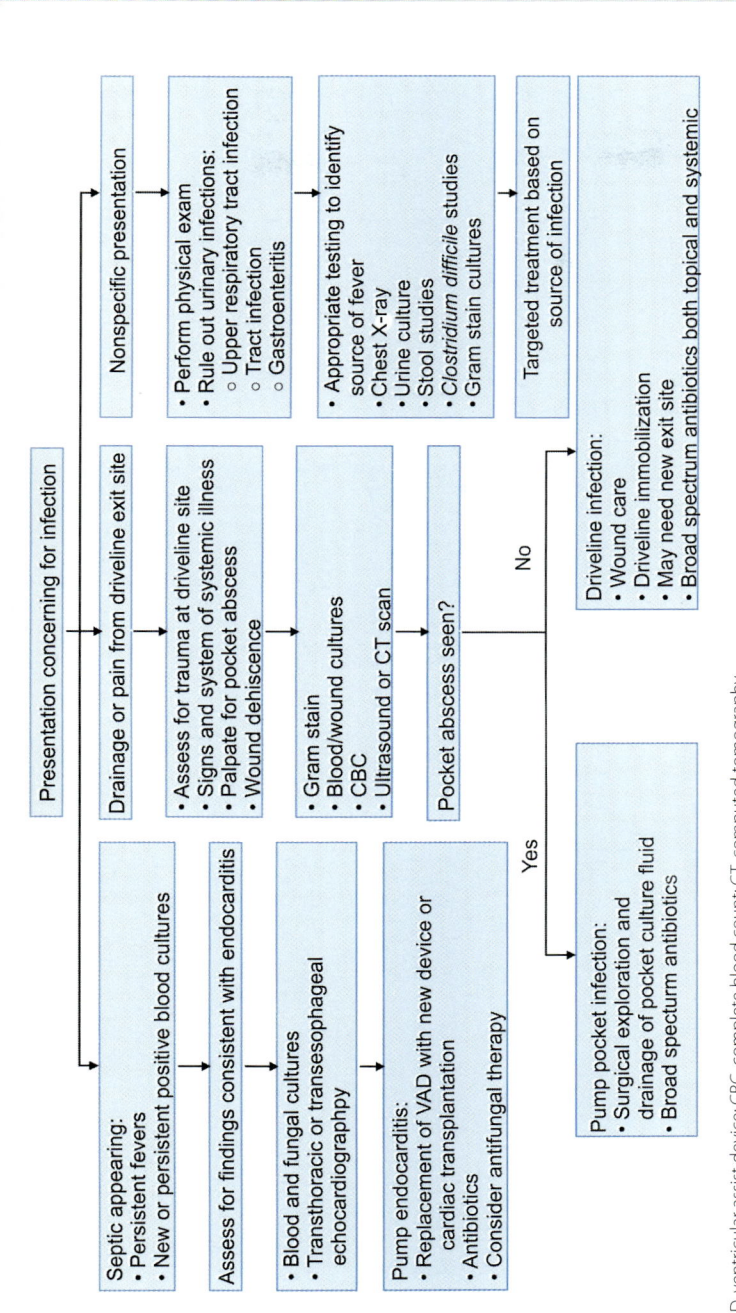

Approach to Left Ventricular Assist Devices and Follow-up...

Presentation concerning for infection

Septic appearing:
- Persistent fevers
- New or persistent positive blood cultures

Assess for findings consistent with endocarditis

- Blood and fungal cultures
- Transthoracic or transesophageal echocardiograhpy

Pump endocarditis:
- Replacement of VAD with new device or cardiac transplantation
- Antibiotics
- Consider antifungal therapy

Drainage or pain from driveline exit site

- Assess for trauma at driveline site
- Signs and system of systemic illness
- Palpate for pocket abscess
- Wound dehiscence

- Gram stain
- Blood/wound cultures
- CBC
- Ultrasound or CT scan

Pocket abscess seen?

Yes → **Pump pocket infection:**
- Surgical exploration and drainage of pocket culture fluid
- Broad spectrum antibiotics

No → **Driveline infection:**
- Wound care
- Driveline immobilization
- May need new exit site
- Broad spectrum antibiotics both topical and systemic

Nonspecific presentation

- Perform physical exam
- Rule out urinary infections:
  ○ Upper respiratory tract infection
  ○ Tract infection
  ○ Gastroenteritis

- Appropriate testing to identify source of fever
- Chest X-ray
- Urine culture
- Stool studies
- *Clostridium difficile* studies
- Gram stain cultures

Targeted treatment based on source of infection

VAD, ventricular assist device; CBC, complete blood count; CT, computed tomography.

ALGORITHM 4: Approach to patient with suspected left ventricular assist device infection

Algorithms in Heart Failure

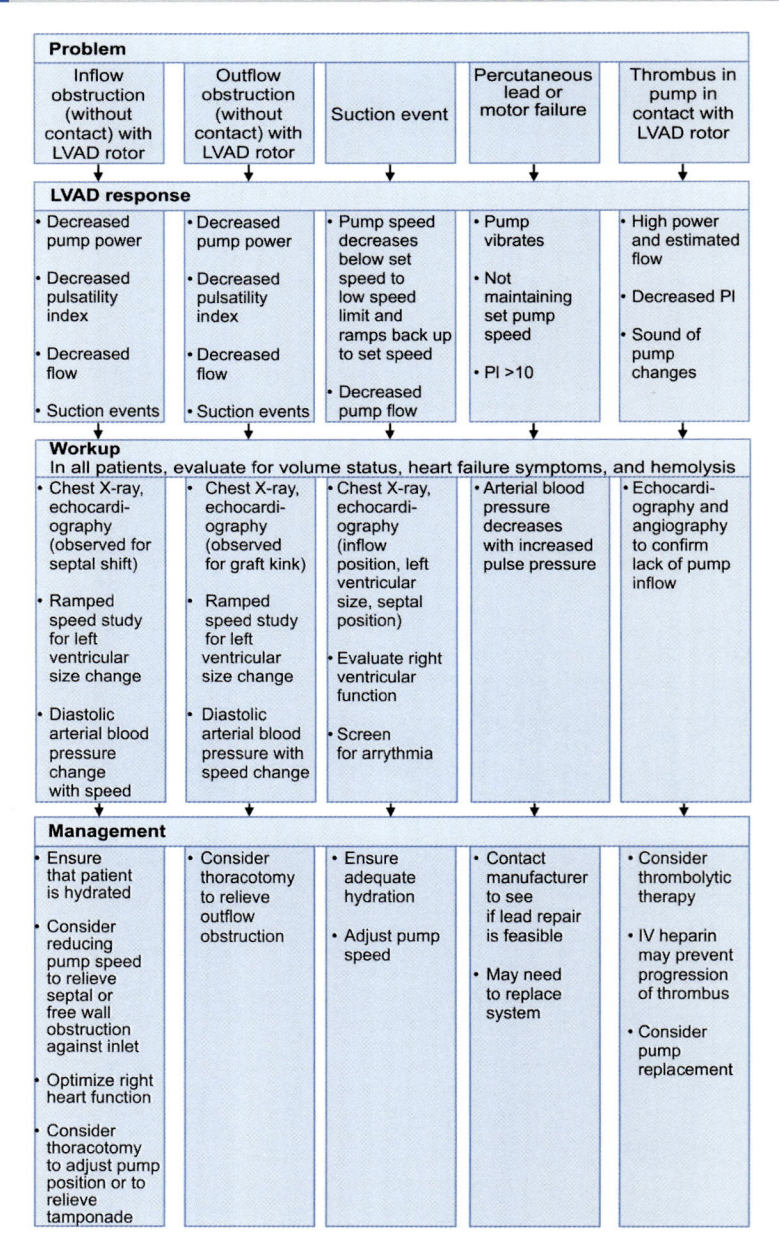

Problem				
Inflow obstruction (without contact) with LVAD rotor	Outflow obstruction (without contact) with LVAD rotor	Suction event	Percutaneous lead or motor failure	Thrombus in pump in contact with LVAD rotor

LVAD response				
• Decreased pump power • Decreased pulsatility index • Decreased flow • Suction events	• Decreased pump power • Decreased pulsatility index • Decreased flow • Suction events	• Pump speed decreases below set speed to low speed limit and ramps back up to set speed • Decreased pump flow	• Pump vibrates • Not maintaining set pump speed • PI >10	• High power and estimated flow • Decreased PI • Sound of pump changes

Workup				
In all patients, evaluate for volume status, heart failure symptoms, and hemolysis				
• Chest X-ray, echocardiography (observed for septal shift) • Ramped speed study for left ventricular size change • Diastolic arterial blood pressure change with speed	• Chest X-ray, echocardiography (observed for graft kink) • Ramped speed study for left ventricular size change • Diastolic arterial blood pressure with speed change	• Chest X-ray, echocardiography (inflow position, left ventricular size, septal position) • Evaluate right ventricular function • Screen for arrythmia	• Arterial blood pressure decreases with increased pulse pressure	• Echocardiography and angiography to confirm lack of pump inflow

Management				
• Ensure that patient is hydrated • Consider reducing pump speed to relieve septal or free wall obstruction against inlet • Optimize right heart function • Consider thoracotomy to adjust pump position or to relieve tamponade	• Consider thoracotomy to relieve outflow obstruction	• Ensure adequate hydration • Adjust pump speed	• Contact manufacturer to see if lead repair is feasible • May need to replace system	• Consider thrombolytic therapy • IV heparin may prevent progression of thrombus • Consider pump replacement

LVAD, left ventricular assist device; PI, pulsatility index.

ALGORITHM 5: Troubleshooting common problems in left ventricular assist devices

Left Ventricular Suction Event

Suction and associated flow events are most commonly a result of low left ventricular filling pressures or left ventricular free wall excursion into the left ventricular inflow cannula. This can occur if the pump speed is higher than the volume available to the LVAD. This may be due to dehydration or less commonly if the pump speed is set too high. In patients with a suction event, echocardiography and chest X-ray is indicated to evaluate for inflow cannula position and left ventricular size. Evaluation for arrhythmia should be considered as both a cause and effect of suction events. Right ventricular dysfunction can also impair preload to the inflow cannula. Treatment can include hydration or adjustment of pump speed.

Ventricular Arrhythmias

Patients with cardiomyopathy and, especially, ischemic cardiomyopathy, are susceptible to ventricular tachycardia (VT) or ventricular fibrillation (VF). Ventricular tachycardia or VF is a marker for increased mortality risk. Ventricular tachycardia or VF as a result of a suction event should be considered. Most patients have implantable cardioverter-defibrillators to allow antitachycardia pacing and some require VT radiofrequency ablation.

Pump Thrombus

Thrombus in the pump can affect speed, power, flow and pulsatile index. Etiologies include an embolic capture of thrombus into the device or growth of thrombus from prior deposits. In patients who are hemodynamically stable, heparin drip, or thrombolysis may resolve the clinical syndrome. If the device function is significantly affected by the presence of thrombus, LVAD replacement should be considered.

CONCLUSION

Identification of appropriate LVAD candidates as well as risk stratification is essential for counseling and referral for heart failure patients. Comorbidities must be identified at the time of referral and addressed prior to implantation. Routine ongoing care considerations as well as acute management considerations should be made known to healthcare teams that may encounter LVAD patients.

KEY POINTS

Preoperative selection and optimization

preoperative selection of patients should include consideration of the following:

- Surgical risk
- Dependable home support
- Adherence to medication and therapeutic regimen

Preoperative optimization of comorbid conditions should include:

- Nutritional status
- Optimize right heart function
- Appropriately timing anticoagulation and correcting coagulopathy

Patients with valvular disease:

- Mechanical aortic valve should be replaced with a bioprosthetic valve
- Aortic insufficiency, mitral regurgitation, mitral stenosis, and tricuspid regurgitation should be addressed during the time of surgery

Anatomic shunting should be evaluated for and corrected if necessary prior to procedure

Preoperative prealbumin level should be greater than 15 mg/dL prior to implant surgery.

Ongoing management

- Mean arterial pressure should be targeted to 70–90 mmHg
- Early echocardiography is recommended to guide management of right ventricular function
- Anticoagulation in patients with pulsatile pumps necessitates use of warfarin at a goal international normalized ratio of 1.5–2.5. In patients with axial, continuous pumps, aspirin should be added
- Patients with fever or leukocytosis should be scrutinized with high suspicion for systemic infection or pump endocarditis.

Troubleshooting

- Left ventricular assist device (LVAD) function assessments should include pump speed, power, pulsatile index, and estimated flow
- Ventricular arrhythmia in patients with LVAD should include consideration of a suction event of the left ventricular free wall or septum
- New onset hemolysis during LVAD support should lead to assessment for pump thrombosis.

SUGGESTED READINGS

1. Bedi M, Kormos R, Winowich S, McNamara DM, Mathier MA, Murali S. Ventricular arrhythmias during left ventricular assist device support. Am J Cardiol. 2007;99(8):1151-3.
2. Bennett MK, Roberts CA, Dordunoo D, Shah A, Russell SD. Ideal methodology to assess systemic blood pressure in patients with continuous-flow left ventricular assist devices. J Heart Lung Transplant. 2010;29(5):593-4.
3. Epstein AE, DiMarco JP, Ellenbogen KA, Estes NA, Freedman RA, Gettes LS, et al. 2012 ACCF/AHA/HRS focused update incorporated into the ACCF/AHA/HRS 2008 guidelines for device-based therapy of cardiac rhythm abnormalities: a report of the American College of Cardiology Foundation/American Heart Association Task Force on Practice Guidelines and the Heart Rhythm Society. J Am Coll Cardiol. 2013;61(3):e6-75.
4. Goldstein DJ, John R, Salerno C, Silvestry S, Moazami N, Horstmanshof D, et al. Algorithm for the diagnosis and management of suspected pump thrombus. J Heart Lung Transplant. 2013;32(7):667-70.
5. Hasin T, Marmor Y, Kremers W, Topilsky Y, Severson CJ, Schirger JA, et al. Readmissions after implantation of axial flow left ventricular assist device. J Am Coll Cardiol. 2013;61(2):153-63.
6. Holdy K, Dembitsky W, Eaton LL, Chillcott S, Stahovich M, Rasmusson B, et al. Nutrition assessment and management of left ventricular assist device patients. J Heart Lung Transplant. 2005;24(10);1690-6.
7. Kirklin JK, Naftel DC, Kormos RL, Stevenson LW, Pagani FD, Miller MA, et al. Second INTERMACS annual report: more than 1,000 primary left ventricular assist device implants. J Heart Lung Transplant. 2010;29(1):1-10.
8. Lietz K, Long JW, Kfoury AG, Slaughter MS, Silver MA, Milano CA, et al. Outcomes of left ventricular assist device implantation as destination therapy in the post-REMATCH era: implications for patient selection. Circulation. 2007;116:497-505.
9. Lockard KL, DeGore L, Schwarm P, Winowich S, O'Shea G, Siegenthaler M, et al. Lack of Improvement in Prealbumin at Two Weeks Predicts a Poor Outcome after Mechanical Circulatory Support. J Heart Lung Transplant. 2009;28(2):S66.
10. Mano A, Fujita K, Uenomachi K, Kazama K, Katabuchi M, Wada K, et al. Body mass index is a useful predictor of prognosis after left ventricular assist system implantation. J Heart Lung Transplant. 2009;28(5):428-33.
11. Simon D, Fischer S, Grossman A, Downer C, Hota B, Heroux A, et al. Left ventricular assist device-related infection: treatment and outcome. Clin Infect Dis. 2005;40(8):1108-15.
12. Slaughter MS, Pagani FD, Rogers JG, Miller LW, Sun B, Russell SD, et al. Clinical management of continuous-flow left ventricular assist devices in advanced heart failure. J Heart Lung Transplant. 2010;29(4 Suppl):S1-39.
13. Wilson SR, Givertz MM, Stewart GC, Mudge GH Jr. Ventricular assist devices the challenges of outpatient management. J Am Coll Cardiol. 2009;54(18):1647-59.

CHAPTER 27

How to Approach Palliative and End-of-life Care?

Tiny Jaarsma, Anna Strömberg

INTRODUCTION

While the disease trajectory of each heart failure (HF) patient is different, a pattern of gradual decline is likely, punctuated by episodes of acute deterioration and, eventually, a seemingly unexpected death or death owing to progressive HF. Across the course of the illness, most HF patients will go through several phases which can be marked by different goals for treatment and care and different issues in communication. Open and clear communication is vital to ensure good quality of care during the disease trajectory of the HF patients, their family, and caregivers. Ineffective communications on prognosis and needs of patients can increase anxiety and uncertainty in patients affecting their outcomes.

Implementing palliative care for people with HF does not need to be based on risk of death prediction, but on recognition that the patients with HF palliative care needs. Palliative care services should be integrated with cardiological ones along the whole disease trajectory (parallel care). Prognostication is not needed to implement palliative care, but can be valuable for planning end-of-life care.

PLANNING CARE IN THE DIFFERENT PHASES OF THE HEART FAILURE TRAJECTORY

Although the HF trajectory is unpredictable and there are no clear boundaries between phases, it is important to realize that as the

How to Approach Palliative and End-of-life Care?

disease progresses; the goals of treatment should be re-evaluated, as previous aims can become unrealistic and reflect false hope.

Preferences from patients and family members during the HF trajectory include:
- Good communication with healthcare providers:
  - Respect
  - Comprehensive information
  - Guidance on how to respond to a medical emergency
  - Discuss prognosis
  - Time to deal with practical matters regarding end-of-life
- Recognizing and adressing physical needs:
  - Control of HF symptoms
- Adressing psychosocial needs:
  - Loss of social contacts
  - Increased dependency on others
- Respect and address spiritual needs.

Descisions and advanced planning with regard to palliative care and end-of-life care discussions should be documented, regularly reviewed, and routinely communicated to all those involved in the patient's care (Algorithm 1).

Healthcare providers should make sure that:
- Patient and care giver preferences are followed wherever possible
- Patients may choose not to or not be in a position express preferences, e.g., due to symptoms of depression or cognitive impairment
- Patient and caregiver preferences may change as health status and other circumstances alter, and should regularly be reviewed.

Stage 1

Diagnosis and First Contacts with Healthcare Providers, Treatment Initiation and Stabilization: Chronic Phase (Fig. 1)

For most patients with HF, start a disease trajectory after diagnosis, with a relatively stable primary phase needing routine chronic disease management. Since palliative care as defined by the World Health Organization as care focusing on symptom relief and spiritual and psychosocial support from diagnosis to the end-of-life, the palliative care communication and planning should start already when a patient is diagnosed with HF, often the main responsibility of patient care is in the primary care.

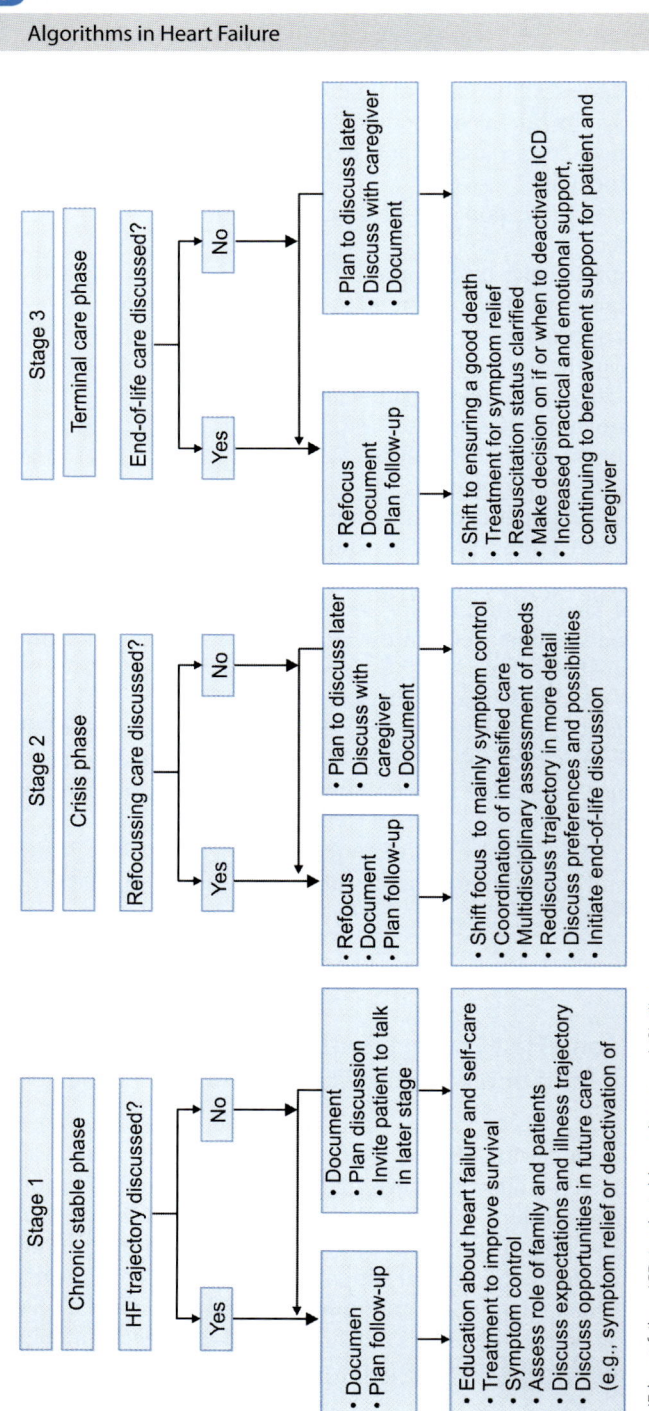

Algorithms in Heart Failure

Stage 1
Chronic stable phase

HF trajectory discussed?

- **Yes**
  - Documen
  - Plan follow-up
  - Education about heart failure and self-care
  - Treatment to improve survival
  - Symptom control
  - Assess role of family and patients
  - Discuss expectations and illness trajectory
  - Discuss opportunities in future care (e.g., symptom relief or deactivation of

- **No**
  - Document
  - Plan discussion
  - Invite patient to talk in later stage

Stage 2
Crisis phase

Refocussing care discussed?

- **Yes**
  - Refocus
  - Document
  - Plan follow-up
  - Shift focus to mainly symptom control
  - Coordination of intensified care
  - Multidisciplinary assessment of needs
  - Rediscuss trajectory in more detail
  - Discuss preferences and possibilities
  - Initiate end-of-life discussion

- **No**
  - Plan to discuss later
  - Discuss with caregiver
  - Document

Stage 3
Terminal care phase

End-of-life care discussed?

- **Yes**
  - Refocus
  - Document
  - Plan follow-up

- **No**
  - Plan to discuss later
  - Discuss with caregiver
  - Document

- Shift to ensuring a good death
- Treatment for symptom relief
- Resuscitation status clarified
- Make decision on if or when to deactivate ICD
- Increased practical and emotional support, continuing to bereavement support for patient and caregiver

HF, heart failure; ICD, implantable cardioverter-defibrillator.

ALGORITHM 1: In planning discussions of the heart failure trajectory and end of life with heart failure patients and their families

How to Approach Palliative and End-of-life Care?

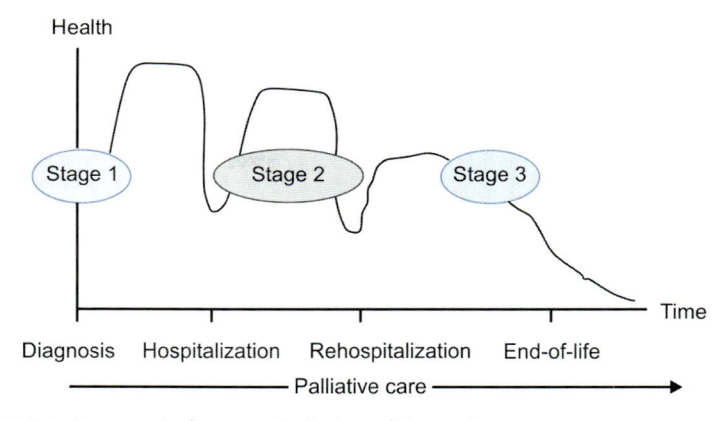

FIG. 1: Focus and refocus care in the heart failure trajectory

Focus of Treatment and Care

- Goals of care include active monitoring, guideline based therapy to prolong survival, symptom control, self-care, patient and caregiver education
- Patients are given comprehensive education of their condition including treatment options, self-care, and prognosis
- Regular monitoring and appropriate review according to national guidelines and local protocols
- Determine and discuss the role of the family or caregivers
- Discuss what the patients expects and wishes and what to do in case of an acute or slow deterioration
- Discuss issues around cardiac resynchronization therapy or implantable cardioverter defibrillator (ICD) in case of implantation.

Stage 2

Hospitalization or Rehospitalization (Crisis Phase) and Refocusing (Fig. 1)

Being admitted to hospital due to deteriorating HF is an indicator that the prognosis of the patient worsened. Therefore, palliative care needs to be refocused including more education on monitoring and management of symptoms of deterioration, e.g., daily weighing and symptom control and flexible diuretic intake in case of congestion. Patients and their families often need psychosocial support from healthcare professionals to handle the physical and psychosocial aspects of the HF syndrome and HF self-care.

Focus of Treatment and Care

- The goal of care shifts increasingly to maintaining optimal symptom control and quality of life
- A key professional might be identified in the clinic or the community to co-ordinate care and liaise between specialist HF, palliative care, and other services
- A holistic, multidisciplinary assessment of patient and caregiver needs takes place
- Opportunities to discuss prognosis and the likely course of the illness in more detail are provided by professionals, including recommendation for completing an advance care plan
- Out-of-hours services are documented in care plans in the event of acute deterioration.

Stage 3

Further Deterioration and Terminal Care Phase: Intensify Care (Fig. 1)

Patients suffering from repeated hospitalizations have a very poor prognosis. They often suffer from several handicapping symptoms, have a decreased quality of life, and more depressive symptoms. At this stage of medical and device treatment, psychosocial support, and educational initiatives need to be intensified. Clinical indicators include, despite maximal treatment, renal impairment, hypotension, persistent edema, fatigue, and cachexia.

Somewhere after this stage, the patients with HF enter the terminal phase. The care then needs to be intensified and home-based care is often the most convenient alternative for the patient and his/her family. However, home-based palliative care services are not available for patients with HF to the same extent as cancer patients.

Focus of Treatment and Care

- Goals for treatment are shifting to ensure a good death and dignity without agony and suffering
- Heart failure treatment for symptom control is continued and resuscitation status clarified, documented, and communicated to all care providers

- An integrated care pathway for the dying may be introduced to structure care planning
- Increased practical and emotional support for carers is provided, continuing to bereavement support
- Issues to consider include:
  - Is home an appropriate environment to die?
  - Is (night) sedation needed?
  - Is dietary advice needed?
  - What regimen is still needed and which interventions or drugs can be discontinued?
  - Who will regularly assess the patient conditions and advice on the need for a change in treatment?
  - What is the resuscitation status of the patient and document do not resuscitate if relevant (discuss with family and carers)
- Treatment for symptoms needs to be considered and might include opioids for dyspnea and pain; oxygen for dyspnea; stimulants for fatigue; benzodiazepines or counseling for anxiety; lower extremity strengthening for fatigue and dyspnea; continuous positive airway pressure or oxygen for sleep-disordered breathing; and antidepressants
- Comfort measures include:
  - Medication is assessed and nonessentials discontinued
  - There is a protocol on subcutaneous drugs (pain, agitation, nausea)
- Review ICD and other devices; if appropriate plan deactivation.

CONCLUSION

Palliative care focuses on symptom relief and spiritual and psychosocial support from diagnosis to the end of life.

Communication and planning should start already early in the HF trajectory and care should be adjusted and refocused in different stages. Decisions and advanced planning with regard to palliative care and end-of-life care discussions should be documented, regularly reviewed, and routinely communicated to all those involved in the patient's care. This includes an assessment of understanding and needs, planning for the future, including advance directives, discussing the potential need for device withdrawal and symptom management.

Algorithms in Heart Failure

KEY POINTS

- ❏ Patient and caregiver preferences may change as health status and other circumstances alter, and should regularly be reviewed
- ❏ Even with an unpredictable trajectory, it is vital to regularly evaluate the goals of treatment and care as previous goals can become unrealistic and reflect false hope
- ❏ Open and clear communication is vital to ensure good quality of care during the disease trajectory of the heart failure patients, their family and caregivers.

SUGGESTED READINGS

1. Clayton JM, Hancock KM, Butow FN, Tattersall MH, Currow DC; Adler J, et al. Clinical practice guidelines for communicating prognosis and end-of-life issues with adults in the advanced stages of a life-limiting illness, and their caregivers. Med J Aust. 2007;186;(12 Suppl):S77, S79, S83-108.
2. Goodlin SJ. Palliative Care in congestive heart failure. J Am Coll Cardiol. 2009;54(5):386-96.the A
3. Low J, Pattenden J, Candy B, Beattie JM, Jones L. Palliative care in advanced heart failure: an international review of the perspectives of recipients and health professionals on care provision. J Card Fail. 2011;17(3):231-52.
4. Lawrie I, Kite S. Communication in heart failure. In: Johnson M, Lehman R, Twycross R (Eds). Heart Failure and Palliative Care: A Team Approach, 1st edition. UK: Oxford; 2006.
5. Jaarsma T, Beattie JM, Ryder M, Rutten FH, McDonagh T, Mohacsi P, et al. Palliative care in heart failure: a position statement from the palliative care workshop of the Heart Failure Association of the European Society of Cardiology. Eur J Heart Fail. 2009;11(5):433-43.
6. Scottish Partnership for Palliative Care. (2008). Living and dying with advanced heart failure: a palliative care approach. [online] Available from www.palliativecarescotland.org.uk/content/publications/HF-final-document.pdf. [Accessed November, 2014].

SECTION 6

Cardiomyopathies: Practical Recommendations to Diagnosis and Management

28
CHAPTER

Hypertrophic Cardiomyopathy

Christian Prinz, Lothar Faber, Alan S Maisel

INTRODUCTION

The prevalence of hypertrophic cardiomyopathy (HCM) is estimated to be one case per 500–1,000 in the overall population. The hallmark of this cardiomyopathy is an excessive thickening of the left ventricular myocardium, occasionally, also of the right ventricular myocardium, without any other identifiable causes such as arterial hypertension or valve disease. It is possible to distinguish two phenotypes of HCM. Most common HCM is the hypertrophic obstructive cardiomyopathy (HOCM, 70%) in which there is left ventricular outflow tract obstruction. Less commonly the hypertrophic nonobstructive cardiomyopathy phenotype (HNCM) is present.

CLINICALLY IMPORTANT PATHOPHYSIOLOGICAL PRINCIPLES

Algorithm 1 demonstrates clinically important pathophysiological principles in HCM.

CLINICAL OBSERVATIONS AND SYMPTOMS

Patients may be completely asymptomatic or severely restricted by the disease. Classical findings in history or on clinical examination are dyspnea and angina pectoris under stress. Furthermore, dizziness, palpitations, and occasionally, syncope are common. The

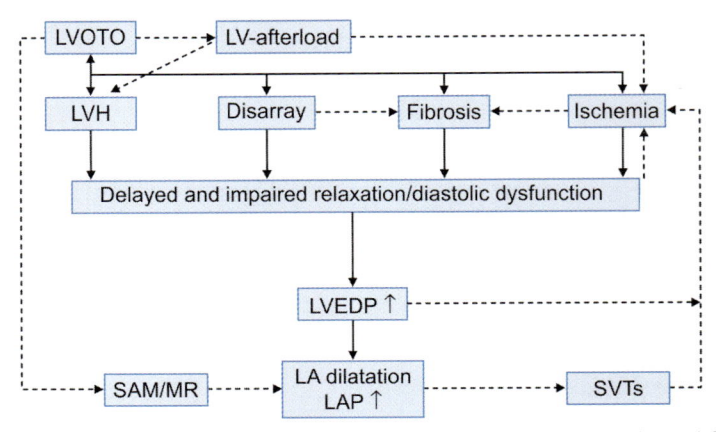

```
┌───────┐      ┌─────────────┐
│ LVOTO │------│ LV-afterload│----------------------------┐
└───┬───┘      └──────┬──────┘                            │
    │    ╲            │                                   │
    ▼     ╲           ▼           ▼            ▼          │
┌───────┐  ┌─────────┐    ┌──────────┐   ┌──────────┐    │
│  LVH  │  │ Disarray│----│ Fibrosis │---│ Ischemia │◄---┤
└───┬───┘  └────┬────┘    └────┬─────┘   └────┬─────┘    │
    │           │              │              │          │
    ▼           ▼              ▼              ▼          │
┌─────────────────────────────────────────────────┐      │
│ Delayed and impaired relaxation/diastolic dysfunction │ │
└───────────────────────┬─────────────────────────┘      │
                        ▼                                │
                  ┌──────────┐                           │
                  │ LVEDP ↑  │---------------------------┤
                  └─────┬────┘                           │
                        ▼                                ▼
┌──────────┐      ┌─────────────┐              ┌──────────┐
│ SAM/MR   │------│ LA dilatation│-------------│  SVTs    │
└──────────┘      │   LAP ↑     │              └──────────┘
                  └─────────────┘
```

LVOTO, left ventricular outflow tract obstruction; LVH, left ventricular hypertrophy; LV, left ventricular; LVEDP, left ventricular end-diastolic pressure; SAM, systolic anterior movement; MR, mitral regurgitation; LAP, left atrial pressure; SVTs, supraventricular tachycardias.

ALGORITHM 1: Clinically important pathophysiological principles causing diastolic dysfunction in hypertrophic cardiomyopathy

most devastating symptom remains sudden cardiac death (SCD) caused by malignant arrhythmias. Routine management includes, therefore, repeated risk stratification.

DIAGNOSTIC ALGORITHMS

Physical Examination

The physician should first take a detailed clinical history of the patients pertaining to signs and symptoms and possible risk factors for SCD (see algorithm later). Furthermore, a detailed physical examination should be performed. In all patients the physician should be aware of the stigmata of systemic diseases, occasionally associated with left ventricular hypertrophy such as Noonan syndrome (facial dysmorphia) or Anderson-Fabry disease (typical maculopapular skin lesions) since these disorders may require specific therapeutic approaches.

Electrocardiography

Most HCM patients (75–95%) show unspecific electrocardiography changes (e.g., signs for left ventricular hypertrophy, hyper-voltage, pseudo-infarct Q waves). However, a normal electrocardiogram (ECG) never excludes the presence of HCM.

Echocardiographic Evaluation

Echocardiography should be performed in all patients with HCM (also using of axis views) since a maximal wall thickness of greater than 30 mm is an established risk marker for SCD. Doppler echocardiography can be used to quantify the severity of left ventricular outflow tract obstruction and to calculate the pressure gradients. The severity of mitral regurgitation can be assessed by Doppler echocardiography. As indirect but reliable sign, an enlargement of the left atrium reflects ventricular relaxation disturbances. Furthermore, a flattening of the EF slope of the anterior mitral leaflet, and a reduction or prolongation of the rapid filling phase all indicates diastolic ventricular dysfunction. Also on echocardiography attention must be paid to signs for cardiac storage disorders or myocardial hypertrophy due to secondary causes such as valve diseases.

USE OF OTHER IMAGING MODALITIES

In patients with insufficient acoustic window, maximal wall thicknesses and determination of the left ventricular muscle mass can also be determined by using cardiac magnetic resonance imaging or cardiac tomography. Myocardial scars and myocardial fibrosis can be detected by using late gadolinium-enhanced cardiac magnetic resonance imaging. Recent reports indicate that there may be a causal relationship between the extent of fibrosis and the risk of ventricular arrhythmias.

USE OF BIOMARKERS

The authors recommend baseline assessment of B-type natriuretic peptide (BNP) or N-terminal proBNP in HCM patients with clinical signs and symptoms of heart failure. B-type natriuretic peptide levels can be used for therapy guidance and to assess the success of medical therapy in decompensated patients.

Until now, the role of biomarkers for the detection of myocardial fibrosis in HCM remains unclear. Probably in the future, clinical management and risk stratification will be changed by integrating biomarkers for the detection of myocardial fibrosis in HCM.

EXERCISE TESTS

Spiroergometry should be performed to determine the objective workload capacity in patients with HCM. This method also provides information about blood pressure response at rest and under load (risk stratification) and provides information about therapeutic success.

Rhythm Diagnostics

Established risk stratification requires a 48-hour (ambulatory) Holter ECG recording to detect nonsustained ventricular tachycardia (nsVT). In the last years, invasive electrophysiological examination has become less important. The authors only carry out this type of recording for specific instances (for example, suspicion of concomitant Wolff-Parkinson-White syndrome).

Invasive Diagnostics

In order to exclude or verify coexistent coronary sclerosis, to evaluate the vascular supply to the septum prior to planned septal ablation, and to verify prognostically relevant myocardial bridging, the authors recommend invasive diagnostics. Myocardial storage diseases (amyloidosis) should be excluded by myocardial biopsies. Elevated end-diastolic left ventricular pressure is usually an expression of a lack of distensibility and a sign for diastolic dysfunction.

Molecular Genetics

Evaluating first degree relatives for the presence of HCM is recommended. If genetic diagnostics are not possible, adolescents between 12 years and 18 years of age should be examined annually, and adults over 18 years of age every 5 years, using echocardiography.

THERAPEUTIC ALGORITHMS

In HCM, physical endurance activity should be performed in the aerobic range (abstaining from high performance sports, athletics, or competitive sports). However, the authors recommend not a general prohibition on sports. Smoking should be avoided and alcohol should not be ingested since outflow tract obstruction can be aggravated by reduction of afterload and cause arrhythmias. The

Hypertrophic Cardiomyopathy

earlier indication for infective endocarditis prophylaxis with HOCM has since been qualified.

RISK STRATIFICATION

Treatment of high-risk HCM patients with implantable cardioverter defibrillator (ICD) has proven to prevent SCD (Algorithm 2).

Until now, five major risk factors have been identified. High-risk patients with greater than or equal to two risk factors are considered to have an annual SCD rate of approximately 4%. The single risk factors are:

- There is a positive family history of premature SCD caused by HCM in about 25% of the affected families (<45 years of age)
- Documented nsVT is a sensitive marker for increased risk of suffering SCD
- Syncope at rest or during exercise is an important risk marker for all age groups
- An abnormal blood pressure response during exercise is defined as an increase in the systolic blood pressure of less than 20 mmHg from the baseline value. A progressive fall in blood pressure during exercise or a fall in the systolic value by 20 mmHg after an initial increase, particularly in younger patients (<40 years of age) is also assessed as being associated with risk
- Extreme left ventricular hypertrophy with wall thicknesses greater than 30 mm is also associated with risk.

The authors consider two first degree risk markers to be an indication for primary prophylactic ICD implantation. An individual decision must be made for patients with one first degree

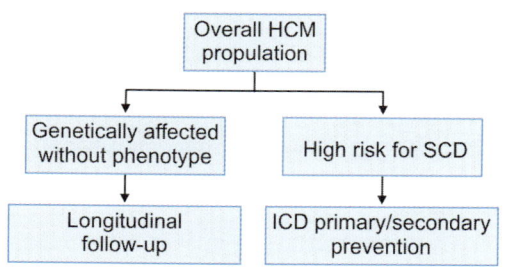

HCM, hypertrophic cardiomyopathy; SCD, sudden cardiac death; ICD, implantable cardioverter defibrillator.

ALGORITHM 2: Importance of identifying hypertrophic cardiomyopathy patients at high risk for sudden cardiac death. Such patients should be treated by an implantable cardioverter defibrillator. All other patients should undergo longitudinal follow-up

TABLE 1: Identification at risk hypertrophic cardiomyopathy patients for implantation with an implantable cardioverter defibrillator

First degree risk factors	Definition
Positive family history of SCD	Cases with SCD <45 years
Recurrent syncope	≥2 incidents
Left ventricular hypertrophy	≥30 mm at any side in the left ventricle
Abnormal BPR during exercise	Increase <20 mmHg or fall >20 mmHg
Nonsustained VT in Holter ECG	≥3 consecutive QRS complexes with HR ≥120 beats/min

Second degree risk factors	Definition
Atrial fibrillation/atrial flutter	Any form
Left atrial dilatation	>45 mm (M-Mode echo)
High LVOT gradient at rest, evidence of myocardial ischemia during exercise	>80 mmHg (CW-Doppler)
Early manifestation of HCM	<30 years of age
Myocardial bridging near the LAD	In younger patients (<45 years)
Marked fibrosis in cardiac MRI	Fibrosis ≥2 segments in 17 segment model of the left ventricle

HCM, hypertrophic cardiomyopathy; ICD, implantable cardioverter defibrillator; SCD, sudden cardiac death; BPR, blood pressure response; VT, ventricular tachycardia; ECG, electrocardiogram; LVOT, left ventricular outflow tract; MRI, magnetic resonance imaging; HR, heart rate; CW-Doppler, continuous wave-Doppler; LAD, left descending artery.

risk marker. Second degree risk factors may provide additional support for decisions (Table 1). A previously survived cardiac arrest or documentation of sustained ventricular tachycardia is clear indications for an ICD implantation.

Table 1 gives an algorithm to identify at-risk HCM patients for implantation with an implantable cardioverter defibrillator (ICD). If two first degree risk factors are present, an ICD should be implanted. In case of one present risk factor, an individualized approach should be used. Presence or absence of second risk factors may be helpful for decision making.

Asymptomatic Patients

In asymptomatic patients, there is no clear indication for pharmacotherapy due to an absence of data. For pathophysiological considerations, the authors advise initiating pharmacotherapy using β-blockers. The role of an upstream medical therapy to prevent myocardial fibrosis including statins, ω-3 polyunsaturated fatty acids or aldosterone receptor blockers remains unclear until now. However, risk evaluation should be performed precisely in this group of patients. The authors recommend strict control of any coexistent arterial hypertension (reduction of the myocardial growth stimulus) which is of particular importance.

Symptomatic Hypertrophic Nonobstructive Cardiomyopathy Phenotype Patients

Beta-blockers or verapamil-type calcium antagonists should be used for rate control due to the ubiquitous presence of diastolic dysfunction in HCM (Algorithm 3). In patients with signs of congestion or concomitant hypertension, the authors recommend the use of diuretics and angiotensin converting enzyme inhibitors (ACEIs) or angiotensin receptor antagonists. It is important to perform a tight monitoring because the authors and others observed in individual cases induction of an outflow tract obstruction in patients who were initially recorded as having HNCM. If atrial fibrillation occurs, patients develop oftentimes with loss of an active ventricular filling a considerable drop in output and are at higher risk of cardiac embolic events. The authors recommend the prompt use of anticoagulants.

Symptomatic Hypertrophic Obstructive Cardiomyopathy Patients

Taking pathophysiology into account, agents for the reduction of preload or afterload (such as nitrate, ACEIs, and nifedipine-type calcium antagonists) should be avoided in HOCM due to possible aggravation of the outflow tract obstruction gradients. Therefore, therapy of coexistent arterial hypertension may be difficult. Also positive inotropic drugs such as digitalis preparations should not be used. The authors prefer and recommend the use of β-blockers which prolong diastole and improve, therefore, diastolic left ventricular filling. Furthermore, they reduce obstruction of the outflow tract due to a negative inotropic effect. If β-blockers are not well-tolerated or are not sufficiently effective, a switch to verapamil-type calcium antagonists is possible. In case of severe coexisting arterial hypertension diuretics and/or central α-blockers can be used in order to avoid exacerbation of the left ventricular outflow tract obstruction.

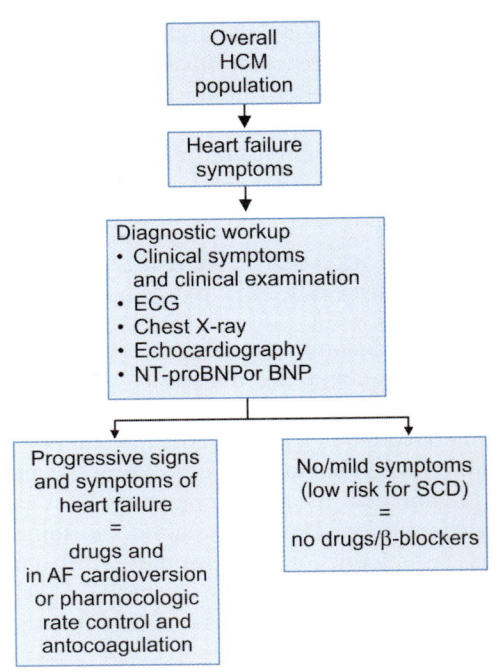

Algorithms in Heart Failure

```
┌─────────────┐
│  Overall    │
│   HCM       │
│ population  │
└──────┬──────┘
       ▼
┌─────────────┐
│Heart failure│
│  symptoms   │
└──────┬──────┘
       ▼
┌─────────────────────┐
│ Diagnostic workup   │
│ • Clinical symptoms │
│   and clinical      │
│   examination       │
│ • ECG               │
│ • Chest X-ray       │
│ • Echocardiography  │
│ • NT-proBNP or BNP  │
└──────┬──────────────┘
       │
   ┌───┴────┐
   ▼        ▼
```

| Progressive signs and symptoms of heart failure = drugs and in AF cardioversion or pharmacologic rate control and antocoagulation | No/mild symptoms (low risk for SCD) = no drugs/β-blockers |

HCM, hypertrophic cardiomyopathy; ECG, electrocardiogram; NT-proBNP, N-terminal pro-B-type natriuretic peptide; BNP, B-type natriuretic peptide; SCD, sudden cardiac death; AF, atrial fibrillation.

ALGORITHM 3: The chart shows an algorithm for the Treatment of HCM patients affected by heart failure symptoms. However, each patient needs an individualized therapeutically approach

Beyond medical therapy, septal myectomy using the Morrow procedure was the standard therapy for many years for patients with HOCM who cannot be adequately treated using pharmacotherapy (Algorithm 4). During this procedure, a part of the hypertrophied basal septum will be excised which leads to a thinning of the remaining septum to 5–8 mm. This procedure has success rates of more than 90%. The authors recommend the procedure in patients with symptoms corresponding to New York Heart Association class III and a gradient greater than 50 mmHg (at rest or provocation). Literature reports about a perioperative mortality in experienced centers of approximately 1–2%. The rate of complete atrioventricular blocks is postoperatively about 2–5%.

Another therapeutically approach uses pacemaker stimulation in order to reduce the obstruction of the left ventricular outflow

Hypertrophic Cardiomyopathy

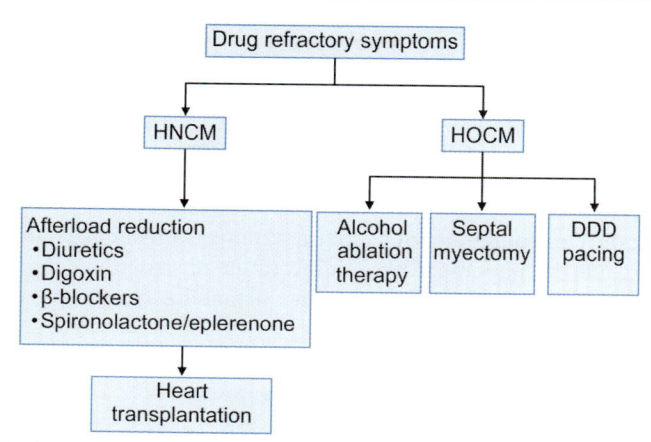

```
                    Drug refractory symptoms
                    /                        \
                 HNCM                        HOCM
                   |                    /     |      \
    Afterload reduction           Alcohol  Septal   DDD
      • Diuretics                 ablation myectomy pacing
      • Digoxin                   therapy
      • β-blockers
      • Spironolactone/eplerenone
                   |
               Heart
           transplantation
```

HOCM, hypertrophic obstructive cardiomyopathy; HNCM, hypertrophic nonobstructive cardiomyopathy; DDD, dual-chamber.

ALGORITHM 4: Treatment of hypertrophic obstructive cardiomyopathy patients. It is important to recognize that the therapy between patients with obstruction and without obstruction differs due to the different therapeutically possibilities

tract. First euphoric results to this technique in the 1990s had to be relativized since more recent studies have demonstrated a significant placebo effect.

Since the introduction of percutaneous septal ablation therapy (known as percutaneous tansluminal septal myocardial ablation, transcoronary ablation of septal hypertrophy, acetylsalicylic acid or aspirin or erythropoiesis-stimulating agents), the range of therapeutic options for symptomatic HOCM patients was expanded. During the procedure, 1–3 mL of 96% ethanol are injected into one of the septal branches supplying the hypertrophied myocardium which causes acute regional contractile dysfunction and will lead to a thinning of the hypertrophied myocardium over the long term. Success rates of this iatrogenic chemical necrosis with a clear reduction or elimination of the obstruction is achieved in 90% of all cases. Recent data demonstrated that the mortality associated with the procedure is similar to that for myectomy (1–2%) in experienced centers. Implantation of pacemakers due to high-grade AV blocks initially occurred in up to 30% of patients but this complication could be reduced in established centers to significantly lower values of up to 5%.

After myectomy or septal ablation, the recommend continuing pharmacotherapy (β-blockers, calcium antagonists) to prevent progression of the underlying disease.

CONCLUSION

Hypertrophic cardiomyopathy (HCM) is the most common hereditary disease of the heart. Risk stratification regarding the need for prophylactic implantation of an implantable cardiac defibrillator (ICD) is crucial. Pharmacotherapy follows the treatment of patients with heart failure with a normal ejection fraction (HFNEF). Surgical myectomy and percutaneous septal ablation are nowadays standard treatments in patients with outflow tract obstruction (HOCM). Goals for treatment should be a near-normal life expectancy and a highly satisfactory quality of life.

KEY POINTS

- Treatment of hypertrophic cardiomyopathy requires continuous monitoring in, or in collaboration with, specialized centers
- Every patient, even asymptomatic patients, should undergo adequate risk stratification in terms of the risk of sudden cardiac death, with subsequent implantable cardioverter defibrillator implantation if required
- Symptomatic treatment of patients with hypertrophic non-obstructive cardiomyopathy corresponds to specific treatment of heart failure
- For symptomatic hypertrophic obstructive cardiomyopathy, septal ablation and septal myectomy are now comparable procedures. The choice of method depends on an individual approach.

SUGGESTED READINGS

1. Gersh BJ, Maron BJ, Bonow RO, Dearani JA, Fifer MA, Link MS, et al. 2011 ACCF/AHA guideline for the diagnosis and treatment of hypertrophic cardiomyopathy: executive summary: a report of the American College of Cardiology Foundation/American Heart Association task Force on Practice Guidelines. Circulation. 2011;124:2761-96.
2. Maron BJ, McKenna WJ, Danielson GK, Kappenberger LJ, Kuhn HJ, Seidman CE, et al. American College of Cardiology/European Society of Cardiology Clinical Expert Consensus Document on Hypertrophic Cardiomyopathy: a report of the American College of cardiology Foundation Task Force on Clinical Expert Consensus Documents and the European Society of Cardiology Committee for Practice Guidelines. Eur Heart J. 2003;24:1965-91.
3. Prinz C, Farr M, Hering D, Horstkotte D, Faber L. The diagnosis and treatment of hypertrophic cardiomyopathy. Dtsch Arztebl Int. 2011;108:209-15.
4. Prinz C, Farr M, Laser KT, Esdorn H, Piper C, Horstkotte D, et al. Determining the role of fibrosis in hypertrophic cardiomyopathy. Expert Rev Cardiovasc Ther. 2013;11:495-504.

CHAPTER 29

Takotsubo Syndrome

Andrew C Morley-Smith, Alexander R Lyon

INTRODUCTION

Takotsubo syndrome (TTS) is an increasingly recognized, but still underdiagnosed cause of reversible acute cardiomyopathy. Takotsubo syndrome was first described in Japan, and named takotsubo after the left ventricle's resemblance to the Japanese fisherman's octopus trap at ventriculography. Also known as stress cardiomyopathy or "broken heart syndrome," it is a clinical syndrome mimicking acute ST elevation myocardial infarction (STEMI), but in the absence of causative obstructive coronary artery disease. Catecholamine surge is the etiological cornerstone in TTS, with serum levels at presentation significantly elevated compared both to resting levels in the same patient and to levels in comparable patients with acute ischemic heart failure. As such TTS is usually triggered by an event causing sympathetic activity with catecholamine release that induces characteristic patterns of left ventricular wall motion abnormalities with systolic dysfunction. The classic pattern of marked apical hypokinesis with compensatory basal hyperkinesia is now recognized as one phenotypic subtype, with basal and mid-ventricular variants also recognized with increasing frequency. Whatever the form it takes, the changes typically resolve completely, at least macroscopically, in a period of days to weeks, depending on the severity of the acute abnormalities. This chapter sets out the key aspects of clinical assessment and management of patients with TTS, basing discussion around easy-access algorithms. Takotsubo syndrome is a recently recognized entity and so there is still little evidence on

Algorithms in Heart Failure

FIG. 1: Risk factors for Takotsubo syndrome

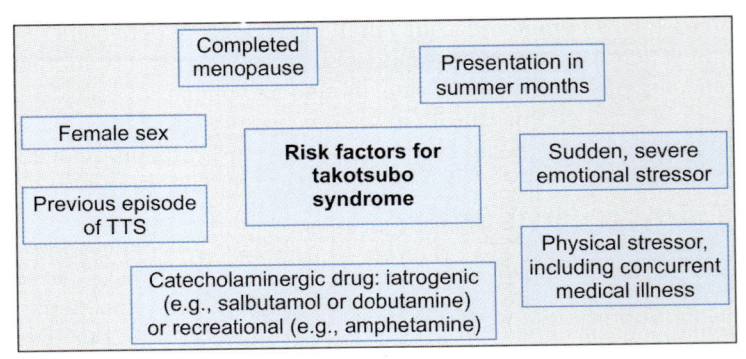

Risk factors for takotsubo syndrome:
- Completed menopause
- Presentation in summer months
- Female sex
- Sudden, severe emotional stressor
- Previous episode of TTS
- Physical stressor, including concurrent medical illness
- Catecholaminergic drug: iatrogenic (e.g., salbutamol or dobutamine) or recreational (e.g., amphetamine)

TTS, Takotsubo syndrome.

which to base management rationale. This discussion is based on available evidence, current consensus, and the viewpoint of the authors.

About 1–2% of patients with suspected acute coronary syndrome (ACS) are eventually diagnosed with TTS, and postmenopausal women account for 70–90% of reported cases. Takotsubo syndrome is uncommon (<3% of cases) in those under 50 years. Unlike ACS and other atherosclerosis related conditions, presentation is more common in the summer months, and lacks the early morning peak associated with plaque rupture events. Typically, there is a history of recent emotional event (26.8%; e.g., bereavement, major argument, gambling losses), physical stress (37.8%; e.g., exhausting work, asthma attack, neuromuscular crisis), or a combination (e.g., suicide attempt), though in a significant minority, no preceding stressor can be identified (34.3%; Gianni et al., 2006). Iatrogenic causes are also recognized, including various drugs, induction of general anesthetic, adrenaline administration, and dobutamine stress echocardiography. From a medicolegal perspective, there is suspicion that physical restraint or electrical stunning (e.g., Taser weapons) might also trigger the condition (Fig. 1).

Most patients with TTS present to the emergency department, often arriving by ambulance with suspected ACS heralded by acute chest pain (67.8%) and/or dyspnea (17.8%), and sometimes with ventricular arrhythmia or cardiogenic shock (1.5 and 4.2%, respectively; Gianni et al., 2006). There will be risk factors as described in figure 1. On bedside assessment, particular suspicion could be brought by description of symptoms typical for ACS in the context of a precipitating stressful event, particularly in postmenopausal women. Clinically, patients show signs of

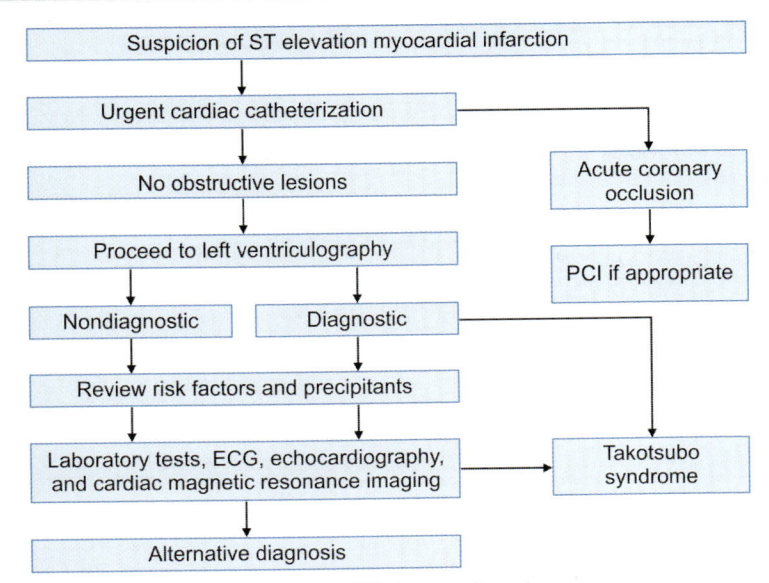

```
┌─────────────────────────────────────────────────┐
│  Suspicion of ST elevation myocardial infarction │
└─────────────────────────────────────────────────┘
                      ↓
┌─────────────────────────────┐
│  Urgent cardiac catheterization │──────────┐
└─────────────────────────────┘          ↓
          ↓                      ┌──────────────────┐
┌──────────────────────┐         │ Acute coronary   │
│ No obstructive lesions │        │ occlusion        │
└──────────────────────┘         └──────────────────┘
          ↓                               ↓
┌─────────────────────────────┐  ┌──────────────────┐
│ Proceed to left ventriculography │  │ PCI if appropriate │
└─────────────────────────────┘  └──────────────────┘
       ↓            ↓
┌──────────────┐ ┌──────────────┐
│ Nondiagnostic │ │  Diagnostic   │
└──────────────┘ └──────────────┘
                      ↓
┌─────────────────────────────────────┐
│ Review risk factors and precipitants │
└─────────────────────────────────────┘
                      ↓
┌─────────────────────────────────────────┐   ┌──────────────┐
│ Laboratory tests, ECG, echocardiography, │──▶│  Takotsubo   │
│ and cardiac magnetic resonance imaging   │   │  syndrome    │
└─────────────────────────────────────────┘   └──────────────┘
                      ↓
┌──────────────────────┐
│ Alternative diagnosis │
└──────────────────────┘
```

PCI, percutaneous coronary intervention; ECG, electrocardiography.

ALGORITHM 1: Initial assessment of patients with Takotsubo syndrome

sympathetic overdrive with profound sweatiness, hypertension, and anxiety. The electrocardiography (ECG) is abnormal, often with ST segment elevation or, later, deep T wave inversion. This is accompanied by QTc prolongation which can predispose to arrhythmia and should be monitored closely. Coronary angiography is important, and subsequent ventriculography, echocardiography, and cardiac magnetic resonance imaging (CMR) help to complete the diagnosis and assess for cardiac complications (Algorithm 1).

Diagnostic criteria based on expert consensus have been proposed by both the Mayo Clinic (Prasad et al., 2008) and a Swedish group (Omerovic, 2011). In practice, a nuanced clinical judgement is often required (Algorithm 2). Some cases will be obviously TTS with clear stress precipitant, normal coronary arteries, marked apical hypokinesis on ventriculography and echocardiography, and no late gadolinium enhancement on CMR. But many are less clear. Clinical experience and multidisciplinary discussion are required in the acute phase to resolve the diagnostic dilemma and decide initial management. Follow-up at 6 weeks often resolves these unclear cases, as in greater than 90% of TTS, the dysfunction and patchy CMR late gadolinium enhancement will have resolved by this time.

Patients should be admitted to an acute cardiac or medical unit. Continuous cardiac ECG monitoring is important due to the

Algorithms in Heart Failure

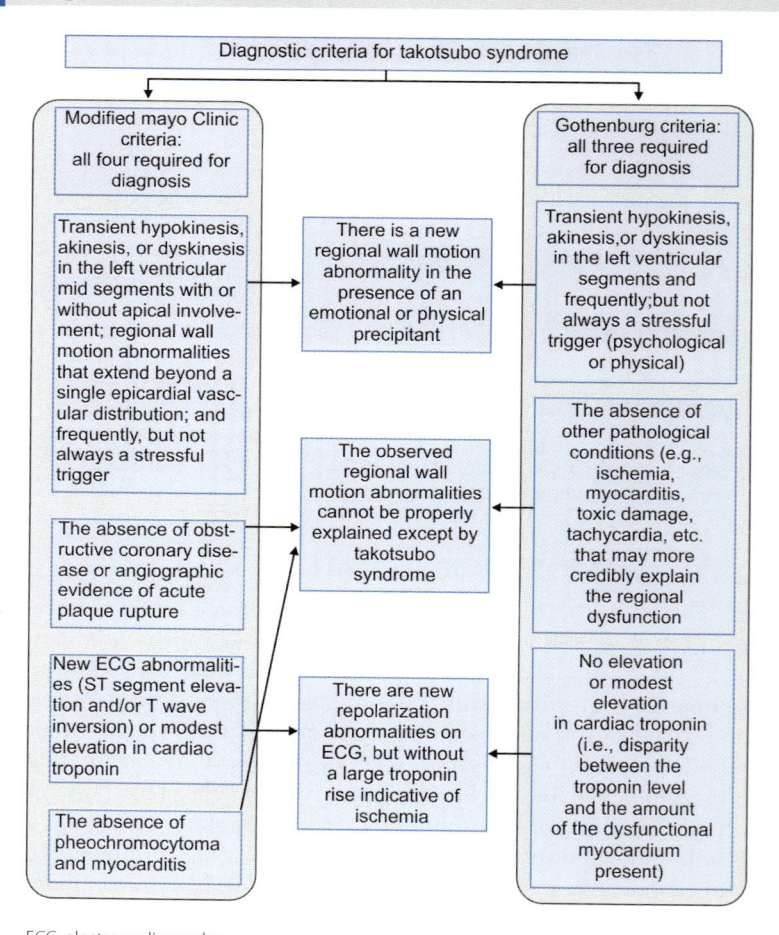

```
                    Diagnostic criteria for takotsubo syndrome
```

Modified mayo Clinic criteria: all four required for diagnosis

- Transient hypokinesis, akinesis, or dyskinesis in the left ventricular mid segments with or without apical involvement; regional wall motion abnormalities that extend beyond a single epicardial vascular distribution; and frequently, but not always a stressful trigger
- The absence of obstructive coronary disease or angiographic evidence of acute plaque rupture
- New ECG abnormalities (ST segment elevation and/or T wave inversion) or modest elevation in cardiac troponin
- The absence of pheochromocytoma and myocarditis

Shared criteria (center):
- There is a new regional wall motion abnormality in the presence of an emotional or physical precipitant
- The observed regional wall motion abnormalities cannot be properly explained except by takotsubo syndrome
- There are new repolarization abnormalities on ECG, but without a large troponin rise indicative of ischemia

Gothenburg criteria: all three required for diagnosis

- Transient hypokinesis, akinesis, or dyskinesis in the left ventricular segments and frequently; but not always a stressful trigger (psychological or physical)
- The absence of other pathological conditions (e.g., ischemia, myocarditis, toxic damage, tachycardia, etc. that may more credibly explain the regional dysfunction
- No elevation or modest elevation in cardiac troponin (i.e., disparity between the troponin level and the amount of the dysfunctional myocardium present)

ECG, electrocardiography.

ALGORITHM 2: Comparison of diagnostic criteria for Takotsubo syndrome

risk of acute arrhythmias, particularly in the setting of significantly prolonged QTc interval. Contrast echocardiography and CMR in the early phase post gadolinium will exclude left ventricular thrombus, and the late post gadolinium phase will provide further evidence to exclude myocardial infarction (Algorithm 3). Once STEMI has been excluded, antiplatelet and anticholesterol drugs can be reviewed for discontinuation. Systemic anticoagulation should be initiated if left ventricular thrombus is confirmed. Mild cases with rapid symptomatic improvement may require no therapy and early discharge. Patients with persistent symptoms

Takotsubo Syndrome

Clinical diagnosis of takotsubo syndrome

Acute management priorities

- **ECG:** check QTc–is continuous ECG monitoring required?
- **Care environment:** is the patient at high risk of complications?
- **Shock:** is there evidence of cardiogenic shock?
- **CMR:** confirm diagnosis, exclude LV thrombus, and establish baseline for follow-up
- **Echocardiography:** assess degree of LV dysfunction and exclude LVOTO
- **Drug therapy (1):** can antiplatelets and anticholesterol drugs be stopped?
- **Drug therapy (2):** introduce heart failure drugs if warranted, e.g., ACE inhibitors and β-blocker; consider anticoagulation if thrombus present
- **Triggers:** any evidence of coexistent conditions, e.g., pheochromocytoma

Follow-up management priorities

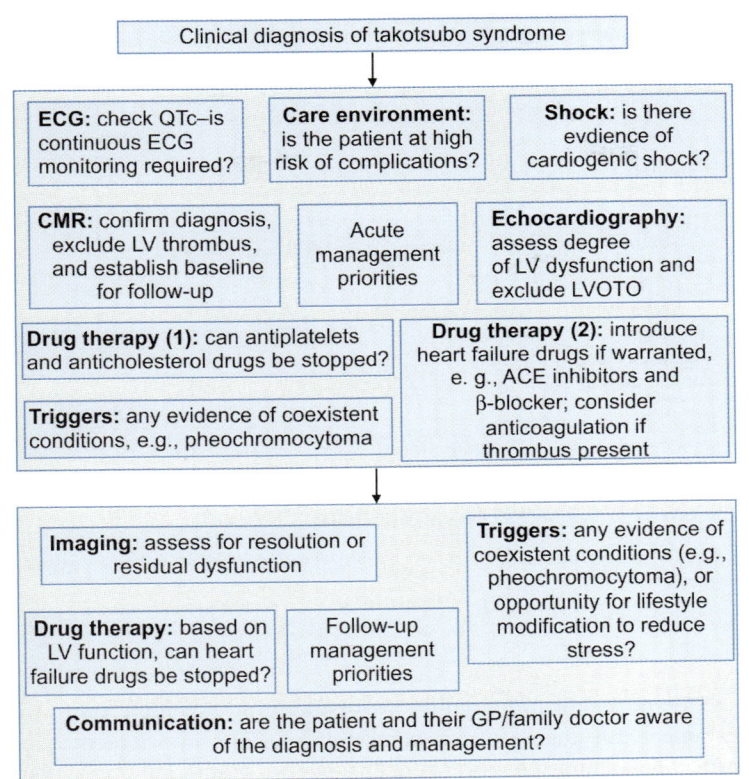

- **Imaging:** assess for resolution or residual dysfunction
- **Triggers:** any evidence of coexistent conditions (e.g., pheochromocytoma), or opportunity for lifestyle modification to reduce stress?
- **Drug therapy:** based on LV function, can heart failure drugs be stopped?
- **Communication:** are the patient and their GP/family doctor aware of the diagnosis and management?

ECG, electrocardiography; CMR, cardiac magnetic resonance imaging; LV, left ventricular; LVOTO, left ventricular outflow tract obstruction; ACE, angiotensin converting enzyme; GP, general practitioner

ALGORITHM 3: Management of Takotsubo syndrome

and left ventricular dysfunction often warrant conventional heart failure therapy with graded introduction of angiotensin converting enzyme (ACE) inhibitors and β-blockers licensed for heart failure. Takotsubo syndrome with severe hemodynamic instability provides unique challenges and is given in algorithm 4. In the recovery phase, it is appropriate to introduce standard heart failure therapy as hemodynamics allow including ACE inhibitors, β-blockers, and potentially an aldosterone receptor antagonist. Takotsubo syndrome can be the herald for an underlying medical condition, such as pheochromocytoma or intracranial pathologies, and consideration should be given to appropriate screening especially if the patient is young, male, or has an atypical pattern of wall motion abnormality.

Algorithms in Heart Failure

```
┌─────────────────────────────────────────────────────┐
│    Takotsubo syndrome with cardiogenic shock        │
└─────────────────────────────────────────────────────┘
                         ↓
┌─────────────────────────────────────────────────────┐
│         Continuous hemodynamic monitoring           │
└─────────────────────────────────────────────────────┘
                         ↓
┌─────────────────────────────────────────────────────┐
│   Immediate echocardiography to assess for LVOTO    │
└─────────────────────────────────────────────────────┘
            ↓                              ↓
      ┌──────────┐                   ┌──────────┐
      │ Present  │                   │  Absent  │
      └──────────┘                   └──────────┘
            ↓                       ↓           ↓
  ┌──────────────┐          ┌──────────┐  ┌──────────┐
  │  Cautious β  │          │ High PVR │  │ Low PVR  │
  │  blockade and│          └──────────┘  └──────────┘
  │  consider RV │                ↓
  │ apical pacing│          ┌──────────┐
  └──────────────┘          │IV nitrates│
            ↓                └──────────┘
            ↓                     ↓            ↓
  ┌─────────────────────────────────────────────────┐
  │                  Levosimendan                   │
  └─────────────────────────────────────────────────┘
                         ↓
  ┌─────────────────────────────────────────────────┐
  │          Mechanical circulatory support         │
  └─────────────────────────────────────────────────┘
```

⇨ Persistent cardiogenic shock

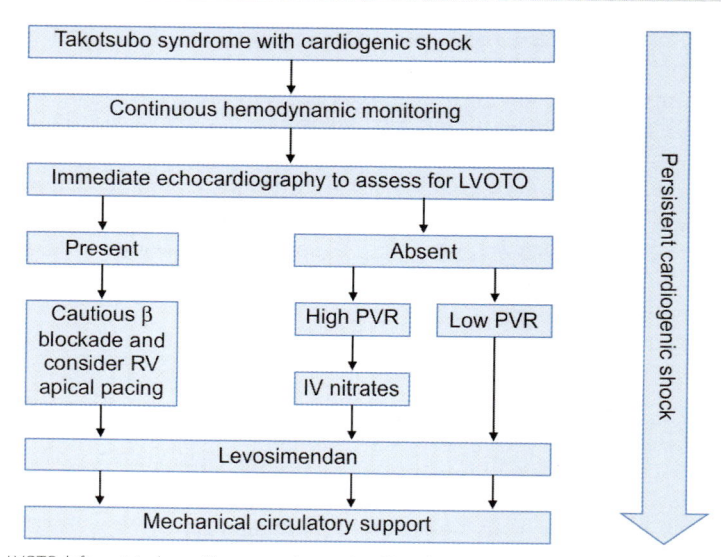

LVOTO, left ventricular outflow tract obstruction; RV, right ventricular; PVR, pulmonary vascular resistance.

ALGORITHM 4: Management of Takotsubo syndrome complicated by cardiogenic shock

Urgent echocardiographic assessment is essential both to establish the degree of left ventricular systolic impairment and crucially to define the presence or absence of dynamic left ventricular outflow tract obstruction (LVOTO). If present, β-blockers should be cautiously introduced to prolong diastolic filling time and increase in left ventricular end-diastolic volume, reducing the left ventricular outflow gradient and improving cardiac output, and electrical pacing of the right ventricular apex could be considered. In this situation, and in cases where the low cardiac output is associated with low pulmonary vascular resistance, afterload reduction with intravenous nitrates and ACE inhibitors can be detrimental and should be avoided. The decision to use "sympathomimetic drugs for positive inotropy" is challenging and counterintuitive in TTS. Given its etiology, further activation of catecholamine receptors or their downstream molecular pathways might worsen the left ventricular dysfunction. In addition, dobutamine infusion may worsen dynamic LVOTO, and many cases of dobutamine induced TTS have been described during stress protocols. In contrast, levosimendan is a positive inotrope that acts to sensitize cardiac myofilaments to calcium. Recent data shows levosimendan is safe to use in patients with TTS, and in our animal model, it was shown to be effective rescue from cardiogenic shock (Paur et al., 2012). Though further studies are necessary to define its role, levosimendan is our recommendation for inotropic drug therapy in TTS with cardiogenic shock. However, given its limited availability, medical practitioners may be forced to resort to alternatives (e.g., noradrenaline) as the only available inotrope until transfer to a tertiary center. In patients with refractory cardiogenic shock and deteriorating multiorgan failure, mechanical circulatory support should be considered (e.g., with venoarterial extracorporeal membrane oxygenation or ventricular assist device).

CONCLUSION

Takotsubo syndrome is a unique and intriguing syndrome that still frequently eludes diagnosis. Our understanding of TTS has increased exponentially over the past decade, with much greater clarity in approach to its diagnosis and best management. Ultimately, however, there remains only a partial awareness of TTS's true incidence in the emergency department or in the catheter laboratory, and sparse clinical evidence for how to manage these patients. Coordinated epidemiological and pathophysiological studies will improve recognition, shed light on its mechanisms, and validate the theoretical and animal models that form the basis of our practice today. The Heart Failure Association of the European Society recently published a position statement which provides a structured approach to the diagnosis and management of patients hospitalised with TTS.

KEY POINTS

- Takotsubo syndrome is an acute, reversible process, most often seen in postmenopausal women and triggered by sudden catecholamine surge from an emotional or physical stress
- The presentation is suggestive of acute ST elevation myocardial infarction, but at cardiac catheterization, the coronary arteries are normal, and ventriculography shows a left ventricle resembling a Japanese octopus trap, or takotsubo
- There is a spectrum of disease from mild chest pain to refractory cardiogenic shock
- Management is aimed at supporting the hemodynamics until the abnormalities have resolved, employing mechanical circulatory support if necessary
- Acute complications are common, and approximately 5–10% cases are serious. However, prognosis is excellent in those surviving to discharge and the majority of patients make a complete recovery.

SUGGESTED READINGS

1. Eitel I, von Knobelsdorff-Brenkenhoff F, Bernhardt P, Carbone I, Muellerleile K, Aldrovandi A, et al. Clinical characteristics and cardiovascular magnetic resonance findings in stress (takotsubo) cardiomyopathy. JAMA. 2011;306(3):277-86.
2. Gianni M, Dentali F, Grandi AM, Sumner G, Hiralal R, Lonn E. Apical ballooning syndrome or takotsubo cardiomyopathy: a systematic review. Eur Heart J. 2006;27(13):1523-9.
3. Kurisu S, Inoue I, Kawagoe T, Ishihara M, Shimatani Y, Nakamura S, et al. (2004). Time course of electrocardiographic changes in patients with tako-tsubo syndrome: comparison with acute myocardial infarction with minimal enzymatic release. Circ J. 2004;68(1):77-81.
4. Lyon AR, Bossone E, Schneider B, et al. Current state of knowledge on Takotsubo syndrome: a Position Statement from the Taskforce on Takotsubo Syndrome of the Heart Failure Association of the European Society of Cardiology. Eur J Heart Fail. 2016;18(1): p. 8-27.
5. Madhavan M, Borlaug BA, Lerman A, Rihal CS, Prasad A. Stress hormone and circulating biomarker profile of apical ballooning syndrome (Takotsubo cardiomyopathy): insights into the clinical significance of B-type natriuetic peptide and troponin levels. Heart, 2009;95(17):1436-41.
6. Madhavan M, Rihal CS, Lerman A, Prasad A. Acute heart failure in apical ballooning syndrome (TakoTsubo/stress cardiomyopathy): clinical correlates and Mayo Clinic risk score. J Am Coll Cardiol. 2011; 57(12):1400-1.
7. Naruse Y, Sato A, Kasahara K, Makino K, Sano M, Takeuchi Y, et al. The clinical impact of late gadolinium enhancement in Takotsubo cardiomyopathy: serial analysis of cardiovascular magnetic resonance images. J Cardiovasc Magn Reson. 2011;13:67.
8. Nguyen TH, Neil CJ, Sverdlov AL, Mahadavan G, Chirkov YY, Kucia AM, et al. N-terminal pro-brain natriuretic protein levels in takotsubo cardiomyopathy. Am J Cardiol. 2011;108(9):1316-21.
9. Omerovic E. How to think about stress-induced cardiomyopathy? – Think "out of the box"! Scand Cardiovasc J. 2011;45(2):67-71.
10. Paur H, Wright PT, Sikkel MB, Tranter MH, Mansfield C, O'Gara P, et al. High levels of circulating epinephrine trigger apical cardiodepression in a β2-adrenergic receptor/Gi-dependent manner: a new model of Takotsubo cardiomyopathy. Circulation. 2012;126(6): 697-706.
11. Prasad A, Lerman A, Rihal CS. Apical ballooning syndrome (Tako-Tsubo or stress cardiomyopathy): a mimic of acute myocardial infarction. Am Heart J. 2008;155(3):408-17.
12. Wright PT, Tranter MH, Morley-Smith AC, Lyon AR. Pathophysiology of takotsubo syndrome: temporal phases of cardiovascular responses to extreme stress. Circ J. 2014;78(7):1550-8.

CHAPTER 30

Myocarditis

Michel Noutsias

INTRODUCTION

The diagnosis "myocarditis" comprises both acute myocarditis and its chronic sequelae, inflammatory cardiomyopathy (DCMI) as an acknowledged specific cardiomyopathy entity, being defined as cardiac dysfunction in association with myocarditis. Transition of acute myocarditis to chronic dilated cardiomyopathy (DCM) occurs in approximately 21% of the patients within a follow-up time of 33 months. Epidemiological data on acute myocarditis and DCM are summarized in table 1. Dilated cardiomyopathy is the leading indication for heart transplantation.

PATHOGENESIS

Polymerase chain reaction (PCR) investigations revealed comparable detection frequencies of a given repertoire of viral genomes [parvovirus B19 (B19V), human herpes virus type 6 and type 7,

TABLE 1: Epidemiological data on myocarditis and dilated cardiomyopathy

Disease	Data
Acute myocarditis	Incidence: 0.17/1,000 man-years
Dilated cardiomyopathy	Incidence: 0.02/1,000 man-years
	Prevalence: 131 cases per 10^6 persons/year
Sudden cardiac death	Myocarditis can be histologically confirmed in 10–20% of adult sudden cardiac death cases age <35 years

Epstein-Barr virus (EBV), adenovirus, and enterovirus] in endomyocardial biopsies (EMB) from both acute myocarditis and chronic DCM patients, thereby suggesting viral persistence in this continuum. Notwithstanding these important insights, a comprehensive analysis encompassing all the known infectious agents and further conditions which have been associated with the onset of acute myocarditis and DCM (Table 2) is not available thus far.

TABLE 2: Infectious agents, toxic agents, and conditions associated with acute myocarditis, inflammatory cardiomyopathy, and dilated cardiomyopathy*

Infectious agents	
Viruses	Adenovirus, arbovirus, arenavirus, coxsackievirus (especially CBV), cytomegalovirus, dengue virus, echovirus, encephalomyocarditis virus, enterovirus, EBV, flavivirus, hepatitis A, B, and C viruses, herpes simplex virus, herpes zoster virus, HIV, HHV-6, influenza virus, junin virus, lymphocytic choriomeningitis virus, lyssavirus, measles virus, mumps virus, B19V, poliomyelitis virus, rabies virus, respiratory syncytial virus, rubella virus, rubeola virus, vaccinia virus, varicella-zoster virus, variola virus, yellow fever virus
Bacteria	Actinomyces, *Borrelia* sp., *Brucella* sp., *Chlamydia pneumoniae*, *Chlamydophila psittaci*, *Clostridium tetani*, *Corynebacterium diphtheriae*, *Coxiella burnetii*, *Francisella tularensis*, *Haemophilus influenzae*, *Legionella pneumophila*, *Leptospira*, *Neisseria gonorrhoea*, *Meningococcus*, *Mycobacterium tuberculosis*, *Mycoplasma pneumoniae*, *Pneumococcus*, *Rickettsiae*, *Salmonella typhi*, *Serratia marcescens*, *Staphylococcus*, *Streptococcus pneumoniae*, *Streptococcus pyogenes*, *Treponema pallidum*, *Tropheryma whippelii*, *Vibrio cholerae*
Fungi	*Actinomyces* sp., aspergillus, blastomyces, candida, coccidioides, cryptococcus, histoplasma, mucormycosis, nocardia, *Sporothrix schenckii*
Protozoa	Ascaris, *Entamoeba histolytica*, echinococcosis, leishmaniasis, helminthic diseases, malaria, *Paragonimus westermani*, *Schistosoma* species, *Strongyloides stercoralis*, *Taenia solium*, *Trichinella spiralis*, *Toxoplasma gondii*, trichinosis, *Trypanosoma cruzi*, sleeping sickness or African trypanosomiasis, visceral larva migrans, *Wuchereria bancrofti*

Continued

Continued

Toxic conditions	
Animal toxic agents	Bee stings, wasp stings, scorpion bites, snake bites, spider bites
Medication	Acetazolamide, amitriptyline, aminophylline, amphotericin B, amphetamines, ampicillin, benzodiazepines, bumetanide, carbamazepine, catecholamines, cefaclor, cephalosporins, chemotherapeutics (especially anthracyclines), chloramphenicol, chlorthalidone, clozapine, colchicine, cocaine, cyclophosphamide, cyclosporine, dobutamine, ethanol, fluorouracil, furosemide, hemetine, hydralazine, hydrochlorothiazide, interleukin-2, isoniazid, lidocaine, lithium, metolazone, methyldopa, methysergide, nitroprusside, oxyphenbutazone, para-aminosalicylic acid, penicillin, phenindione, phenylbutazone, phenytoin, reserpine, spironolactone, sulfadiazine, sulfamethoxypyridine, sulfisoxazole, sulfonylureas, streptomycin, tetracycline, thiazides, triazolam, trastuzumab, tricyclic antidepressants
Physical conditions	Catecholamines, various cytokines (i.e., tumor necrosis factor, interleukin-2), electric shock, hyperpyrexia, radiation, sepsis
Toxic agents	Alcohol, arsenic, carbon monoxide, copper, diverse inhalants, iron, lead, lithium, phosphorus, tetanus toxoid
Cardiac involvement in systemic disorders	Celiac disease, Churg-Strauss syndrome, collagen vascular diseases, inflammatory bowel disease, diabetes mellitus, hypereosinophilia, Kawasaki's disease, myasthenia gravis, polymyositis, sarcoidosis, scleroderma, systemic lupus erythematosus, thyrotoxicosis, Wegener's granulomatosis

*The table is not deemed to present all known or suspected associations with acute myocarditis, inflammatory cardiomyopathy, and dilated cardiomyopathy completely. In parts, the associations are based on case reports only, and a robust "proof of principle" causative relationship or pathogenic pathway is not established.

EBV, Epstein–Barr virus; HIV, human immunodeficiency virus; HHV-6, human herpes virus type 6; B19V, parvovirus B19; CBV, coxsackie B virus.

The three-phase model of coxsackie B virus (CBV) induced murine myocarditis, which has been derived from experimental insights, may be in broadly valid also for the intricate processes involved in human virus induced myocarditis. As summarized in figure 1, the initial viral infection induces the acute myocardial inflammation during acute myocarditis, followed by the subacute phase, during which complex virus-host interactions are decisively

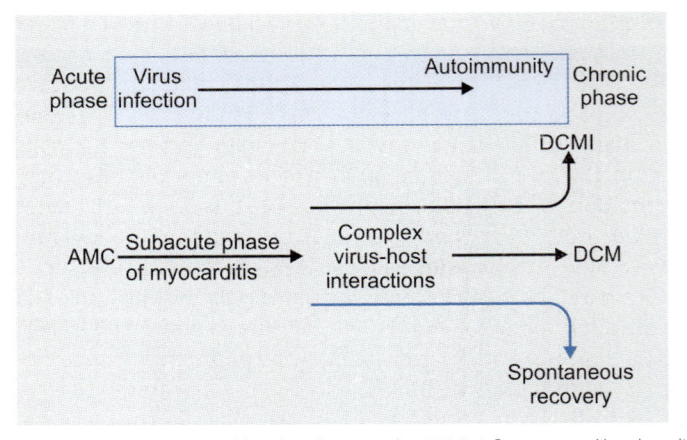

```
Acute  | Virus              Autoimmunity     | Chronic
phase  | infection    ────────────────────▶  | phase
                                     DCMI
                                      ↑
          Subacute phase    Complex
AMC  ───────────────────▶   virus-host  ──────▶ DCM
          of myocarditis    interactions
                                      ↓
                                 Spontaneous
                                  recovery
```

AMC, acute myocarditis; DCM, dilated cardiomyopathy; DCMI, inflammatory dilated cardiomyopathy.

FIG. 1: Pathogenesis of virus induced acute myocarditis, and its transition to either inflammatory cardiomyopathy or dilated cardiomyopathy or to spontaneous resolution

involved in the further evolution of the disease: either complete or partial spontaneous recovery and healing of myocarditis, or manifestation of the chronic sequelae, DCM and DCMI (with immunohistologal detectable low level intramyocardial inflammation), respectively. The intricate pathways of the network involved in the subacute phase include individual susceptibility to viral persistence, adaptive and innate immune response patterns, the evolution of anticardiac-autoimmunity evoked by viral infection (i.e., by molecular mimicry), and genetic determinants of these interactions. After the subacute phase, maladaptive general heart failure pathways gain importance in the chronic stage of the disease, and superimpose to the cardiodepressive effects of the detrimental immune regulation, and of relevant viral persistence. Inflammatory cardiomyopathy is characterized by low level intramyocardial inflammation, accompanied by low level persistence of viral loads in the absence of viremia.

CLINICAL PRESENTATION

Acute myocarditis patients can present with a diverse spectrum of clinical scenarios: with an acute myocardial infarction (AMI) like situation, chest discomfort, arrhythmias, acute heart failure, palpitations, syncope or sudden cardiac death (SCD) (Fig. 2). Acute myocarditis patients may report an antecedent (days to few weeks) flu-like illness with respiratory or gastrointestinal tract infection before the onset of acute myocarditis symptoms. However, acute myocarditis may be missed frequently due to subclinical presentation. In acute myocarditis with preserved ejection fraction (MCpEF), regional wall motion abnormalities, diastolic dysfunction, wall edema, and pericardial effusions may be detected by echocardiography and by cardiac magnetic resonance imaging (CMR). Acute myocarditis with reduced ejection fraction (MCrEF) is dominated by heart failure symptoms (i.e., dyspnea on exertion or at rest, peripheral edema), and presents as new onset DCM. The clinical findings comprise cardiomegaly, pulmonary congestion or edema, and pleural effusions in chest X-ray. Furthermore, systolic and diastolic dysfunction, left ventricular dilatation or biventricular dilatation, and occasionally, left ventricular thrombi can be confirmed by echocardiography. The most severe presentation of MCrEF is acute fulminant myocarditis (AFMC), requiring inotropic support with high doses of catecholamines. Both MCpEF and MCrEF can present with various types of electrocardiography (ECG) abnormalities [right or left bundle branch block, ST segment depression, Q waves and T wave inversions, atrioventricular (AV)-block] and rhythm disturbances on Holter monitoring (sinus tachycardia or bradycardia, supraventricular extrasystoles, atrial fibrillation or flutter, and ventricular tachycardia, flutter or fibrillation). Acute myocarditis is a frequent cause of SCD, especially, in age less than 35 years, and is often associated with strenuous physical exertion.

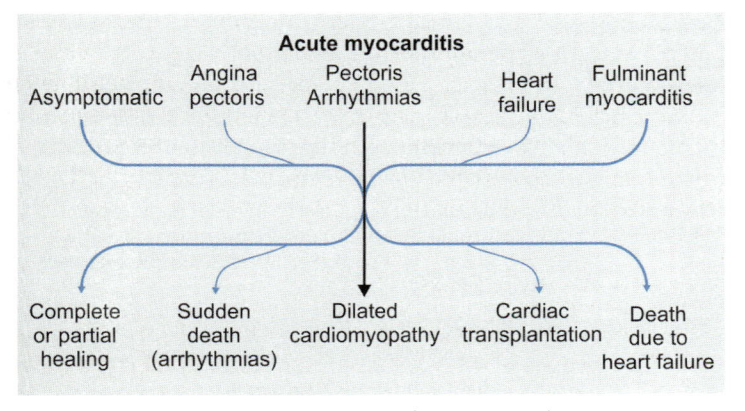

FIG. 2: Clinical presentation and outcomes of acute myocarditis

PROGNOSIS

Highly heterogeneous clinical courses have been observed after acute myocarditis, spanning from complete or partial healing, to chronic DCM, the need for cardiac transplantation, and fatal outcomes due to SCD and terminal heart failure (Fig. 2). Transition of acute myocarditis to DCM or DCMI has been reported in approximately 20% of the patients, occasionally accompanied by recurrent myocarditis events. After acute myocarditis, transplantation free survival has been determined as 78% within a mean follow-up of 59 ± 42 months. The 5-year survival rate of histologically confirmed myocarditis and idiopathic DCM patients is comparable (56% vs. 54%, respectively).

The initial left ventricular ejection fraction (LVEF), left ventricular end-diastolic pressure, and left ventricular end-diastolic diameter (LVEDD) have no independent prognostic relevance in acute myocarditis. Recent research has elucidated the prognostic relevance of several clinical, CMR, and EMB parameters for MCrEF patients, which are summarized in table 3.

TABLE 3: Conditions or factors with prognostic relevance for acute myocarditis, inflammatory cardiomyopathy, and dilated cardiomyopathy

Factor/condition	Prognostic data
AFMC	While 93% of the AFMC patients were alive at 11 years follow-up time; HR for death or cardiac transplantation: 0,10; 95% CI: 0.01–0.88, only 45% of the acute myocarditis patients with lymphocytic, nonfulminant myocarditis were alive
Immunohistological proof of myocarditis/DCMI	Independent prognostic parameter for adverse outcome (SCD, indication for heart transplantation, and refractory end-stage heart failure; HR: 3.46; 95% CI: 1.39–8.62; p = 0.008)
NYHA III-IV	Independent prognostic parameters for adverse outcome (SCD, indication for heart transplantation and refractory end-stage heart failure; HR: 3.20; 95% CI: 1.36–7.57; p = 0.008)
Absence of β-blockers	Independent prognostic parameter for adverse outcome (SCD, indication for heart transplantation, and refractory end-stage heart failure; HR: 0.43; 95% CI: 0.21–0.91; p = 0.027)
QRS duration ≥120 ms	Independent prognostic parameter for adverse outcome (HR: 2.83; 95% CI: 1.07–7.49; p = 0.012)
MAP <87 mmHg	Independent prognostic parameter for adverse outcome (HR: 2.58; 95% CI: 1.26–5.08; p <0.001)

Continued

Continued

Factor/condition	Prognostic data
Sinus rhythm >78/min	Associated with poor outcome (HR: 2.92, 95% CI: 1.02–8.29; p = 0.045)
LGE (CMR)	Independent prognostic factor for adverse outcome (HR: 3.4; 95% CI: 1.26–9); LGE fraction of >4.4% of left ventricular mass independent of LVEF; LGE best predictor for SCD (HR: 12.8; p <0.01)

AFMC, acute fulminant myocarditis; CMR, cardiovascular magnetic resonance imaging; LGE, late gadolinium enhancement; MAP, mean arterial blood pressure; SCD, sudden cardiac death; HR, hazard ratio; CI, confidence interval; LVEF, left ventricular ejection fraction; NYHA, New York Heart Association; DCMI, inflammatory dilated cardiomyopathy.

DIAGNOSIS

Endomyocardial Biopsy Technique

Endomyocardial biopsy can be obtained by venous or arterial percutaneous approach from the right ventricular septum or from the left ventricle. Left ventricular EMB may yield more diagnostic results compared to RV-EMB, however, the highest diagnostic yields were achieved by biventricular EMB procedures. Complications of EMBs obtainment are fairly rare in experiences centers, and serious periprocedural complications have been reported less than 0.5%.

Histology of Endomyocardial Biopsy

The histological Dallas criteria can differentiate between "active" (interstitial infiltrates with myocytolysis with or without fibrosis; Fig. 3) and borderline myocarditis (increased infiltrates with or without fibrosis). However, this histological approach is hampered by low sensitivity, the substantial sampling error, and a high interobserver variability. Moreover, the Dallas criteria have no prognostic or therapeutic value (immunosuppression). Nonetheless, histological EMB evaluation is essential for the diagnosis of further specific pathologies [i.e., giant cell myocarditis (GCMC), sarcoidosis, myocardial storage diseases].

Immunohistology of Endomyocardial Biopsy

Immunohistology enables the specific detection, quantification, and phenotypic characterization. Moreover, endothelial cell adhesion molecule (CAM) expression has evolved to a further cornerstone of the immunohistological EMB assessment for myocarditis and DCMI. Two immunohistological diagnostic concepts are available: greater than 7.0 $CD3^+/CD2^+$ lymphocytes/

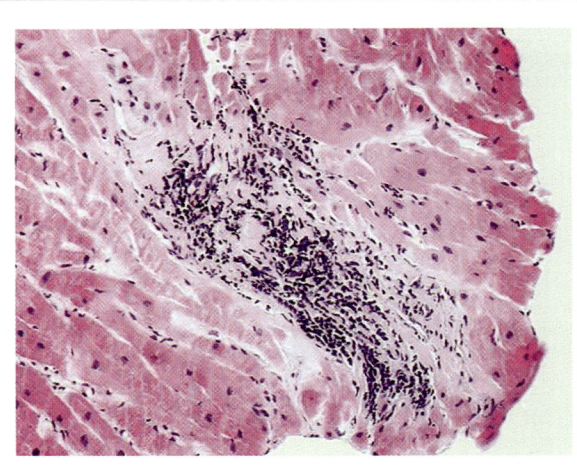

FIG. 3: Histological proof of myocarditis. Focal lymphomononuclear infiltrates with adjacent myocytolysis (active myocarditis; original magnification x200)

mm myocardial tissue area and concurrent abundance of several CAMs, and furthermore greater than 14.0 leukocytes/mm^2 with facultative CAMs abundance. Intramyocardial inflammation can be detected in approximately 50% of the acute myocarditis and DCM patients using these immunohistological concepts. A synopsis summarizing the features of histology and immunohistology is presented in table 4. Representative findings of immunohistological EMB stainings are demonstrated in figure 4.

Virological Analyses of Endomyocardial Biopsy

It is assumed that the majority of acute myocarditis cases are induced by viral infections in the western world, often preceded by gastrointestinal or respiratory tract infections. Serological viral analyses are not reflecting PCR detection of viral genomes in EMB. Contemporary analyses of EMB comprise detection of genomes by PCR, determination of viral loads, and viral genotype detection by sequencing. The disease specificity of coxsackievirus or enterovirus has been confirmed by meta-analysis, and enterovirus or CBV infection is associated with adverse prognosis confirmed in several investigations. However, recent prospective studies failed to confirm any prognostic relevance of the PCR detection of viral genomes (including, i.e., B19V, human herpes virus type 6, adenovirus, EBV). The lack of differentiation of irrelevant chronic viral genome persistence ("bioportfolio"), especially for B19V, may be of paramount importance in this setting.

TABLE 4: Comparison of the histological evaluation of myocarditis and of the immunohistological evaluation of inflammatory cardiomyopathy

Factors	Histological evaluation of myocarditis (Dallas Criteria)	Immunohistological evaluation of inflammatory cardiomyopathy
Interobserver variability	High	Not precisely known, but expected to be substantially lower, especially using DIA
Sampling error	High	Not precisely known, but expected to be substantially lower
Variability of detection of inflammation	High	Lower
Specific identification and quantification of infiltrates	Impossible	Feasible
Phenotypic characterization of infiltrates	Impossible	Broad phenotypic characterization feasible (i.e., T-lymphocytes, CTLs, macrophages, specific activation markers)
Evaluation of CAMs expression	Impossible	Feasible
Prognostic relevance	No prognostic relevance	Patients with immunohistologically proven DCMI have a worse prognosis
Clinical relevance	No discrimination of DCM patients who benefit from immunosuppression	Patients with immunohistologically proven DCMI benefit from immunosuppressive treatment

CAM, cell adhesion molecule; DCM, dilated cardiomyopathy; DIA, digital image analysis ; CTLs, cytotoxic T cells; DCMI, inflammatory cardiomyopathy

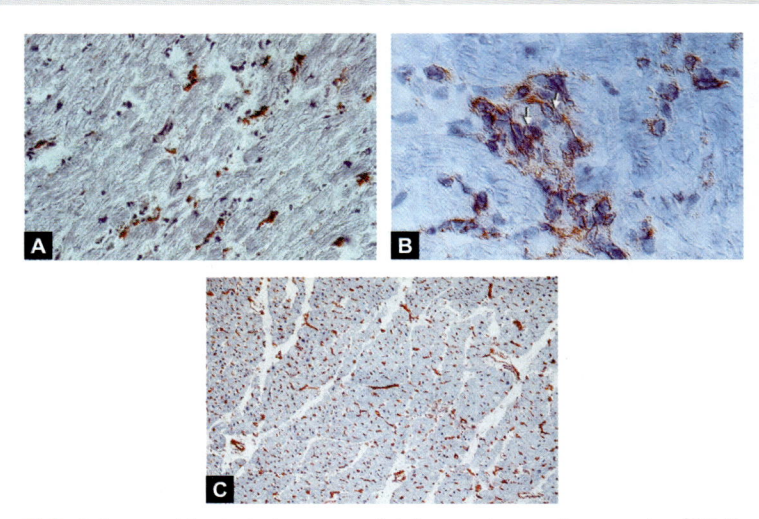

FIG. 4: Immunohistological aspects of inflammatory cardiomyopathy (DCMI). **A,** Diffuse infiltration pattern of lymphocyte function associated antigen-1[+] lymphocytes in DCMI (original magnification x400); **B,** focal infiltration pattern of perforin[+] cytotoxic T-lymphocytes in DCMI, encircling and entering (white arrows) a cross-sectioned cardiomyocyte, suggesting myocytolysis (original magnification x630); **C,** homogeneous intercellular adhesion molecule-1 abundance in DCMI (original magnification x200)

Cardiac Magnetic Resonance Imaging Diagnosis of Myocarditis

Cardiac magnetic resonance, has evolved to a well-acknowledged diagnostic tool for myocarditis. The consensus "Lake Louise" criteria require at least two of the following three parameters to be present:
1. At least one late gadolinium enhancement (LGE) focus with nonischemic regional distribution
2. Early gadolinium enhancement ratio between myocardium and skeletal muscle in gadolinium-enhanced T1-weighted images
3. Regional or global myocardial signal intensity increase in T2-weighted images.

Further findings may be left ventricular dysfunction, pericardial effusion, and left ventricular thrombus.

Late gadolinium enhancement plays a major diagnostic role in CMR analyses. In acute myocarditis and DCM, the LGE pattern is typically subepicardial, has no association to ischemic regional distribution, and is often present in the lateral wall

Myocarditis

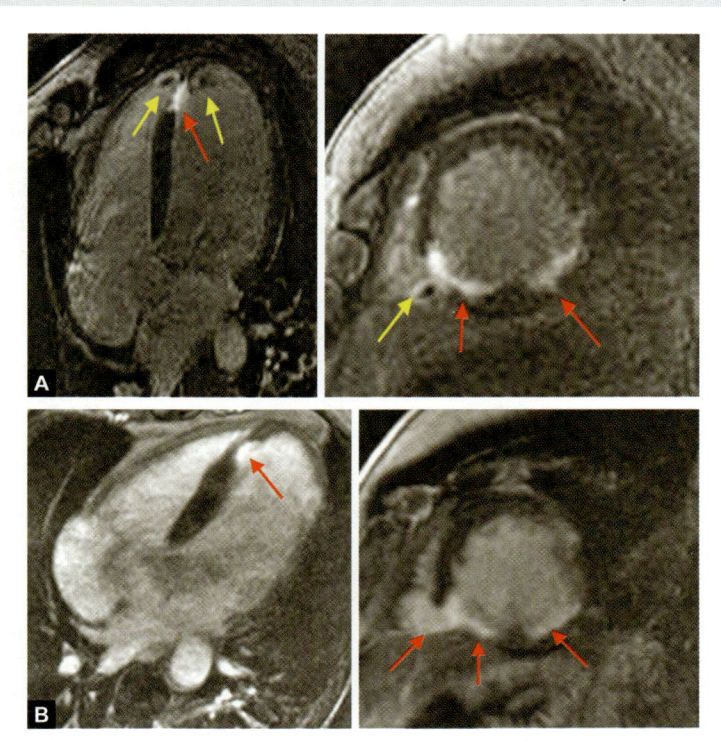

FIG. 5: Dynamics of cardiac magnetic resonance imaging findings in myocarditis. **A,** Magnetic resonance imaging (MRI) in the acute phase of acute myocarditis with reduced ejection fraction with left ventricular ejection fraction (LVEF): 17% in a 39-year-old male patient. Late gadolinium enhancement (LGE) in the apical, inferoseptal, and inferolateral segments (red arrows), as well as thrombi in the right and left ventricle (yellow arrows). **B,** follow-up MRI 8 weeks after the initial presentation; LVEF improved to 38%. Persisting LGE in the apical, inferoseptal, and inferolateral segments (red arrows), indicating left ventricular scar formation. The left ventricular thrombi were not detectable at this stage under anticoagulation

and midventricular within the septum. Endomyocardial biopsy diagnostics and CMR detected LGE have a high synergy, and myocarditis is unlikely in patients without LGE. The natural course of LVEF, inflammation, and/or fibrosis can be evidenced by CMR non invasively (Fig. 5).

Autoantibodies

A variety of autoantibodies targeting various myocardial structures has been described for acute myocarditis and DCM patients. The detectability of anticardiac autoantibodies has been associated with adverse prognosis in acute myocarditis patients. The immunoglobulin G3 (IgG3) fraction of antibodies might be more especially important for adverse outcomes of DCM. However, disease specificity and the "proof of principle" status are controversial for most of these anticardiac antibodies. An interesting model postulated binding of autoantibodies to the Fc receptor of the cardiomyocytes, which thereby induce negative inotropic effects, and eventually contribute to heart failure.

TREATMENT

Clinical Management and Conventional Heart Failure Treatment; Sudden Cardiac Death Prevention

For MCpEF, the general prognosis is good, and no controlled study is available that favors specific treatment. Symptomatic heart failure treatment with angiotensin converting enzyme (ACE) inhibitor or angiotensin receptor blockers (ARB), diuretics, β-blockers, and/or ivabradine (for heart rates >78/min) may be considered, nitrates to improve angina pectoris symptoms, may be considered.

Heart failure guidelines equally apply to MCrEF and DCM, including heart failure medication, cardiac resynchronization, assist devices, and cardiac transplantation as ultima ratio. Identified potential cardiotoxic agents (i.e., alcohol, anthracyclines) should be discontinued. In cases with pericardial effusion (myopericarditis), specific management and treatment should follow the respective recommendations.

In AFMC patients, LVEF often improves dramatically, and LVEDD decreases, and may even normalize under heart failure regimens, with an excellent long-term outcome as compared to lymphocytic myocarditis with mildly or moderately impaired LVEF. Mechanical support [i.e., left ventricular assist device, extracorporeal membrane oxygenation, Impella) may be necessary to bridge this critical status.

Acute myocarditis or DCM patients should be followed regularly by clinical assessment and noninvasive examinations, including echocardiography and CMR. Especially, in cases with deterioration of left ventricular function parameters, or with failure of improvement despite complete heart failure medication (i.e., within 2 weeks), EMB should be obtained in these patients and subjected to contemporary diagnostic EMB techniques. Immunomodulatory treatment should be considered, especially, in such cases not responding to standard congestive heart failure

(CHF) care, preferably in experiences centers and/or in the framework of multicenter controlled studies or registries.

Sudden cardiac death prevention in the context of acute myocarditis primarily applies to MCrEF; however, SCD can occur in MCpEF patients as well. Absence of strenuous physical activity is recommended during the first weeks after acute myocarditis regardless of LVEF to avoid SCD. Primary SCD prevention by implantable cardioverter defibrillator (ICD) implantation is not recommended in MCrEF of less than 3 months duration, since LVEF can improve substantially during the natural course under CHF medication. The wearable cardioverter defibrillator (WCD) is recommended to bridge the period of 3 months after newly diagnosed DCM. The WCD also prevents from the dilemma of premature ICD implantations in MCrEF.

These diagnostic and disease management pathways have been summarized and illustrated in algorithm 1.

Genetic counseling and noninvasive cardiological screening (ECG) is advisable in patients with familial DCM and their first degree relatives.

Immunomodulatory Treatment

In general, the natural course of acute myocarditis has to be awaited under conventional heart failure regimens. Endomyocardial biopsy must be especially considered in MCrEF patients, and are mandatory in cases suggestive of GCMC. Several immunomodulatory studies have shown beneficial effects in selected patient groups with chronic DCM (usually with persisting heart failure with reduced ejection fraction ≥6 months after first presentation). Recent clinical research has vigorously enriched our knowledge on diagnosis, prognosis, and immunomodulatory modalities of myocarditis patients. However, the results of multicenter controlled trials are needed to foster this evidence.

Immunosuppression

In subjects with high grade AV block or ventricular tachycardia, GCMC can be suspected. For histologically diagnosed GCMC, immunosuppression with corticosteroids and azathioprine, or anti-CD3 antibodies has a class Ib indication, significantly reducing mortality, morbidity, need for cardiac transplantation, and the giant cell infiltrates (Fig. 6).

Immunosuppression is no therapeutic option in histologically confirmed myocarditis (Dallas criteria), in the negligence of viral

Algorithms in Heart Failure

```
                          Clinically suspected myocarditis
                                       │
                          Exclusion of CAD and of further secondary causes
                                       │
        ┌──────────────────────────────┼──────────────────────────────┐
        │                              │                              │
MCrEF <45%; cardiogenic shock   MCREF LVEF <45%;              MCPEF LVEF ≥45%
        │                        hemodynamic stable
        │                              │
Circulatory support           ┌────────┴────────┐
• Pharmacological       WCP if LVEF ≤35%    CHF treatment; CMR;
• Mechanical (ECMO,          │              further prognostic parameters
  LVAD, Impella)       LVEF at 90 days ≤35%       │
• Heart transplantation      │               ┌────┴────┐
        │                ICD implantation   CMR        CMR negative:
   ┌────┴────┐                              positive:   MC unlikely
No recovery  Recovery                       MC suspected    │
   │                                            │        ┌──┴──┐
  EMB                                  CHF treatment;  Recovery  No EMB
   │                                   follow-up ECG,
Giant cell MC, eosinophilic            echocardiography, CMR
MC, sarcoidosis                             │
   │                                   No sustained recovery
Immunosuppression                           │
                                           EMB
   │  Further deterioration                 │
   │  Hemodynamic instability         Consider immunomodulation
   │
No specific EMB diagnosis  ← Hemodynamic instability
   │
Further deterioration
   │
• Mechanical circulatory
  support (LVAD/Bi-VAD;
  Impella)
• Heart transplantation
```

ALGORITHM 1: Proposed algorithm of diagnosis and treatment of patients with clinically suspected myocarditis

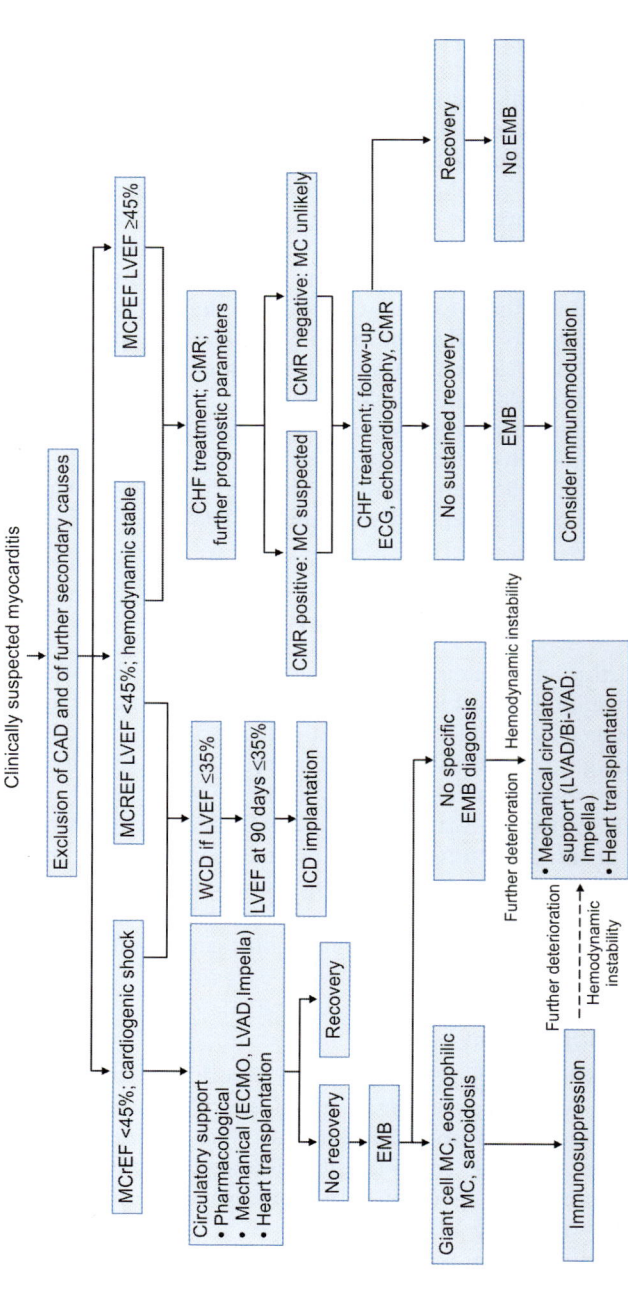

CAD, coronary artery disease; CMR, cardiac magnetic resonance imaging; EMB, endomyocardial biopsy; ICD, implantable cardioverter defibrillator; LVAD, left ventricular assist device; LVEF, left ventricular ejection fraction; MCpEF, acute myocarditis with preserved ejection fraction; MCrEF, acute myocarditis with reduced ejection fraction; WCD, wearable cardioverter defibrillator; ECG, electrocardiography; ECMO, extracorporeal membrane oxygenation.

Myocarditis

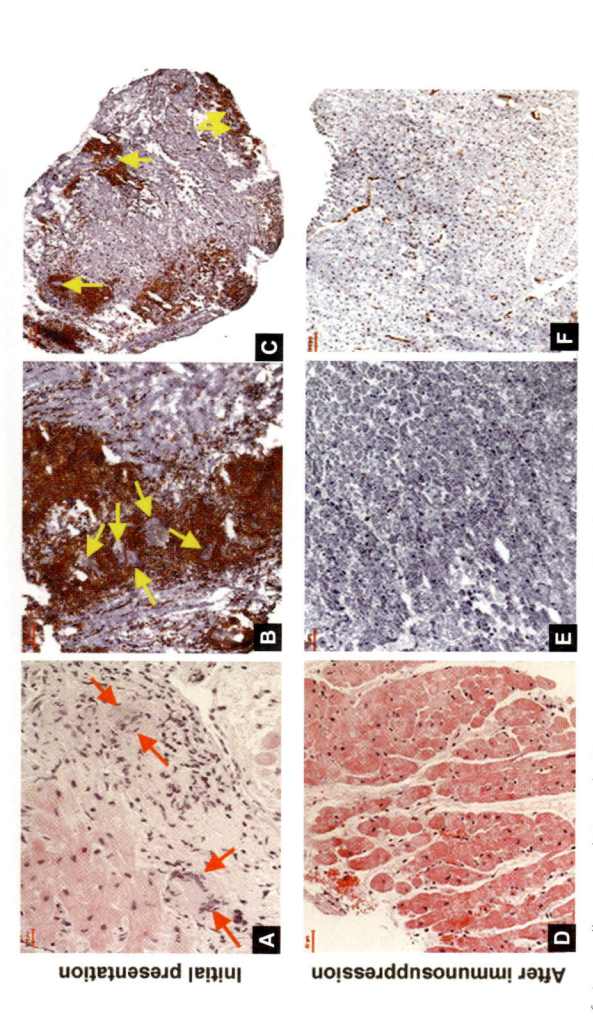

FIG 6: Resolution of giant cell myocarditis under immunosuppression. Histological and immunohistological findings of endomyocardial biopsies (EMBs) at the initial EMBs (panels A–C) and after immunosuppression (panels D–F) in a female 51-year-old patient presenting with acute myocarditis with reduced ejection fraction, left ventricular ejection fraction 26%, and polymorphic nonsustained ventricular tachycardias. **A,** Histology (hematoxylin and eosin staining) demonstrated focal lymphocytic infiltration and multinucleated giant cells (red arrows; x400); **B,** immunohistological staining of focal CD11a/lymphocyte function associated antigen-1+ (LFA-1) lymphocytes with giant cells (yellow arrows; x200); **C,** focal intercellular adhesion molecule-1 (ICAM-1) abundance pronounced in areas adjacent to giant cells (yellow arrows; x200); **D,** histology in the follow-up EMBs 6 months after immunosuppression, devoid of any giant cells (x200); **E,** normal LFA-1+ infiltration in the follow-up EMBs after immunosuppression (x200) **F,** baseline ICAM-1 expression in the follow-up EMBs a immunosuppression (x100)

genome detection. However, immunosuppression has proven beneficial effects in patients with immunohistologically confirmed myocarditis (DCMI) in two single-center randomized investigations, with exclusion of viral genome persistence in one of these studies.

Antiviral Immunomodulation with Interferon

Interferon (IFN)-β is crucially involved in the antiviral immune response in experimental CBV-induced myocarditis. The available single-center experience on the antiviral efficacy of IFN-β (6-months treatment) revealed elimination of enteroviral (n = 15) and adenoviral genomes (n = 7) in DCMI patients, and shown to improve long-term prognosis of EV-positive patients. However, IFN-β treatment failed to confirm beneficial effects in DCM patients with B19V persistence.

Immunoadsorption

The favorable hemodynamic results of immunoadsorption (IA) in DCM patients have been confirmed in several single-center investigations, and can be ascribed to multiple mechanisms: removal of autoantibodies, decrease of lymphocytic infiltration and CAM expression, and decreased oxidative stress. The effects of IA may be partly due to the restoration of immunoglobulins with 0.5 g/kg polyclonal IgG after IA. Approximately 40% of the IA treated patients show improvement of hemodynamic and clinical parameters, lasting for greater than 2.5 years after treatment, and IA contributes to a significant reduction of hospitalization and morbidity. Distinct myocardial gene expression profiles and cardiodepressant autoantibodies may be helpful to differentiate DCM patients who will likely and favorably respond to IA. A randomized multicenter IA trial for DCM patients is ongoing (NCT00558584).

CONCLUSION

For myocarditis, heterogeneous clinical presentations and outcomes have been observed. The clinical treatment of myocarditis follows general heart failure guidelines. Recent investigations have identified several conditions that are associated with adverse prognosis, which are important cornerstones for the identification of patients at increased risk. The wearable cardioverter defibrillator may be especially important for myocarditis to prevent from sudden cardiac death, bridging the highly dynamic initial phase of reduced LVEF. Cardiac magnetic resonance imaging has gained substantial importance for the non-invasive diagnosis of myocarditis. Recurrent pericardial effusions are responsive to non-steroidal anti-inflammatory drugs and/or colchicine. Concurrent EMB investigations encompassing histology, immunohistology and virological analyses, are pertinent for the definitive diagnosis of myocarditis. Endomyocardial biopsy are especially indicated in myocarditis patients with reduced LVEF and/or life-threatening arrhythmias, suggestive of giant-cell myocarditis, which is a proven indication for immunosuppression. Several immunomodulatory studies have shown beneficial effects in selected patient groups, characterized primarily by EMB results. Recent clinical research has vigorously enriched our knowledge on diagnosis, prognosis, and immunomodulatory modalities of myocarditis patients, and has partly disenchanted this intriguing conundrum. However, the results of multicenter controlled trials are needed to foster this evidence.

KEY POINTS

- Acute myocarditis patients can present with a diverse spectrum of clinical scenarios
- Acute myocarditis with preserved systolic left ventricular ejection fraction and acute myocarditis with reduced left ventricular ejection fraction (MCrEF) should be differentiated
- Highly heterogeneous clinical courses have been observed after acute myocarditis, spanning from complete or partial healing, to chronic dilated cardiomyopathy (DCM), and fatal outcomes
- Contemporary diagnostics of endomyocardial biopsies (EMB) comprise histology and immunohistology for myocarditis, and molecular biological virus detection techniques
- Cardiac magnetic resonance imaging (CMR) has evolved as valuable noninvasive diagnostic approach for the detection of myocarditis and follow-up analyses. Late gadolinium enhancement detected by CMR has a high synergy with EMB diagnostics, and has prognostic relevance
- Heart failure guidelines equally apply to MCrEF and DCM
- Obtainment of EMB must be considered in MCrEF patients who do not improve in more than weeks after initiation of heart failure treatment

Continued

Continued

- ❑ For histologically diagnosed giantcell myocarditis, immuno-suppression with corticosteroids and azathioprine, or anti-CD3 antibodies has a class Ib indication
- ❑ Several immunomodulatory studies have shown beneficial effects in selected patient groups with chronic DCM, partly with specified EMB diagnostic results (immunosuppression in immunohistologically confirmed inflammatory cardiomyopathy; antiviral interferon-β treatment in *Enterovirus* positive patients). Immunoadsorption contributes to sustained improvement of left ventricular ejection fraction, decrease of intramyocardial inflammation, and decline of hospitalization and morbidity. However, the results of multicenter controlled trials must be awaited to foster this evidence.

SUGGESTED READINGS

1. Abdel-Aty H, Boye P, Zagrosek A, Wassmuth R, Kumar A, Messroghli D, et al. Diagnostic performance of cardiovascular magnetic resonance in patients with suspected acute myocarditis: comparison of different approaches. J Am Coll Cardiol. 2005;45(11):1815-22.
2. Ackerman MJ, Priori SG, Willems S, Berul C, Brugada R, Calkins H, et al. HRS/EHRA expert consensus statement on the state of genetic testing for the channelopathies and cardiomyopathies: this document was developed as a partnership between the Heart Rhythm Society (HRS) and the European Heart Rhythm Association (EHRA). Europace. 2011;13(8):1077-109.
3. Al-Khatib SM, Hellkamp A, Curtis J, Mark D, Peterson E, Sanders GD, et al. Nonevidence-based ICD implantations in the United States. JAMA. 2011;305(1):43-9.
4. Andersson B, Caidahl K, Waagstein F. Idiopathic dilated cardiomyopathy among Swedish patients with congestive heart failure. Eur Heart J. 1995;16(1):53-60.
5. Aretz HT. Myocarditis: the Dallas criteria. Hum Pathol. 1987;18(6):619-24.
6. Assomull RG, Prasad SK, Lyne J, Smith G, Burman ED, Khan M, et al. Cardiovascular magnetic resonance, fibrosis, and prognosis in dilated cardiomyopathy. J Am Coll Cardiol. 2006;48(10):1977-85.
7. Baboonian C, Treasure T. Meta-analysis of the association of enteroviruses with human heart disease. Heart. 1997;78(6):539-43.
8. Baccouche H, Mahrholdt H, Meinhardt G, Merher R, Voehringer M, Hill S, et al. Diagnostic synergy of non-invasive cardiovascular magnetic resonance and invasive endomyocardial biopsy in troponin-positive patients without coronary artery disease. Eur Heart J. 2009;30(23):2869-79.
9. Baccouche H, Mahrholdt H, Meinhardt G, Merher R, Voehringer M, Hill S, et al. Diagnostic synergy of non-invasive cardiovascular magnetic resonance and invasive endomyocardial biopsy in troponin-positive patients without coronary artery disease. European Heart journal. 2009;30(23):2869-79.
10. Basso C, Calabrese F, Corrado D, Thiene G. Postmortem diagnosis in sudden cardiac death victims: macroscopic, microscopic and molecular findings. Cardiovascular research. 2001;50(2):290-300.

Myocarditis

11. Burke AP, Farb A, Virmani R, Goodin J, Smialek JE. Sports-related and nonsports-related sudden cardiac death in young adults. Am Heart J. 1991;121(2 Pt 1):568-75.
12. Caforio AL, Calabrese F, Angelini A, Tona F, Vinci A, Bottaro S, et al. A prospective study of biopsy-proven myocarditis: prognostic relevance of clinical and aetiopathogenetic features at diagnosis. Eur Heart J. 2007;28(11):1326-33.
13. Chen YS, Yu HY, Huang SC, Chiu KM, Lin TY, Lai LP, et al. Experience and result of extracorporeal membrane oxygenation in treating fulminant myocarditis with shock: what mechanical support should be considered first? J Heart Lung Transplant. 2005;24(1):81-7.
14. Chung MK, Szymkiewicz SJ, Shao M, Zishiri E, Niebauer MJ, Lindsay BD, et al. Aggregate national experience with the wearable cardioverter-defibrillator: event rates, compliance, and survival. J Am Coll Cardiol. 2010;56(3):194-203. 20620738.
15. Cooper LT, Baughman KL, Feldman AM, Frustaci A, Jessup M, Kühl U, et al. The role of endomyocardial biopsy in the management of cardiovascular disease: a scientific statement from the American Heart Association, the American College of Cardiology, and the European Society of Cardiology. Circulation. 2007;116(19):2216-33.
16. Cooper LT, Baughman KL, Feldman AM, Frustaci A, Jessup M, Kühl U, et al. The role of endomyocardial biopsy in the management of cardiovascular disease: a scientific statement from the American Heart Association, the American College of Cardiology, and the European Society of Cardiology. Circulation. 2007;116(19):2216-33.
17. Cooper LT, Berry GJ, Shabetai R. Idiopathic giant-cell myocarditis--natural history and treatment. Multicenter Giant Cell Myocarditis Study Group Investigators. N Eng J Med. 1997;336(26):1860-6.
18. Cooper LT, Hare JM, Tazelaar HD, Edwards WD, Starling RC, Deng MC, et al. Usefulness of immunosuppression for giant cell myocarditis. Am J Cardiol. 2008;102(11):1535-9.
19. Cooper LT, Jr., Berry GJ, Shabetai R. Idiopathic giant-cell myocarditis--natural history and treatment. Multicenter Giant Cell Myocarditis Study Group Investigators. N Engl J Med. 1997;336(26):1860-6.
20. Cooper LT. Myocarditis. N Engl J Med. 2009;360(15):1526-38.
21. Corrado D, Basso C, Thiene G. Sudden cardiac death in young people with apparently normal heart. Cardiovascular research. 2001;50(2):399-408.
22. D'Ambrosio A, Patti G, Manzoli A, Sinagra G, Di Lenarda A, Silvestri F, et al. The fate of acute myocarditis between spontaneous improvement and evolution to dilated cardiomyopathy: a review. Heart. 2001;85(5):499-504.
23. D'Ambrosio A, Patti G, Manzoli A, Sinagra G, Di Lenarda A, Silvestri F, et al. The fate of acute myocarditis between spontaneous improvement and evolution to dilated cardiomyopathy: a review. Heart. 2001;85(5):499-504.
24. Dec GW, Waldman H, Southern J, Fallon JT, Hutter AM, Palacios I. Viral myocarditis mimicking acute myocardial infarction. J Am Coll Cardiol. 1992;20(1):85-9.
25. Deonarain R, Cerullo D, Fuse K, Liu PP, Fish EN. Protective role for interferon-beta in coxsackievirus B3 infection. Circulation. 2004;110(23):3540-3.
26. Di Lenarda A, Pinamonti B, Mestroni L, Salvi A, Sabbadini G, Gregori D, et al. The natural history of dilated cardiomyopathy: a review of the Heart Muscle Disease Registry of Trieste. Ital Heart J Suppl. 2004;5(4):253-66. Come e cambiata la storia naturale della cardiomiopatia dilatativa. Una revisione del Registro delle Malattie del Miocardio di Trieste.
27. Dorffel WV, Wallukat G, Dorffel Y, Felix SB, Baumann G. Immunoadsorption in idiopathic dilated cardiomyopathy, a 3-year follow-up. Int J Cardiol. 2004;97(3):529-34.
28. Fabre A, Sheppard MN. Sudden adult death syndrome and other non-ischaemic causes of sudden cardiac death. Heart. 2006;92(3):316-20.
29. Fauchier L, Babuty D, Poret P, Casset-Senon D, Autret ML, Cosnay P, et al. Comparison of long-term outcome of alcoholic and idiopathic dilated cardiomyopathy. Eur Heart J. 2000;21(4):306-14.

30. Feldman AM, McNamara D. Myocarditis. N Eng J Med. 2000;343(19):1388-98.
31. Felix SB, Staudt A, Dorffel WV, Stangl V, Merkel K, Pohl M, et al. Hemodynamic effects of immunoadsorption and subsequent immunoglobulin substitution in dilated cardiomyopathy: three-month results from a randomized study. J Am Coll Cardiol. 2000;35(6):1590-8.
32. Felix SB, Staudt A. Non-specific immunoadsorption in patients with dilated cardiomyopathy: mechanisms and clinical effects. Int J Cardiol. 2006;112(1):30-3.
33. Felix SB, Staudt A. Non-specific immunoadsorption in patients with dilated cardiomyopathy: mechanisms and clinical effects. Int J Cardiol. 2006;112(1):30-3.
34. Friedrich MG, Sechtem U, Schulz-Menger J, Holmvang G, Alakija P, Cooper LT, et al. Cardiovascular magnetic resonance in myocarditis: A JACC White Paper. J Am Coll Cardiol. 2009;53(17):1475-87.
35. Friedrich MG, Sechtem U, Schulz-Menger J, Holmvang G, Alakija P, Cooper LT, et al. Cardiovascular magnetic resonance in myocarditis: A JACC White Paper. J Am Coll Cardiol. 2009;53(17):1475-87.
36. Friedrich MG, Strohm O, Schulz-Menger J, Marciniak H, Luft FC, Dietz R. Contrast media-enhanced magnetic resonance imaging visualizes myocardial changes in the course of viral myocarditis. Circulation. 1998;97(18):1802-9.
37. Frustaci A, Chimenti C, Calabrese F, Pieroni M, Thiene G, Maseri A. Immunosuppressive therapy for active lymphocytic myocarditis: virological and immunologic profile of responders versus nonresponders. Circulation. 2003;107(6):857-63.
38. Frustaci A, Russo MA, Chimenti C. Randomized study on the efficacy of immunosuppressive therapy in patients with virus-negative inflammatory cardiomyopathy: the TIMIC study. European Heart journal. 2009;30(16):1995-2002.
39. Frustaci A, Russo MA, Chimenti C. Randomized study on the efficacy of immunosuppressive therapy in patients with virus-negative inflammatory cardiomyopathy: the TIMIC study. European heart journal. 2009;30(16):1995-2002.
40. Fujioka S, Kitaura Y, Ukimura A, Deguchi H, Kawamura K, Isomura T, et al. Evaluation of viral infection in the myocardium of patients with idiopathic dilated cardiomyopathy. J Am Coll Cardiol. 2000;36(6):1920-6.
41. Gatmaitan BG, Chason JL, Lerner AM. Augmentation of the virulence of murine coxsackie-virus B-3 myocardiopathy by exercise. J Experiment Med. 1970;131(6):1121-36.
42. Grogan M, Redfield MM, Bailey KR, Reeder GS, Gersh BJ, Edwards WD, et al. Long-term outcome of patients with biopsy-proved myocarditis: comparison with idiopathic dilated cardiomyopathy. J Am Coll Cardiol. 1995;26(1):80-4.
43. Grun S, Schumm J, Greulich S, Wagner A, Schneider S, Bruder O, et al. Long-term follow-up of biopsy-proven viral myocarditis: predictors of mortality and incomplete recovery. J Am Coll Cardiol. 2012;59(18):1604-15.
44. Gutberlet M, Spors B, Thoma T, Bertram H, Denecke T, Felix R, et al. Suspected chronic myocarditis at cardiac MR: diagnostic accuracy and association with immunohistologically detected inflammation and viral persistence. Radiology. 2008;246(2):401-9.
45. Hauck AJ, Kearney DL, Edwards WD. Evaluation of postmortem endomyocardial biopsy specimens from 38 patients with lymphocytic myocarditis: implications for role of sampling error. Mayo Clinic proceedings. 1989;64(10):1235-45.
46. Hershberger RE, Lindenfeld J, Mestroni L, Seidman CE, Taylor MR, Towbin JA. Genetic evaluation of cardiomyopathy--a Heart Failure Society of America practice guideline. J Card Fail. 2009;15(2):83-97.
47. Herskowitz A, Ahmed-Ansari A, Neumann DA, Beschorner WE, Rose NR, Soule LM, et al. Induction of major histocompatibility complex antigens within the myocardium of patients with active myocarditis: a nonhistologic marker of myocarditis. J Am Coll Cardiol. 1990;15(3):624-32.

Myocarditis

48. Holzmann M, Nicko A, Kühl U, Noutsias M, Poller W, Hoffmann W, et al. Complication rate of right ventricular endomyocardial biopsy via the femoral approach: a retrospective and prospective study analyzing 3048 diagnostic procedures over an 11-year period. Circulation. 2008;118(17):1722-8.
49. Hufnagel G, Pankuweit S, Richter A, Schonian U, Maisch B. The European Study of Epidemiology and Treatment of Cardiac Inflammatory Diseases (ESETCID). First epidemiological results. Herz. 2000;25(3):279-85.
50. Hunt SA, Baker DW, Chin MH, Cinquegrani MP, Feldmanmd AM, Francis GS, et al. ACC/AHA Guidelines for the Evaluation and Management of Chronic Heart Failure in the Adult: Executive Summary A Report of the American College of Cardiology/American Heart Association Task Force on Practice Guidelines (Committee to Revise the 1995 Guidelines for the Evaluation and Management of Heart Failure): Developed in Collaboration With the International Society for Heart and Lung Transplantation; Endorsed by the Heart Failure Society of America. Circulation. 2001;104(24):2996-3007.
51. Imazio M, Adler Y. Management of pericardial effusion. Eur Heart J. 2013;34(16):1186-97.
52. Kadish A, Goldberger J. Selecting patients for ICD implantation: are clinicians choosing appropriately? JAMA. 2011;305(1):91-2.
53. Kanzaki Y, Terasaki F, Okabe M, Hayashi T, Toko H, Shimomura H, et al. Myocardial inflammatory cell infiltrates in cases of dilated cardiomyopathy as a determinant of outcome following partial left ventriculectomy. Japanese Circ J. 2001;65(9):797-802.
54. Kao AC, Krause SW, Handa R, Karia D, Reyes G, Bianco NR, et al. Wearable defibrillator use in heart failure (WIF): results of a prospective registry. BMC Cardiovasc Dis. 2012;12(1):123.
55. Karavidas A, Lazaros G, Noutsias M, Matzaraki V, Danias PG, Pyrgakis V, et al. Recurrent coxsackie B viral myocarditis leading to progressive impairment of left ventricular function over 8years. Int J Cardiol. 2011;151(2):e65-7.
56. Karjalainen J, Heikkila J. Incidence of three presentations of acute myocarditis in young men in military service. A 20-year experience. Eur Heart J. 199920(15):1120-5.
57. Kindermann I, Kindermann M, Kandolf R, Klingel K, Bultmann B, Muller T, et al. Predictors of outcome in patients with suspected myocarditis. Circulation. 2008;118(6):639-48.
58. Kindermann I, Kindermann M, Kandolf R, Klingel K, Bultmann B, Muller T, et al. Predictors of outcome in patients with suspected myocarditis. Circulation. 2008;118(6):639-48.
59. Knebel F, Bohm M, Staudt A, Borges AC, Tepper M, Jochmann N, et al. Reduction of morbidity by immunoadsorption therapy in patients with dilated cardiomyopathy. Int J Cardiol. 2004;97(3):517-20.
60. Kuethe F, Lindner J, Matschke K, Wenzel JJ, Norja P, Ploetze K, et al. Prevalence of parvovirus B19 and human bocavirus DNA in the heart of patients with no evidence of dilated cardiomyopathy or myocarditis. Clin Infect Dis. 2009;49(11):1660-6.
61. Kuethe F, Sigusch HH, Hilbig K, Tresselt C, Gluck B, Egerer R, et al. Detection of viral genome in the myocardium: lack of prognostic and functional relevance in patients with acute dilated cardiomyopathy. Am Heart J. 2007;153(5):850-8.
62. Kuhl U, Lassner D, von Schlippenbach J, Poller W, Schultheiss HP. Interferon-Beta improves survival in enterovirus-associated cardiomyopathy. J Am Coll Cardiol. 2012;60(14):1295-6.
63. Kuhl U, Lassner D, von Schlippenbach J, Poller W, Schultheiss HP. Interferon-Beta improves survival in enterovirus-associated cardiomyopathy. J Am Coll Cardiol. 2012;60(14):1295-6.
64. Kühl U, Noutsias M, Seeberg B, Schultheiss HP. Immunohistological evidence for a chronic intramyocardial inflammatory process in dilated cardiomyopathy. Heart. 1996;75(3):295-300.
65. Kühl U, Pauschinger M, Bock T, Klingel K, Schwimmbeck CP, Seeberg B, et al. Parvovirus B19 infection mimicking acute myocardial infarction. Circulation. 2003;108(8):945-50.

Algorithms in Heart Failure

66. Kühl U, Pauschinger M, Noutsias M, Seeberg B, Bock T, Lassner D, et al. High prevalence of viral genomes and multiple viral infections in the myocardium of adults with "idiopathic" left ventricular dysfunction. Circulation. 2005;111(7):887-93.
67. Kühl U, Pauschinger M, Seeberg B, Lassner D, Noutsias M, Poller W, et al. Viral persistence in the myocardium is associated with progressive cardiac dysfunction. Circulation. 2005;112(13):1965-70.
68. Kühl U, Schultheiss HP. Treatment of chronic myocarditis with corticosteroids. Eur Heart J. 1995;16(Suppl O):168-72.
69. Lauer B, Niederau C, Kuhl U, Schannwell M, Pauschinger M, Strauer BE, et al. Cardiac troponin T in patients with clinically suspected myocarditis. Journal of the American College of Cardiology. 1997;30(5):1354-9.
70. Lehrke S, Lossnitzer D, Schob M, Steen H, Merten C, Kemmling H, et al. Use of cardiovascular magnetic resonance for risk stratification in chronic heart failure: prognostic value of late gadolinium enhancement in patients with non-ischaemic dilated cardiomyopathy. Heart. 2011;97(9):727-32.
71. Lehrke S, Lossnitzer D, Schob M, Steen H, Merten C, Kemmling H, et al. Use of cardiovascular magnetic resonance for risk stratification in chronic heart failure: prognostic value of late gadolinium enhancement in patients with non-ischaemic dilated cardiomyopathy. Heart. 2011;97(9):727-32.
72. Mahfoud F, Gartner B, Kindermann M, Ukena C, Gadomski K, Klingel K, et al. Virus serology in patients with suspected myocarditis: utility or futility? Eur Heart J. 2011;32(7):897-903.
73. Mahfoud F, Ukena C, Kandolf R, Kindermann M, Bohm M, Kindermann I. Blood pressure and heart rate predict outcome in patients acutely admitted with suspected myocarditis without previous heart failure. J Hypertens. 2012;30(6):1217-24.
74. Mahon NG, Madden BP, Caforio AL, Elliott PM, Haven AJ, Keogh BE, et al. Immunohistologic evidence of myocardial disease in apparently healthy relatives of patients with dilated cardiomyopathy. J Am Coll Cardiol. 2002;39(3):455-62.
75. Mahrholdt H, Goedecke C, Wagner A, Meinhardt G, Athanasiadis A, Vogelsberg H, et al. Cardiovascular magnetic resonance assessment of human myocarditis: a comparison to histology and molecular pathology. Circulation. 2004;109(10):1250-8.
76. Mahrholdt H, Wagner A, Judd RM, Sechtem U, Kim RJ. Delayed enhancement cardiovascular magnetic resonance assessment of non-ischaemic cardiomyopathies. Eur Heart J. 2005;26(15):1461-74.
77. Maisch B, Bültman B, Factor S, Sekiguchi M, McKenna WJ, Richardson PJ, et al. World Heart Federation consensus conferences definition of inflammatory cardiomyopathy (myocarditis): report from two expert committees on histology and viral cardiomyopathy. Heartbeat. 1999;4:3-4.
78. Maisch B, Camerini F, Schultheiss HP. Immunosuppressive therapy for myocarditis. N Eng J Med. 1995;333(25):1713.
79. Maisch B, Pankuweit S, Karatolios K, Ristic AD. Invasive techniques--from diagnosis to treatment. Rheumatology (Oxford, England). 2006;45(Suppl 4):iv32-8.
80. Maisch B, Portig I, Ristic A, Hufnagel G, Pankuweit S. Definition of inflammatory cardiomyopathy (myocarditis): on the way to consensus. A status report. Herz. 2000;25(3):200-9.
81. Maisch B, Seferovic PM, Ristic AD, Erbel R, Rienmuller R, Adler Y, et al. Guidelines on the diagnosis and management of pericardial diseases executive summary. The Task force on the diagnosis and management of pericardial diseases of the European society of cardiology. Eur Heart J. 2004;25(7):587-610.
82. Makaryus AN, Revere DJ, Steinberg B. Recurrent reversible dilated cardiomyopathy secondary to viral and streptococcal pneumonia vaccine-associated myocarditis. Cardiology in review. 2006;14(4):e1-4.

83. Mason JW, O'Connell JB, Herskowitz A, Rose NR, McManus BM, Billingham ME, et al. A clinical trial of immunosuppressive therapy for myocarditis. The Myocarditis Treatment Trial Investigators. N Eng J Med. 1995;333(5):269-75.
84. McCarthy RE, Boehmer JP, Hruban RH, Hutchins GM, Kasper EK, Hare JM, et al. Long-term outcome of fulminant myocarditis as compared with acute (nonfulminant) myocarditis. The New England journal of medicine. 2000;342(10):690-5.
85. Norja P, Hokynar K, Aaltonen LM, Chen R, Ranki A, Partio EK, et al. Bioportfolio: lifelong persistence of variant and prototypic erythrovirus DNA genomes in human tissue. Proceedings of the National Academy of Sciences of the United States of America. 2006;103(19):7450-3.
86. Noutsias M, Hohmann C, Pauschinger M, Schwimmbeck PL, Ostermann K, Rode U, et al. sICAM-1 correlates with myocardial ICAM-1 expression in dilated cardiomyopathy. International journal of cardiology. 2003;91(2-3):153-61.
87. Noutsias M, Kühl U, Lassner D, Gross U, Pauschinger M, Schultheiss HP, et al. Parvovirus B19-associated active myocarditis with biventricular thrombi--results of endomyocardial biopsy investigations and cardiac magnetic resonance imaging. Circulation. 2007;115(13): e378-80.
88. Noutsias M, Pankuweit S, Maisch B. Myocarditis, cardiac tamponade, and pericarditis. In: Tubaro M, Danchin N, Filippatos G, Goldstein P, Vranckx P, Zahger D (Eds). The ESC Textbook of Acute and Intensive Cardiac Care. Oxford: Oxford University Press; 2010. pp. 565-77.
89. Noutsias M, Pauschinger M, Gross U, Lassner D, Schultheiss HP, Kuhl U. Giant-cell myocarditis in a patient presenting with dilated cardiomyopathy and ventricular tachycardias treated by immunosuppression: a case report. Int J Cardiol. 2008;128(2):e58-9.
90. Noutsias M, Pauschinger M, Ostermann K, Escher F, Blohm JH, Schultheiss H, et al. Digital image analysis system for the quantification of infiltrates and cell adhesion molecules in inflammatory cardiomyopathy. Med Sci Monit. 2002;8(5):MT59-71.
91. Noutsias M, Pauschinger M, Schultheiss H, Kühl U. Phenotypic characterization of infiltrates in dilated cardiomyopathy - diagnostic significance of T-lymphocytes and macrophages in inflammatory cardiomyopathy. Med Sci Monit. 2002;8(7):CR478-87.
92. Noutsias M, Pauschinger M, Schultheiss HP, Kuhl U. Cytotoxic perforin+ and TIA-1+ infiltrates are associated with cell adhesion molecule expression in dilated cardiomyopathy. Eur J Heart Fail. 2003;5(4):469-79.
93. Noutsias M, Pauschinger M, Schultheiss HP, Kühl U. Advances in the immunohistological diagnosis of inflammatory cardiomyopathy. Eur Heart J Suppl. 2002;4:I54-I62.
94. Noutsias M, Seeberg B, Schultheiss HP, Kühl U. Expression of cell adhesion molecules in dilated cardiomyopathy: evidence for endothelial activation in inflammatory cardiomyopathy. Circulation. 1999;99(16):2124-31.
95. Noutsias M, Seeberg B, Schultheiss HP, Kühl U. Expression of cell adhesion molecules in dilated cardiomyopathy: evidence for endothelial activation in inflammatory cardiomyopathy. Circulation. 1999;99(16):2124-31.
96. Noutsias M. Myocarditis. Heart Failure: the Expert's Approach. New Delhi: Jaypee Brothers Medical Publishers (P) Ltd; 2014. pp. 506-21.
97. Pankuweit S, Moll R, Baandrup U, Portig I, Hufnagel G, Maisch B. Prevalence of the parvovirus B19 genome in endomyocardial biopsy specimens. Hum Pathol. 2003;34(5):497-503.
98. Pankuweit S, Richter A, Ruppert V, Maisch B. Classification of cardiomyopathies and indication for endomyocardial biopsy revisited. Herz. 2009;34(1):55-62.
99. Phillips M, Robinowitz M, Higgins JR, Boran KJ, Reed T, Virmani R. Sudden cardiac death in Air Force recruits. A 20-year review. JAMA. 1986;256(19):2696-9.
100. Richardson P, McKenna W, Bristow M, Maisch B, Mautner B, O'Connell J, et al. Report of the 1995 World Health Organization/International Society and Federation of Cardiology

Task Force on the Definition and Classification of cardiomyopathies. Circulation. 1996;93(5):841-2.
101. Schenk T, Enders M, Pollak S, Hahn R, Huzly D. High prevalence of human parvovirus B19 DNA in myocardial autopsy samples from subjects without myocarditis or dilative cardiomyopathy. J Clin Microbiol. 2009;47(1):106-10.
102. Schenk T, Enders M, Pollak S, Hahn R, Huzly D. High prevalence of human parvovirus B19 DNA in myocardial autopsy samples from subjects without myocarditis or dilative cardiomyopathy. J Clin Microbiol. 2009;47(1):106-10.
103. Schimke I, Muller J, Priem F, Kruse I, Schon B, Stein J, et al. Decreased oxidative stress in patients with idiopathic dilated cardiomyopathy one year after immunoglobulin adsorption. J Am Coll Cardiol. 2001;38(1):178-83.
104. Schultheiss HP, Noutsias M, Kühl U, Pauschinger M. Myocarditis and Viral Cardiomyopathy. In: Camm AJ, Lüscher TF, Serruys PW (Eds). The ESC Textbook of Cardiovascular Medicine. Oxford: Blackwell Publishing Ltd; 2006. pp. 490-501.
105. Shanes JG, Ghali J, Billingham ME, Ferrans VJ, Fenoglio JJ, Edwards WD, et al. Interobserver variability in the pathologic interpretation of endomyocardial biopsy results. Circulation. 1987;75(2):401-5.
106. Staudt A, Bohm M, Knebel F, Grosse Y, Bischoff C, Hummel A, et al. Potential role of autoantibodies belonging to the immunoglobulin G-3 subclass in cardiac dysfunction among patients with dilated cardiomyopathy. Circulation. 2002;106(19):2448-53.
107. Staudt A, Eichler P, Trimpert C, Felix SB, Greinacher A. Fc (gamma) receptors IIa on cardiomyocytes and their potential functional relevance in dilated cardiomyopathy. J Am Coll Cardiol. 2007;49(16):1684-92.
108. Staudt A, Eichler P, Trimpert C, Felix SB, Greinacher A. Fc(gamma) receptors IIa on cardiomyocytes and their potential functional relevance in dilated cardiomyopathy. Journal of the American College of Cardiology. 2007;49(16):1684-92.
109. Staudt A, Schaper F, Stangl V, Plagemann A, Bohm M, Merkel K, et al. Immunohistological changes in dilated cardiomyopathy induced by immunoadsorption therapy and subsequent immunoglobulin substitution. Circulation. 2001;103(22):2681-6.
110. Staudt A, Staudt Y, Dorr M, Bohm M, Knebel F, Hummel A, et al. Potential role of humoral immunity in cardiac dysfunction of patients suffering from dilated cardiomyopathy. J Am Coll Cardiol. 2004;44(4):829-36.
111. Strauer BE, Kandolf R, Mall G, Maisch B, Mertens T, Schwartzkopff B, et al. Myocarditis--cardiomyopathy. Consensus Report of the German Association for Internal Medicine, presented at the 100th annual meeting, Wiesbaden, 13 April 1994. Acta cardiologica. 1996;51(4):347-71.
112. Taylor DO, Stehlik J, Edwards LB, Aurora P, Christie JD, Dobbels F, et al. Registry of the international society for heart and lung transplantation: twenty-sixth official adult heart transplant report-2009. J Heart Lung Transplant. 2009 Oct;28(10):1007-22.
113. Terasaki F, Okabe M, Hayashi T, Fujioka S, Suwa M, Hirota Y, et al. Myocardial inflammatory cell infiltrates in cases of dilated cardiomyopathy: light microscopic, immunohistochemical, and virological analyses of myocardium specimens obtained by partial left ventriculectomy. J Card Surg. 1999;14(2):141-6.
114. Ukena C, Mahfoud F, Kindermann I, Kandolf R, Kindermann M, Bohm M. Prognostic electrocardiographic parameters in patients with suspected myocarditis. Eur J Heart Fail. 2011;13(4):398-405.
115. Warraich RS, Noutsias M, Kazak I, Seeberg B, Dunn MJ, Schultheiss HP, et al. Immunoglobulin G3 cardiac myosin autoantibodies correlate with left ventricular dysfunction in patients with dilated cardiomyopathy: immunoglobulin G3 and clinical correlates. Am Heart J. 2002;143(6):1076-84.

116. Why HJ, Meany BT, Richardson PJ, Olsen EG, Bowles NE, Cunningham L, et al. Clinical and prognostic significance of detection of enteroviral RNA in the myocardium of patients with myocarditis or dilated cardiomyopathy. Circulation. 1994;89(6):2582-9.
117. Wojnicz R, Nowalany-Kozielska E, Wodniecki J, Szczurek-Katanski K, Nozynski J, Zembala M, et al. Immunohistological diagnosis of myocarditis. Potential role of sarcolemmal induction of the MHC and ICAM-1 in the detection of autoimmune mediated myocyte injury. Eur Heart J. 1998;19(10):1564-72.
118. Wojnicz R, Nowalany-Kozielska E, Wojciechowska C, Glanowska G, Wilczewski P, Niklewski T, et al. Randomized, placebo-controlled study for immunosuppressive treatment of inflammatory dilated cardiomyopathy: two-year follow-up results. Circulation. 2001;104(1):39-45.
119. Yilmaz A, Kindermann I, Kindermann M, Mahfoud F, Ukena C, Athanasiadis A, et al. Comparative evaluation of left and right ventricular endomyocardial biopsy: differences in complication rate and diagnostic performance. Circulation. 2010;122(9):900-9.
120. Yilmaz A, Kindermann I, Kindermann M, Mahfoud F, Ukena C, Athanasiadis A, et al. Comparative evaluation of left and right ventricular endomyocardial biopsy: differences in complication rate and diagnostic performance. Circulation. 2010;122(9):900-9.
121. Young JB, Dunlap ME, Pfeffer MA, Probstfield JL, Cohen-Solal A, Dietz R, et al. Mortality and morbidity reduction with Candesartan in patients with chronic heart failure and left ventricular systolic dysfunction: results of the CHARM low-left ventricular ejection fraction trials. Circulation. 2004;110(17):2618-26.
122. Zagrosek A, Abdel-Aty H, Boye P, Wassmuth R, Messroghli D, Utz W, et al. Cardiac magnetic resonance monitors reversible and irreversible myocardial injury in myocarditis. JACC. 2009;2(2):131-8.
123. Zagrosek A, Abdel-Aty H, Boye P, Wassmuth R, Messroghli D, Utz W, et al. Cardiac magnetic resonance monitors reversible and irreversible myocardial injury in myocarditis. Jacc. 2009;2(2):131-8.
124. Zagrosek A, Wassmuth R, Abdel-Aty H, Rudolph A, Dietz R, Schulz-Menger J. Relation between myocardial edema and myocardial mass during the acute and convalescent phase of myocarditis--a CMR study. J Cardiovasc Magn Reson. 2008;10(1):19.
125. Zee-Cheng CS, Tsai CC, Palmer DC, Codd JE, Pennington DG, Williams GA. High incidence of myocarditis by endomyocardial biopsy in patients with idiopathic congestive cardiomyopathy. J Am Coll Cardiol. 1984;3(1):63-70.
126. Zimmermann O, Rodewald C, Radermacher M, Vetter M, Wiehe JM, Bienek-Ziolkowski M, et al. Interferon beta-1b therapy in chronic viral dilated cardiomyopathy--is there a role for specific therapy? J Card Fail. 2010;16(4):348-56.

31
CHAPTER

Acquired Immune Deficiency Syndrome Induced Cardiac Abnormalities and Heart Failure

Khwaja S Alim, Hermineh Aramin, Minal V Patel, Elizabeth Lee

INTRODUCTION

Human immunodeficiency virus (HIV) or acquired immunodeficiency syndrome (AIDS) is a global epidemic. While a majority of these patients still live in Africa. Globally, there are over 1 million children who have acquired this malady, and 1,600 infants born with the infection every day.

The first case of dilated cardiomyopathy in a patient with AIDS was documented in 1986, strongly suggesting the involvement of AIDS in the development of heart muscle disease.

Though many cardiovascular diseases occur due to HIV, some diseases can be caused due to the HIV treatment. Some drugs are used to delay heart diseases yet some drugs such as zidovudine are cardiotoxic. Highly active antiretroviral therapy (HAART) regimens introduction has shown that there is an increase in both peripheral and coronary arterial diseases.

DIAGNOSIS AND TREATMENT OF HEART FAILURE DUE TO HUMAN IMMUNODEFICIENCY VIRUS OR ACQUIRED IMMUNE DEFICIENCY SYNDROME

Human immunodeficiency virus infected patients can develop several cardiac anomalies including myocarditis, dilated cardiomyopathy, right sided heart failure due to pulmonary hypertension, pericardial effusion, and cardiac tamponade, HAART induced metabolic syndrome, and premature coronary artery disease.

Human Immunodeficiency Virus Induced Cardiomyopathy

Dilated cardiomyopathy, in a patient with HIV is strongly associated with advanced stages of the disease. The introduction of HAART, which includes two nucleoside reverse transcriptase inhibitors and one protease inhibitor, has significantly reduced the prevalence of HIV cardiomyopathy in developed countries.

Screening

Two-dimensional echocardiography (2D echo) remains the most valuable screening tool for HIV-related cardiomyopathy. It assesses the two independent predictors of all-cause mortality; left ventricular systolic dysfunction and left ventricular hypertrophy.

Treatment

Treatment of AIDS patient with heart failure is similar to other patients with nonischemic dilated cardiomyopathy.

Medical Therapy

This consisting of angiotensin converting enzyme inhibitors, β-blockers, and diuretics for fluid control.

Device-based Therapy

Cardiac resynchronization therapy should be offered if indicated. In a very carefully selected group of patients with controlled HIV infection (normal CD4 count, undetectable viremia, good compliance, and psychosocial support), on a stable regimen of HAART, and with no active opportunistic infections who suffer from end-stage congestive heart failure refractory to medical management, ventricular assist devices may be considered.

Heart Transplant

This option remains rather limited in this group of population.

Right-sided Heart Failure due to Pulmonary Hypertension

Right ventricular hypertrophy occurs with right heart failure which is usually first diagnosed by screening electrocardiogram, and confirmed by 2D echo and right heart catheterization.

Treatment

The main focus of therapy is to treat the cause of the pulmonary hypertension. Vasodilator agents like epoprostenol have also been used but it is not clear whether they improve the prognosis, and its administration is generally limited to seriously ill patients.

Pericardial Effusion and Cardiac Tamponade

Pericardial effusions may be related to an opportunistic infection or to malignancy but in most of the cases the clear etiology is not found. Survival of AIDS patients with pericardial effusion is significantly shorter than of patients without an effusion. Two-dimensional echo plays a critical role in diagnosing the extent of pericardial effusion, and ruling out life-threatening conditions like cardiac tamponade.

Treatment

Pericardiocentesis is recommended in large poorly tolerated effusions, especially, in presence of cardiac tamponade.

Highly Active Antiretroviral Therapy Induced Cardiovascular Disease

Lipid abnormalities associated with HAART are related to central adiposity and insulin resistance. The annual incidence of myocardial infarction (MI) among HIV infected patients on HAART is 4–7 times higher when compared to the pre-HAART group. The exposure to the protease inhibitor therapy is associated with high risk of MI.

Treatment

Patients should be strongly encouraged to make lifestyle changes including smoking cessation, restriction of alcohol intake, and reduction in dietary fat, as well as increasing exercise.

Protease inhibitor-sparing regimens may be used, but this decision should be deffered to the specialist in HIV medicine.

Lipid lowering medications should be used if nonpharmacological treatment does not work.

Potential drug interactions should be monitored because most statins are metabolized through the cytochrome P450 3A4 pathway. The inhibition of this pathway by protease inhibitors might increase the concentration of statins, with an increase in the risk of skeletal muscle and hepatic toxicity. Pravastatin appears to be the safest agent because it is the least influenced by this pathway.

CONCLUSION

Most of the AIDS related cardiac complications occur in late stages of the disease. Hence, early diagnoses and treatment of this disease with HAART may delay and even prevent these life-threatening conditions.

KEY POINTS

- Human immunodeficiency virus or acquired immunodeficiency syndrome is a global epidemic
- Many cardiovascular diseases occur due to HIV and some may be caused by HIV treatment as some drugs used are cardiotoxic
- Human immunodeficiency virus infected patients can develop several cardiac anomalies including myocarditis, dilated cardiomyopathy, right sided heart failure due to pulmonary hypertension, pericardial effusion, and cardiac tamponade
- Dilated cardiomyopathy, in a patient with HIV is strongly associated with advanced stages of the disease
- Two-dimensional echocardiography remains the most valuable screening tool for HIV-related cardiomyopathy
- Treatment of AIDS patient with heart failure is similar to other patients with nonischemic dilated cardiomyopathy and includes angiotensin converting enzyme inhibitors, β-blockers, and diuretics for fluid control
- Highly active antiretroviral therapy can induced cardiovascular disease and lipid abnormalities
- Along with lifestyle changes, lipid lowering medications should be used
- Protease inhibitor-sparing regimens may be used, but this decision should be deffered to the specialist in HIV medicine

---

SUGGESTED READINGS

1. Aguilar RV, Farber HW. Epoprostenol (prostacyclin) therapy in HIV-associated pulmonary hypertension. Am J Respir Crit Care Med. 2000;162:1846-50.
2. Barbaro G. Cardiovascular manifestations of HIV infection. Circulation. 2002;106:1420-5.
3. Currie PF, Jacob AJ, Foreman AR, Elton RA, Brettle RP, Boon NA. Heart muscle disease related to HIV infection: prognostic implications. BMJ. 1994;309:1605-7.
4. Currier JS. Cardiovascular risk associated with HIV therapy. J Acquir Immune Defic Syndr. 2002;31:S16-23.

5. Dube MP, Sprecher D, Henry WK, Aberg JA, Torriani FJ, Hodis HN, et al. Preliminary guidelines for the evaluation and management of dyslipidemia in adults infected with human immunodeficiency virus and receiving antiretroviral therapy: recommendations of the Adult AIDS Clinical Trial Group Cardiovascular Disease Focus Group. Clin Infect Dis. 2000;31:1216-24.
6. El Hattaoui M, Charei N, Boumzebra D, Aajly L, Fadouach S. Prevalence of cardiomyopathy in HIV infection: prospective study on 158 HIV patients. Med Mal Infect. 2008;38:387-91.
7. Felker GM, Thompson RE, Hare JM, Hruban RH, Clemetson DE, Howard DL, et al. Underlying causes and long-term survival in patients with initially unexplained cardiomyopathy. N Engl J Med. 2000;342:1077-84.
8. Grunfeld C, Kotler DP, Hamadeh R, Tierney A, Wang J, Pierson RN. Hypertriglyceridemia in the acquired immunodeficiency syndrome. Am J Med. 1989;86(1):27-31.
9. Lipshultz SE, Easley KA, Orav EJ, Kaplan S, Starc TJ, Bricker JT, et al. Cardiac dysfunction and mortality in HIV-infected children: The prospective P2C2 HIV Multicenter Study. Pediatric Pulmonary and Cardiac Complications of Vertically Transmitted HIV Infection (P2C2 HIV) Study Group. Circulation. 2000,102:1542-8.
10. Lubega S, Zirembuzi GW, Lwabi P. Heart diseases among children with HIV/AIDS attending the paediatric infectious diseases clinic at Mulago Hospital. Afr Health Sci. 2005;5(3):219-26.
11. Ntsekhe M, Hakim J. Impact of human immunodeficiency virus infection on cardiovascular disease in Africa. Circulation. 2005;112(23):3602-7.
12. Prendergast BD. HIV and cardiovascular medicine. Heart. 2003;89(7):793-800.
13. Prendergast BD. HIV and cardiovascular medicine. Heart. 2003;89:793-800.

32
CHAPTER

New Onset Cardiomyopathy: Biopsy or Magnetic Resonance Imaging and Other Imaging Modalities

Khwaja S Alim, Matt M Kawahara

INTRODUCTION

Cardiomyopathy is a disease of the heart causing cardiac muscle dysfunctional, which could lead to arrhythmias and heart failure.

The main subtypes of cardiomyopathies include dilated, hypertrophic, restrictive, and arrhythmogenic right ventricular cardiomyopathy (ARVC). Dilated cardiomyopathies are characterized by increased left ventricle size. Additionally, increased left ventricular mass and normal or decreased left ventricular wall thickness can be observed. Ischemic cardiomyopathy is a major subtype of dilated cardiomyopathy (DCM). Unique to hypertrophic cardiomyopathy (HCM) is most often a thickening of the left ventricular wall and a decrease in left ventricular cavity size. Restrictive cardiomyopathy (RCM) is characterized by diastolic dysfunction of either or both ventricles and atrial dilation due to restrictive ventricular physiology. Arrhythmogenic right ventricular cardiomyopathy is characterized by the replacement of cardiac myocytes by fibrofatty tissue.

A commonly used diagnostic tool used to identify cardiac muscle dysfunction is cardiac magnetic resonance (CMR) imaging. Cardiac magnetic resonance imaging offers a noninvasive method of observing myocardial tissues for morphological abnormalities.

Cardiac magnetic resonance imaging and endomyocardial biopsy (EMB) each have unique advantages and disadvantages. The main issue is to discuss the utility of both techniques in the diagnosis of cardiomyopathy.

TABLE 1: Various forms of cardiomyopathy

Dilated	Hypertrophic	Restrictive
• Ischemic • Alcoholic • Congestive • Diabetic • Familial dilated • Idiopathic • Peripartum • Primary	• Asymmetric septal • Familial hypertrophic • Hypertrophic nonobstructive • Hypertrophic obstructive • Idiopathic hypertrophic subaortic stenosis	• Idiopathic restrictive • Infiltrative

CARDIOMYOPATHY

Table 1 discusses various forms of cardiomyopathy.

Ischemic Cardiomyopathy

Ischemic cardiomyopathy is caused by a block in the coronary arterial circulation, which leads to myocardial infarction. This is one of the most common causes of DCM. Algorithm 1 shows the approach to diagnosing this type of myopathy.

Nonischemic Cardiomyopathies

These cardiomyopathies are usually inherited conditions which are classified based on ventricular morphology and abnormal function. They are usually inherited as autosomal dominant conditions. They include HCM, DCM, ARVC, left ventricular noncompaction, and RCM. Algorithm 2 shows the approach to diagnosing this type of myopathy.

Hypertrophic Cardiomyopathy

Hypertrophic cardiomyopathy is the most commonly inherited heart condition, and is leading cause of sudden cardiac death in young adults and competitive athletes in the United States. It usually presents as asymmetrical septal hypertrophy.

Dilated Cardiomyopathy

Dilated cardiomyopathy is characterized by left ventricular dilatation and left ventricular ejection fraction less than 50% which can be seen on conventional two-dimensional (2D echo).

New Onset Cardiomyopathy: Biopsy or Magnetic Resonance Imaging...

```
Workup for ischemic cardiomyopathy
              ↓
        Detailed history
              ↓
       Electrocardiogram
              ↓
           2D echo
              ↓
            WMA
           • LVEF
           • Chamber size
           • LVESV
              ↓
         Stress tests
              ↓
Computed tomography coronary
angiogram/cardiac catheterization Other newer
tests
  • CMR
    EDWT <5 mm representing nonviable scar
  • SPECT and PET scans
```

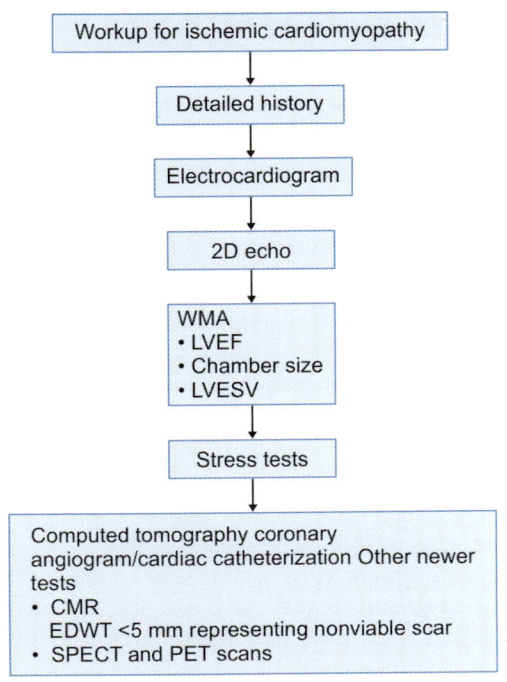

ECG, electrocardiogram; 2D echo, two-dimensional echocardiography; WMA, wall motion abnormality; LVEF, left ventricular ejection fraction; LVESV, left ventricular end-systolic volume; CMR, cardiovascular magnetic resonance; EDWT, end-diastolic wall thickness; SPECT, single photon emission computed tomography; PET, positron emission tomography

ALGORITHM 1: Workup for ischemic cardiomyopathy

Arrhythmogenic Right Ventricular Cardiomyopathy

Arrhythmogenic right-ventricular cardiomyopathy is a condition in which there is myocyte loss and fibrofatty infiltration of the myocardium which leads to an increased susceptibility to arrhythmias and sudden cardiac death.

Left Ventricular Noncompaction

Left ventricular noncompaction is characterized by a heavily trabeculated or spongy appearance of the LV myocardium which is usually first seen on a routine 2D echo. These individuals may progressively develop poor cardiac function, ventricular hypertrophy, and increased risk of thromboembolic events.

Restrictive Cardiomyopathy

Restrictive cardiomyopathy is characterized by increased stiffness of the ventricular chambers, although ventricular wall thickness and systolic function is generally within normal limits. Algorithm 2 shows the approach to diagnosing this type of myopathy.

Infiltrative Cardiomyopathies

Infiltrative cardiomyopathies can cause wide spectrum of inherited and acquired conditions with varying clinical features, and most of these conditions fall under the subgroup of RCM. Algorithm 3 shows the approach to diagnosing this type of myopathy.

Amyloidosis

Amyloidosis is a clinical disorder caused by extracellular deposition of insoluble abnormal fibrils which are derived from aggregation of normally soluble but misfolded protein.

The electrocardiogram (ECG) shows low QRS voltage. This should be the first clue to the diagnosis. Its clinical course is aggressive, with 50% of these patients progressively developing diastolic heart failure with right sided heart failure and fatal arrhythmias.

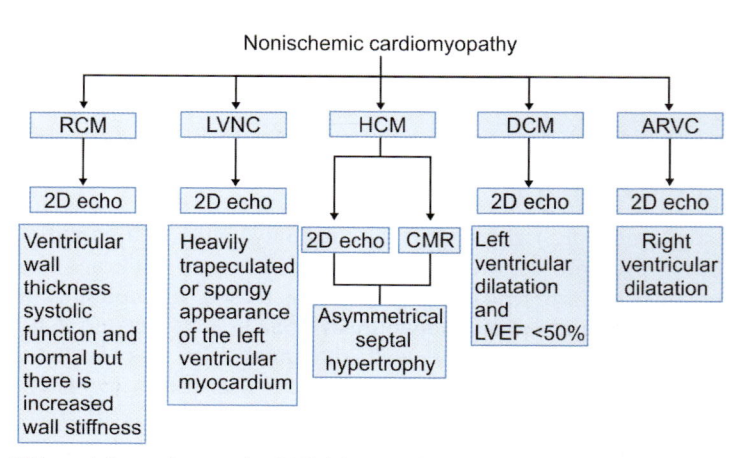

RCM, restrictive cardiomyopathy; LVNC, left ventricular noncompaction; HCM, hypertrophic cardiomyopathy; DCM, dilated cardiomyopathy; ARVC, arrhythmogenic right ventricular cardiomyopathy; LVEF, left ventricular ejection fraction; 2D echo, two-dimensional echocardiography, CMR, cardiac magnetic resonance

ALGORITHM 2: Workup for nonischemic cardiomyopathy

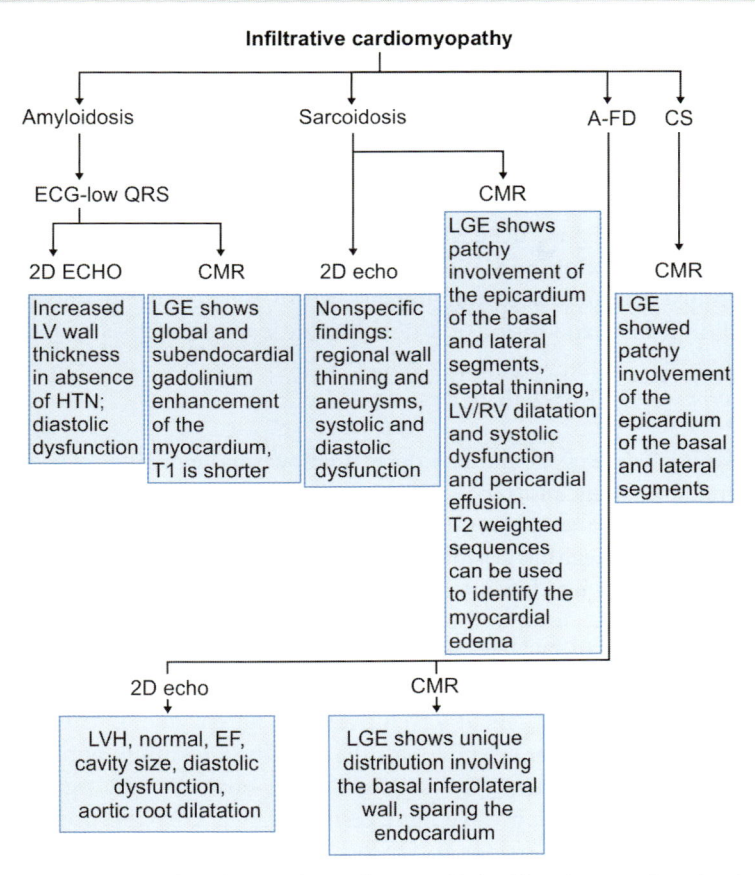

New Onset Cardiomyopathy: Biopsy or Magnetic Resonance Imaging...

Infiltrative cardiomyopathy

- **Amyloidosis**
  - ECG-low QRS
    - 2D ECHO: Increased LV wall thickness in absence of HTN; diastolic dysfunction
    - CMR: LGE shows global and subendocardial gadolinium enhancement of the myocardium, T1 is shorter
- **Sarcoidosis**
  - 2D echo: Nonspecific findings: regional wall thinning and aneurysms, systolic and diastolic dysfunction
  - CMR: LGE shows patchy involvement of the epicardium of the basal and lateral segments, septal thinning, LV/RV dilatation and systolic dysfunction and pericardial effusion. T2 weighted sequences can be used to identify the myocardial edema
- **A-FD**
  - 2D echo: LVH, normal, EF, cavity size, diastolic dysfunction, aortic root dilatation
  - CMR: LGE shows unique distribution involving the basal inferolateral wall, sparing the endocardium
- **CS**
  - CMR: LGE showed patchy involvement of the epicardium of the basal and lateral segments

AF-D, Anderson-Fabry disease; CS, cardiac sarcoidosis; 2D echo, two-dimensional echocardiography; ECG, electrocardiogram; CMR, cardiac magnetic resonance; LGE, late gadolinium enhancement; LV, left ventricle; RT, right ventricle; LVH, left ventricular hypertrophy; HTN, hypertension; EF, ejection fraction.

ALGORITHM 3: Workup for infiltrative cardiomyopathy

The senile systemic amyloidosis (SSA) is associated with increased left ventricular wall thickness but less frequent hemodynamic changes. Its clinical course is also less aggressive than the SAL amyloidosis, although the patients typically have more advanced age and greater morphological abnormalities. The aggressive nature of SAL is attributed to the direct toxic effects of the circulating free light chains that affect the myocardium where as the SSA typically causes infiltrative cardiomyopathy which is less aggressive.

Echocardiogram and CMR imaging show diagnostic features (refer to Algorithm 2).

In the past, the main form of treatment available for these patients was supportive care. But with the relentless research, there are novel therapies that are emerging with promising results. R-1-[6-[R-2-carboxy-pyrrolidin-1-yl]-6-oxo-hexanoyl] pyrrolidine-2-carboxylic acid is a drug which cross-links pairs of SAP molecules *in vivo* resulting in rapid clearance of SAP from the liver and almost complete depletion of plasma SAP. Hence, now all efforts should be made to make a definite and early diagnosis of this disease.

Sarcoidosis

Sarcoidosis is a systemic disorder of unknown etiology which causes granulomatous infiltration of various organs, including the heart. The cardiac sarcoidosis is diagnosed in accordance to the Japanese Ministry of Health and Welfare Guidelines, which includes the use of ECG, CMR, and histopathology.

Anderson-Fabry Disease

Fabry disease is an X-linked condition which has systemic and cardiac manifestations. It develops due to an enzyme deficiency of α-galactosidase, which results in the accumulation of glycosphingolipids in the lysosomes of various cells and organs. Heart is frequently involved and results in myocyte hypertrophy, vacuolation, and regional fibrosis. Currently, the diagnostic criteria are based on genetic mapping, biochemical testing, and EMB.

Myocardial imaging techniques are being explored as non-invasive ways of early screening and diagnosing these patients.

Cardiac Siderosis

Cardiac siderosis develops due to intracellular iron deposition. This causes myocardial damage which ultimately leads to cardiac dysfunction.

Cardiac magnetic resonance T2* is a measure of myocardial relaxation and this is shortened when the excessive hemosidrein stored iron disturbs the magnetic micro-environment, causing decline in the myocardial T2*. This decline in myocardial relaxation is associated with increasing risk of left ventricular dysfunction.

KEY POINTS

- Cardiomyopathy is a disease of the heart causing cardiac muscle dysfunctional, which could lead to arrhythmias and heart failure
- The main subtypes include dilated, hypertrophic, restrictive, and arrhythmogenic right ventricular cardiomyopathy
- Cardiac magnetic resonance imaging is a commonly used diagnostic tool to identify cardiac muscle dysfunction
- Endomyocardial biopsy is also a useful test with its unique advantages and disadvantages.

SUGGESTED READINGS

1. Anderson LJ, Holden S, Davis B, Prescott E, Charrier CC, Bunce NH, et al. Cardiovascular T2-star (T2*) magnetic resonance for the early diagnosis of myocardial iron overload. Eur Heart J. 2001;22:2171-9.
2. Belloni E, De Cobelli F, Esposito A, Mellone R, Perseghin G, Canu T, et al. MRI of cardiomyopathy. AJR Am J Roentgenol. 2008;191:1702-10.
3. Callis TE, Jensen BC, Weck KE, Willis MS. Evolving molecular diagnostics for familial cardiomyopathies: at the heart of it all. Expert Rev Mol Diagn. 2010;10:329-51.
4. Carpenter JP, Pennell DJ. Role of T2* magnetic resonance in monitoring iron chelation therapy. Acta Haematol. 2009;122:146-54.
5. Chimenti C, Pieroni M, Morgante E, Antuzzi D, Russo A, Russo MA, et al. Prevalence of Fabry disease in female patients with late-onset hypertrophic cardiomyopathy. Circulation. 2004;110:1047-53.
6. Cirino AL, Ho C. Familial Hypertrophic Cardiomyopathy Overview. In: Gene Reviews. Seattle: University of Washington; 1993-2012.
7. Davies MJ. The cardiomyopathies: an overview. Heart. 2000;83:469-74.
8. Dickerson JA, Raman SV, Baker PM, Leier CV. Relationship of cardiac magnetic resonance imaging and myocardial biopsy in the evaluation of nonischemic cardiomyopathy. Congest Heart Fail. 2013;19:29-38.
9. Funabashi N, Toyozaki T, Matsumoto Y, Yonezawa M, Yanagawa N, Yoshida K, et al. Images in cardiovascular medicine. Myocardial fibrosis in fabry disease demonstrated by multislice computed tomography: comparison with biopsy findings. Circulation. 2003;107:2519-20.
10. Gillmore JD, Tennent GA, Hutchinson WL, Gallimore JR, Lachmann HJ, Goodman HJ, et al. Sustained pharmacological depletion of serum amyloid P component in patient with systemic amyloidosis. Br J Haematol. 2010;148(5):760-7.
11. Kampmann C, Baehner F, Whybra C, Martin C, Wiethoff CM, Ries M, et al. Cardiac manifestations of Anderson-Fabry disease in heterozygous females. J Am Coll Cardiol. 2002;40:1668-74.
12. Maron BJ, Casey SA, Hauser RG, Aeppli DM. Clinical course of hypertrophic cardiomyopathy with survival to advanced age. J Am Coll Cardiol. 2003,42:882-8.
13. Maron BJ, Towbin JA, Thiene G, Antzelevitch C, Corrado D, Arnett D, et al. Contemporary definitions and classification of the cardiomyopathies: an American Heart Association Scientific Statement from the Council on Clinical Cardiology, Heart Failure and Transplantation Committee; Quality of Care and Outcomes Research and Functional

Genomics and Translational Biology Interdisciplinary Working Groups; and Council on Epidemiology and Prevention. Circulation. 2006;113:1807-16.
14. Merlini G, Westermark P. The systemic amyloidoses: clearer understanding of the molecular mechanisms offers hope for more effective therapies. J Intern Med. 2004;255:159-78.
15. Pepys MB, Herbert J, Hutchinson WL, Tennent GA, Lachmann HJ, Gallimore JR, et al. Targeted pharmacological depletion of serum amyloid P component for treatment of human amyloidosis. Nature. 2002;417(6886):254-9.
16. Pignatelli RH, McMahon CJ, Dreyer WJ, Denfield SW, Price J, Belmont JW, et al. Clinical characterization of left ventricular noncompaction in children: a relatively common form of cardiomyopathy. Circulation. 2003;108:2672-8.
17. Selkoe DJ. Folding proteins in fatal ways. Nature. 2003;426:900-4.
18. Soejima K, Yada H. The work-up and management of patients with apparent or subclinical cardiac sarcoidosis: with emphasis on the associated heart rhythm abnormalities. J Cardiovasc Electrophysiol. 2009;20:578-83.
19. Wood JC, Tyszka JM, Carson S, Nelson MD, Coates TD. Myocardial iron loading in transfusion-dependent thalassemia and sickle cell disease. Blood 2004;103:1934-6.

Index

Page numbers followed by '*f*' and '*t*' indicate figures and tables, respectively.

A

Abciximab 137
Acetazolamide 325
Acquired immune deficiency syndrome induced cardiac abnormalities and heart failure 348
Acute agitation 233
Acute aortic regurgitation 36
Acute coronary syndrome 26, 138
  in patients 134
  medications indicated in 138
  myocarditis 50
Acute Decompensated Heart Failure National Registry 108
Acute fulminant myocarditis 327
Acute heart failure
  disposition 12
    assess initial severity 14
    determining admission location 18
    patient reassessment 16
  evidence-based 15 (algorithm)
  patient 15 (algorithm)
  risk evidence based markers of 13*t*
Acute mitral regurgitation 35
Acute myocardial infarction 326
Acute myocarditis 324
Acute pulmonary
  edema 51, 57
  embolism 9, 26
Acute respiratory
  distress syndrome 57
  failure 50
Acute severe dyspnea 6
Acutely decompensated heart failure 103
Adaptative servoventilation 56
Adaptive-pressure-control 56
Adenoviral genomes 338
Adenovirus 324
Adequate synchrony 55
Advanced
  cardiac imaging studies 69
  cardiovascular imaging 62, 68
  heart failure 277
Alcohol ingestion 161
Aldosterone
  antagonist 126, 137, 214
  secretion 21
Alkylating agents 126
Ambulatory capacity 82
Amiloride 91
Aminophylline 325
Amiodarone 126, 175, 177
Amitriptyline 325
Ampicillin 325
Amyloidosis 72, 242, 271
Anatomic shunt 71
Anderson-Fabry disease 306, 358
Angiotensin converting enzyme inhibitor 137, 138, 186, 153, 155*t*, 209, 237
Anthracyclines 325
Antiarrhythmic
  based upon concomitant heart disease 168 (algorithm)
  drugs 126, 167, 236
  medications 167
  therapy for CHF patients 169
Anticoagulant 138
Anticoagulation 289, 290
  therapy 137
Antidepressants 126
Antifibrotic activity 208
Antineoplastic agents 126
Antipsychotic drugs 126
Antitachycardia pacing 293
Antithrombotic therapy 73
Antiviral immunomodulation with interferon 338
Aortic
  arch 120
  root dissection 36
  stent grafts 63
  valve area 37
Apixaban 164
Approach to initiate beta-blockers in heart failure 155
Arginine vasopressin 120

Algorithms in Heart Failure

Arrhythmia 82
Arrhythmogenic right ventricular
 cardiomyopathy 71, 353
  dysplasia 242
  dysplasia 38
Artificial joint replacements 63
Assessing right atrial pressure 145
 (algorithm)
Assessing shock 144 (algorithm)
Assessment of cardiac function 83
 assessing functional status 83
 management of other
  comorbidities 84
Asthma 156
Asymptomatic
 hypotension 156
 patients 310
Atrial fibrillation
 additional risk factors for 161
 and heart failure 169
 anticoagulation 163
 classification 161
 clinical evaluation 162
  echocardiogram 162
  history and physical
   examination 162
  laboratory tests 162
 clinical presentation 161
 epidemiology 160
 medications to achieve ventricular
  rate control 165
 prognosis 169
 special situation 169
 treatment 163
 restoring and maintaining sinus
  rhythm 165
 ventricular rate control 164
Atrial natriuretic peptide 21
Atrial septal defect 71
Atrioventricular 173
Atrioventricular dissociation 175t

B

Baseline electrocardiogram 133
Benzodiazepines 67, 301, 325
Beta adrenergic agonists 111
Beta-blockers 165
 and proper dosing 156t
 heart failure 153
 verapamil-type calcium
  antagonists 311
Bilevel positive airway pressure 6
Bioelectrical impedance vector
 analysis 41
 device 42f

in the dyspneic patient 41
measurement and results 43f
widespread application 44
Biomarkers
 abnormalities 70, 80
 in acute heart failure 24
Bioprofolio 330
Bisoprolol 156
Bivalirudin 137
Biventricular pacing 195
Blood urea nitrogen 85
Blunt chest trauma 36
Boussignac system 54
Bradycardia 156, 327
Brain natriuretic peptide 80, 81, 85, 133
Bridge to
 decision 279, 280
 transplant 279
Bronchoaspiration 54
Bumetanide 90, 325
Bupropion 126
Burden of atrial fibrillation 271

C

Cachexia 300
Calcium channel blockers 165, 248
Calcium sensitizer levosimendan 108, 117
Candesartan in heart failure: assessment
 of reduction in mortality and
 morbidity 186
Captopril 155
Carbamazepine 126, 325
Carbonic anhydrase inhibitors 91, 98
Cardiac
 amyloidosis 71
 biomarkers 173
 computed tomography 62
 magnetic resonance imaging 317, 353
 masses 70
 output 25
 resynchronization therapy 127, 192, 195, 196t, 197, 203
 sarcoidosis 71
 transplantation 281
Cardiac troponin 217
 clinical use of 224 (algorithm)
 inpatient use of 220
 in hospitalized patients 221
 in outpatients 224
 outpatient use of 222
 possible mechanisms for
  elevated 218
 principles for using 217

Index

special situations 224
Cardiogenic
  dyspnea 45
  shock 25, 51, 60, 143
Cardiomyocytes 182
Cardiomyopathies 143, 150
Cardiomyopathy 70, 354
  forms of 354
    arrhythmogenic right
      ventricular 355
    dilated 354
    hypertrophic 354
    infiltrative 356
    ischemic 354
    left ventricular
      noncompaction 355
    nonischemic 354
    restrictive 356
Cardiopulmonary bypass 34
Cardiorenal rescue study in acute
    decompensated heart failure 99
Cardiorenal syndrome 98, 100, 113
Cardiorespiratory arrest 60
Cardiotoxic chemotherapy 71
Cardiovascular intensive care unit 50
  acute pulmonary edema 50
  cardiogenic shock 50
  cardiorespiratory arrest 50
  postoperative cardiac surgery 50
Cardioversion of hemodynamically
    stable AF 166 (algorithm)
Carotid
  arteries 121
  sinus 120
Carvedilol 156, 165
Catecholamines 325
Catheter ablation 167
Central sleep apnea 267
Cerebral hemorrhage 112
Cerebrovascular disease 13
Characteristics of B-type natriuretic
    peptide and N-terminal
    prohormone B-type natriuretic
    peptide 22*t*
Chest pain 82, 161
Chlorthalidone 126
Chlorthiazide 90
Chronic
  dilated cardiomyopathy 323
  heart failure 133
  obstructive pulmonary disease 51,
    57, 182
  pulmonary obstructive disease 268
  stable angina 132
  treatment of ventricular
    tachycardia 177 (algorithm)
Ciprofloxacin 126
Claustrophobia 54, 67
Clinical
  decision-making in the outpatient
    setting: the use of galectin-3 199
  diagnosis of heart failure 154
    (algorithm)
  management at end-of-life 237
  presentation and outcomes of acute
    myocarditis 327*f*
  use of troponin testing in acute heart
    failure patients 222 (algorithm)
  use of troponin testing 218
    (algorithm)
Clinically suspected myocarditis 336
    (algorithm)
Clopidogrel 136
Cognitive assessment 80
Colchicine 339
Common nonacute coronary syndrome
    etiologies and workup for troponin
    release in acute heart failure
    patients 222 (algorithm)
Comorbidities associated with heart
    failure
  with preserved ejection fraction 183*f*
Comparison of the histological
    evaluation of
  myocarditis and of the
      immunohistological
      evaluation of inflammatory
      cardiomyopathy 331*t*
Compensatory basal hyperkinesia 315
Components of the CHA2DS2–VASC
    scoring system 164
Computed tomographic coronary
    angiogram 133
Congenital heart disease 74
Congestive heart failure 146, 164, 284
  exacerbation 156
Conivaptan 91, 127
Constrictive pericarditis 30, 34, 73
Continuous flow mechanical support in
    advanced heart failure 284
  ongoing management 289
  patient selection 284
Continuous positive airway pressure 54,
    57
Contraindications for
  angiotensin converting enzyme
    inhibitors in heart failure 155*t*
  beta-blockers in heart failure 156
Contrast agents
  hypersensitivity reactions 66
  renal function 66
Controversies 58

Algorithms in Heart Failure

Conventional heart failure treatment 334
Cor pulmonale 26
Coronary artery disease 131, 134
Coxsackie b virus 325
Coxsackievirus 330
Creatinine 85
Crisis phase 299
Cyclophosphamide 126

D

Dabigatran 164
Decompensated chronic valvular heart disease 37
Defibrillators in nonischemic cardiomyopathy treatment evaluation 192
Delivery of intranasal heating 56
Destination therapy 279
Detailed cardiac examination 162
Deterioration and terminal care phase 300
Deventer–Alkmaar heart failure 201
Diabetic ketoacidosis 13
Diagnosis and first contacts with healthcare providers,
   treatment initiation and stabilization: chronic phase 297
Diagnosis of heart failure with preserved ejection fraction
   incorporating echocardiography and biomarkers 185 (algorithm)
Diastolic disfunction 34
Differentiating
   restrictive cardiomyopathy 73
   ventricular tachycardia from other wide complex tachycardias 174 (algorithm)
Digoxin 165
Dilatation of the left ventricular 33
Dilated cardiomyopathy 323, 324, 328, 348, 353
Diltiazem 165
Dilutional hyponatremia 253
Diphenhydramine 66
Direct
   current cardioversion 167
   thrombin inhibitor 136, 138
Diuretic
   optimization strategies evaluation in acute heart failure 96, 100
   resistance 98
   in the hospital
      approach to 89
      different types of diuretics and their sites of action in the nephron 93*f*
      evidence based medicine for using 89
      general concepts 89
      key features of different diuretic classes 92*t*
      landmark randomized control trials on diuretic therapy in acute decompensated heart failure 94*t*
      pharmacokinetics and dosing of diuretics 90*t*
Dobutamine infusion 62, 70, 320
Dofetilide 167, 177
Dopamine 108, 113
Doppler echocardiography 150
Doppler flow patterns 151
Dronedarone 167, 253
Duloxetine 126
Dyskinesia 71
Dyspnea 4, 242
   and pain 301
   categorical examples of the causes of 4
   evaluate 3
   investigations 8
      bioimpedance vector analysis 8
      laboratory investigation 8
      radiology 9
      ultrasound 10
   observation 7
   on exertion 234
   score 4
Dyspneic patients 103

E

Echocardiographic
   evaluation 307
   features 33
   parameters 33
Edema in lower extremities 233
Effective regurgitant orifice 37, 148
Ejection fraction 71
Embolic myocardial infarction 72
Emergency department 21
Emergency heart failure mortality risk grade model 17*t*
Empiric therapy 26
Employ cardiac magnetic resonance imaging 62
Enalapril 155
End-expiratory diameter and respiratory 35

Index

Endomyocardial biopsy 324, 336, 339, 353
  biopsy virological analyses of 330
  histology of 329
  immunohistology of 329
  technique 329
Endothelial cell adhesion molecule 329
Endotracheal intubation 6, 7, 51, 60
Endovascular pacing wires 63
Enoxaparin 137
Enterovirus 324, 330
Epicardial pacing wires 63
Epinephrine 108, 112
Eplerenone 91
  post-acute myocardial infarction heart failure efficacy and survival study 209
Epstein-barr virus 324
Eptifibatide 137
Esmolol 165
European Society of Cardiology 58, 183, 218
Euvolemia 99, 100
Euvolemic 26, 80, 85
Evaluating patients with biomarker abnormalities 72
Evaluation of
  heart failure 62
  left ventricular masses and thrombus 74
Evidence of severe ADHF 13
Excessive intravascular volume depletion 252
Expiratory positive airway pressure 55
Extravascular lung water 39

F

Fabry disease 71
Facial dysmorphia 306
Facial erythema 54
Familial syndromes 70
Fatigue 234, 301
Fibrofatty tissue 353
Flecainide 167
Flow and pulsatile index 293
Fluid retention 80
Focus of treatment and care 300
Fondaparinux 137
Fulminant pneumonia 268
Furosemide 90, 96

G

Gadolinium 70
Galectin-3 81, 199
Galectin-3 levels 205
Galectin-3 to guide therapy 204
Gastric distension 54
General
  nursing assessment of heart failure
    cardiovascular assessment 267
    hypervolemia 242, 266
    hypoperfusion 265
    hypovolemia 267
    lifestyle that can exacerbate symptoms 265
    markers of cardiac rhythm abnormalities 265
    other potential issues 266
    perfusion and oxygen saturation 267
    pulmonary assessment 268
    quality of life 266
    subjective assessment 242
    status 243 (algorithm)
Genetic counseling 335
Genomes 330
Giant-cell myocarditis 339
Glomerular filtration rate and N-terminal pro-brain natriuretic peptide 205 (algorithm)
Glycoprotein IIb/IIIa inhibitor 136
Glycosphingolipids 358
Glycosylated hemoglobin 269
Goal directed medical therapy 284
Guide pericardiocentesis 35

H

Handling of excessive diuresis 98
Harrington rods 63
Healing of myocarditis 326
Healthcare providers 241
Heart failure
  and acute coronary syndrome 131
    clinical approach to 131
    treatment of 135
  assessment and management in nursing homes 232 (algorithm)
  atypical signs and symptoms of 235
  co-ordination of care 235
  diagnostic value 200
  due to human immunodeficiency virus or acquired immune deficiency syndrome 348
  for determining the type of 146 (algorithm)
  frequency of monitoring 233
  from the nursing perspective 241
  in the nursing home setting 231
  management protocol in the nursing home 231

Algorithms in Heart Failure

monitoring
  nursing home residents 232
  signs and symptoms of 234
nonpharmacological
  management 235
patient
  after myocardial infarction 200
  discharge 78
  education 84
  initial patient evaluation 78
  mortality in acute heart failure 200
  mortality in chronic heart failure 201
  pharmacologic management and education 83
  postdischarge management 84
  prognostic value
  rehospitalization in heart failure 201
  symptom management 82
signs and symptoms of 234
step-by-step guidance on initiating 231
with a normal ejection fraction 314
with preserved ejection fraction 34, 181
  diagnosis 182
  management of the patient 181
  pathophysiology 182
  prognosis 187
  treatment 184
with reduced ejection fraction 68
Hemochromatosis 70, 271
Hemodynamics 34
  instability 143
    estimation of intracardiac pressures 145
    regional wall motion abnormalities 144
    significant arrhythmia 13
    valvular function 144
    ventricular systolic function 143
Hepatojugular reflux 96, 268
High flow nasal cannula 56
Highly active antiretroviral therapy 348
  induced cardiovascular disease 350
Histological proof of myocarditis 330f
Holter monitoring 327
Human brain natriuretic peptide 104
Human immunodeficiency virus 348
  induced cardiomyopathy 349
  screening 349
  treatment 349
    device-based therapy 349
    heart transplant 349
    medical therapy 349
Humidification high flow 56
Hydration index 41
Hydrochlorothiazide 126
Hypercapnia 60
Hypercapnic patients 57
Hyperlipidemia 132
Hypertension 82
Hypertonic saline infusion 127
Hypertrophic
  cardiomyopathy 23, 71, 72, 150, 192, 220, 305
    clinical observations and symptoms 305
    clinically important pathophysiological principles 305
    diagnostic 306 (algorithm)
    exercise tests 308
    pathophysiological principles 306 (algorithm)
    patients at high risk for sudden cardiac death 309 (algorithm)
    risk stratification 309
    therapeutic 308 (algorithm)
    treatment of 312 (algorithm)
    use of biomarkers 307
    use of other imaging modalities 307
  obstructive cardiomyopathy 150
Hyponatremia 113, 127
  cyclical nature of 123f
  definitions of 119
  evaluation and treatment of 124
  evaluation of 125
  in heart failure 119
  mechanism 120
  medications that exacerbate 126
  practical approach to 119
  signs of severe 120
  symptoms of mild 120
Hypotension 54

I

Identification of nursing home residents with heart failure and devices 231
Ifosfamide 126
Immunoadsorption 338
Immunohistological aspects of inflammatory cardiomyopathy 332f
Immunohistologically confirmed myocarditis 338
Immunosuppression 335
Impaired exercise tolerance 234

Implantable cardioverter
    defibrillator 63, 178, 192, 192, 197,
    309
  placement 193*t*
  in hypertrophic cardiomyopathy 192
Increased left ventricular wall
    thickness 71
Incremental predictive value 25
Indapamide 90
Indications for
  cardiac resynchronization
    therapy 195 (algorithm)
  mechanical circulatory support 277
Induced nephropathy 66
Infectious agents 324
  animal toxic agents 325
  bacteria 324
  cardiac involvement in systemic
    disorders 325
  fungi 324
  medication 325
  physical conditions 325
  protozoa 324
  toxic agents 325
Infectious agents viruses 324
Infective endocarditis 36
Inferior vena cava 35
Infiltrative cardiomyopathies
  amyloidosis 356
  cardiac siderosis 358
  sarcoidosis 358
Inflammatory cardiomyopathy 324,
    326, 328
Inhalation wheezing 7
Inhibiting cardiac hypertrophy 21
Initiate angiotensin converting enzyme
    inhibitor in heart failure 154
Inotropes 25, 108
  classes of 108
  in acute heart failure 113
  pharmacological properties of 109
  proposed strategy on how to use 114
  selection of the appropriate 115
  when and how to use 108
Inspiratory positive airway pressure 55
Intensive care unit 50
  acute respiratory failure 50
  chronic obstructive pulmonary
    disease 50
  coma 50
  neuromuscular disorders 50
  postoperative high risk
    interventions 50
Interagency Registry for Mechanically
    Assisted Circulatory Support

    patient profiles and timing of
      left ventricular assist device
      support 286
Interdisciplinary healthcare
    providers 235
Interleukin-33 208
Intermediate BNP levels 26
Interventricular septum 151
Intra-aortic balloon
    counterpulsation 113
    pumps 63
Intracellular iron deposition 358
Intracranial pathologies 319
Intramyocardial inflammation 326
Intrathoracic impedance 271
Intravascular
    depletion 99
    volume 25
      depletion 123
Intravenous nitroglycerin 104
Invasive
    angiography 63
    electrophysiologic testing 194
    hemodynamic monitoring 104
    mechanical ventilation 50, 51
      in patients with heart failure 51
Investigation of nontransplant-
    eligible patients who are inotrope
    dependent 279
Ischemic
    disease 143
    heart disease 147, 167
Isoforms 208

J

Japanese Ministry of Health and Welfare
    Guidelines 358
Jet maximum velocities 38
Jugular venous distention 5, 96, 234
Jugular venous pressure 45

K

Kaplan-Meier analysis of the
    risk of death or cardiac
    transplantation 223
Korotkoff sounds 290

L

Lamotrigine 126
Late gadolinium enhancement 332
Left bundle branch block 34, 197
Left ventricular
    assist device versus transplantation
      bridge to 277

decision 280
transplant 279
destination therapy 279
diastolic function 33
dysfunction 122
ejection fraction 143, 197, 281, 328
end-diastolic
diameter 328
volume index 184
filling pressures 34
indications for mechanical
circulatory support 277
outflow tract obstruction 320
systolic dysfunction 164
systolic function 32, 146
transplant 281
patient selection 281
wall thickness 163
Levamisole 126
Levosimendan 112, 115, 320, 321
Lidocaine 175
Lipid lowering therapy 138
Lipid profile 269
Lisinopril 155
Loop diuretics 90
Low cardiac output-hypoperfusion 108
Low molecular weight heparin 136, 138
Lower body mass index 235
Lower extremity swelling 234
Lysosomal storage disorder 71
Lysosomes 358

M

Management of heart failure in an
emergency department setting 29
Mancini and Lietz in selection 281
Mechanical ventilation in acute heart
failure 50
Medication considerations in heart
failure and preserved ejection
fraction, nursing overview of 247t
reduced ejection fraction, nursing
overview of 245t
Melphalan 126
Membrane bound 208
Mental obtundation 265
Metallic implants 63
Methotrexate 126
Metolazone 126
Metoprolol 165
Mid-region pro-atrial natriuretic
peptide 21, 24t
Mid-regional-proadrenomedullin 81
Milrinone 108, 112, 115

Mitral and tricuspid valve
insufficiency 271
Mitral stenosis 30, 148
Mitral-clip procedure 74
Molecular genetics 308
Monoamine oxidase inhibitors 126
Monoclonal antibodies 126
Morphine sulfate 138
Multicenter Automatic Defibrillator
Implantation Trial II 192
with cardiac resynchronization
therapy 203
Multicenter breathing 23
Myocardial
imaging techniques 358
infarction 34, 70, 132
ischemia 117
perfusion 62, 67
Myocarditis 73, 220, 323
autoantibodies 333
cardiac magnetic resonance imaging
diagnosis of 332
clinical presentation 326
diagnosis 329
epidemiological 323
pathogenesis 323
prognosis 328
treatment 334
clinical management 334
immunomodulatory
treatment 335

N

Nasal congestion 54
National Heart, Lung, and Blood
Institute 184
Natriuretic peptides 8, 18, 21, 23, 26, 28,
30, 45, 48, 99, 132, 199
atrial natriuretic peptide and mid-
region pro-atrial natriuretic
peptide, the evidence 24
B-type natriuretic peptide, the
evidence 23
N-terminal pro-B-type natriuretic
peptide: the evidence 23
using natriuretic peptides in the
emergency department 25
Nesiritide 104
Neurohormonal
antagonists 99
blockade medications 214
Neuromuscular
crisis 316
diseases 56

Neutrophil gelatinase-associated lipocalin 81, 85
New onset cardiomyopathy 353
  biopsy 353
  magnetic resonance imaging 353
New York Heart Association 195, 278
Nitroglycerin 138
Nocturia 242, 267
Nocturnal dyspnea 235
Noncardiac origin 132
Noncardiogenic dyspnea 39, 45
Nondihydropyridine calcium channel blocker 138
Noninvasive cardiological screening 335
Noninvasive ventilation 50-52
  advantages and complications of 54
  in acute heart failure 57
  modalities of 54
Nonischemic cardiomyopathy 62
Nonobstructive coronary artery disease 72
Nonosmotic pathway 121
Non-ST elevation myocardial infarction 135, 136, 209
Nonsteroidal anti-inflammatory drugs 100
Noonan syndrome 306
Norepinephrine 108
Nurse consideration at transitions point of care 255
Nurse tips of safety and self-care behaviors at home 258*t*
Nursing management of asymptomatic heart failure 244 (algorithm)
Nursing research opportunities 263

O

Objective assessment related to diagnostic tests 268
  chest radiograph 269
  electrocardiogram 269
  maximal exercise testing 270
  other common diagnostics 271
  serum laboratory 268
  trend data from internal cardiac monitoring 271
  two-dimensional echocardiogram 271
  urinalysis 269
  ventricular function 270
Obstructive sleep apnea 161, 268
Opioids 301
Optivolemic 26
Orthopnea 82, 234, 242

Osmolar iodinated CT contrast agents 66
Oxcarbazepine 126
Oxygen saturation 82

P

Palliative and end-of-life care 296
Paroxysmal AF 161
Paroxysmal nocturnal dyspnea 242, 267
Partial thromboplastin time 289
Patient with suspected left ventricular assist device infection 291 (algorithm)
Peak transtricuspid blood flow velocity 150
Pentostatin 126
Percutaneous coronary intervention 136
Percutaneous left atrial appendage closure devices 74
Pericardial
  disease 143, 149
    acute pericarditis 149
    cardiac tamponade 149
    pericardial effusion 149
  effusion and cardiac tamponade 350
  tamponade 7
  window 149
Pericarditis 149, 161
Peripartum cardiomyopathy 220
Peripheral
  artery disease 164
  edema 252
  pulses 267
  stents 63
Pharmacologic stress test 135
Pheochromocytoma 271, 319
Phosphodiesterase III inhibitors 117
Planning care in the different phases of the heart failure trajectory 296
  discussions of the heart failure trajectory and end of life with heart failure patients and their families 298 (algorithm)
Platinum compounds 126
Pneumonia 7
Pneumothorax 54
Polymerase chain reaction 323
Polypharmacy 84
Positive
  end expiratory pressure 54, 55
  hepatojugular reflux test 266
  intrathoracic pressure 51, 52
  predictive value 24
  troponin test 132

Positron emission tomography 63
Postaortic valve replacement 22
Potassium-sparing diuretics 91
Potential use in clinical decision-making 203
Prasugrel 136
Pre-assesment for mechanical circulatory support 286 (algorithm)
Predisposing conditions 72
Prednisone 66
Premature ventricular contractions 177
Premorbid condition 5
Preoperative assessment for patients undergoing left ventricular assist devices 289
Preprocedural planning 74
Pressure support ventilation 55
Pressure-half time 37
Primary cardiomyopathies 150
Procainamide 175
Propafenone 167
Proportional assist ventilation 56
Prosthetic valve dysfunction 36
Pulmonary
  capillary wedge pressure 21, 35
  congestion 38
  disease 161
  edema 112
  embolus 13
  hypertension 33
  interstitial edema 39
  vascular resistance 115
Pulmonic regurgitation 150
Pulsatility index 290
Pulsus alternans 265
Pursed lip breathing 268

Q

Quality of life 236
Quantification of biventricular volumes 62

R

Radiological left ventricular angiography 153
Radionuclide ventriculography 153, 271
Ramipril 155
Randomized evaluation of mechanical assistance for the treatment of congestive heart failure 280
Regurgitant fractions 74
Regurgitant jet 36, 148
Relaxing arterioles 21
Remifentanil 58
Renal function assessment 82
Renal insufficiency 24
Renal ultrafiltration 113
Renin-angiotensin-aldosterone system 98, 120, 133
Resolution of giant cell myocarditis under immunosuppression 337f
Restrictive cardiomyopathy 73, 353
Rheumatologic diseases 271
Rhythm
  diagnostics 308
  disturbances 327
Rifabutin 126
Right atrial pressure 145
Right heart disease 150
Right ventricle 38
Right ventricular
  akinesia 71
  assist device 277
  dysfunction 71
  function 289
  function 290
  systolic pressure 35
Right-sided heart failure due to pulmonary hypertension 349
Rivaroxaban 164

S

Sarcoidosis 70, 72, 220
Scar distribution 175
Secondary comorbidities 80
Semiquantitative assessment 34
Senile systemic amyloidosis 357
Sepsis 7
Septal occluder devices 63
Serial measurements of galectin-3 202
Serum sodium levels 127
Severe aortic stenosis 22
Severe asthma 57
Severe hyponatremia require hospitalization 127
Shortness of breath 161
Side effects during diuretic therapy
  hypernatremia 99
  hyperuricemia 99
  hypokalemia 99
  ototoxicity 99
Sinus node funny channel inhibitor 246
Sinus or ear pain 54
Sinus tachycardia 327
Sleep-disordered breathing 242, 267
Society of Cardiovascular Patient Care 12
Sodium nitroprusside 104
Sodium valproate 126
Sotalol 167, 177

Index

Spiroergometry 308
Spironolactone 204
Spontaneous chordal rupture 36
ST elevation myocardial infarction 135, 208, 315
ST2
 acute decompensated heart failure 209
 chronic heart failure 213
 in the setting of myocardial infarction or heart failure 210 (algorithm)
 measurement in the inpatient setting 208
Stage D heart failure 278 (algorithm)
ST elevation myocardial infarction and non-ST elevation myocardial infarction 208
Statins 246
Stepwise approach to the acute treatment of sustained ventricular tachycardia 176 (algorithm)
Sternal wires 63
Stress 220
Structural heart disease 70
Sublingual nitroglycerin 135
Subxiphoid view of a pericardial effusion 10f
Sudden cardiac death 192, 194, 306, 326, 334
Sulbactam 126
Supraventricular extrasystoles 327
Sustained arrhythmia 160
Sympathomimetic drugs 320
Symptom management options at end-of-life 238 (algorithm)
Symptomatic hypertrophic
 nonobstructive cardiomyopathy phenotype patients 311
 obstructive cardiomyopathy patients 311
Syncope (less common) 161
Systolic
 anterior motion 150
 blood pressure 13
 failure management overview 285 (algorithm)
Systolic pap 146

T

Tachyarrhythmias 110, 112, 117
Tachyphylaxis 104
Tachypneic 58
Takotsubo syndrome 315
 comparison of diagnostic criteria 318 (algorithm)
 initial assessment of patients 317 (algorithm)
 management of 319, 320 (algorithm)
 risk factors for 316f
Themes in nursing
 assessment of patients' needs 263
 interventions 263
 interventions and outcomes 264
Thermodilution Swan-Ganz catheters 63
Thiazide diuretics 90, 125, 126
Thiazolidinediones 253
Thoracentesis 39
Thoracic ultrasound 45
Three Interventions in Cardiogenic Pulmonary Oedema 58
Thrombolysis in myocardial infarction 136, 137
Thrombolytic therapy 136
Thrombophilia 73
Thyroid function 269
Thyrotoxicosis 161
Ticagrelor 136
Tips on physical activity and exercise 261
Tirofiban 137
Tissue Doppler imaging 34
Tolvaptan 91, 127
 therapy guidelines for initiating 128
Torsemide 90
Torsemide 99
Toxic agents 324
Transaminases 113
Transcatheter aortic valve implantation 74
Transesophageal echocardiography 36, 144, 151
Transient worsening of renal function 101
Transition to end-of-life care 236
Transmitral blood flow velocity 150
Transthoracic echocardiogram 148
Treatment of
 heart failure with preserved ejection fraction 187 (algorithm)
 preserved cardiac function heart failure with an aldosterone antagonist 186
Trending biomarkers 81
Triamterene 91
Tricuspid
 annular plane systolic excursion 38
 regurgitation 71, 268
Tricyclic antidepressants 126
Trimethoprim-sulfamethoxazole 126
Troponin 18, 80

Troubleshooting and monitoring stable device function 290
   common problems in left ventricular assist devices 292 (algorithm)
   left ventricular suction event 293
   pump thrombus 293
   ventricular arrhythmias 293
Typical maculopapular skin lesions 306

U

Ultrasound in the management of acute heart failure 32
Undetectable viremia 349
Unfractionated heparin 136-138
Unstable angina 136, 137
Use of bioelectrical impedance vector analysis in the dyspneic patients 44
Utility of advanced imaging 67

V

Valvular
   disease 143
   disorders 70
   heart disease 73, 147
   regurgitation 148
Vaptan drugs 127
Vascular disease 164
Vasoactive infusions 14
Vasodilators
   in acute heart failure, effects of 103
   induced hypotension 105
   induced management of 106
   recommended dose of 104
Vasopressin
   and heart failure 122
   antagonists 91, 127
Vasopressin role of arginine 122
Vasospasm 72
Vena contracta 36, 37
Venodilation 103
Ventricular
   dimensions and volumes 271
   enlargement 70
   tachyarrhythmias 112, 194
   tachycardia 70, 74, 172, 293
      clinical presentation 172
      initial evaluation 173
         electrocardiogram 173
         imaging 173
         ischemic evaluation 175
      prognosis 178
      treatment 175
         acute 175
         chronic 176
   wall stress 22
   wall stretch 133
Ventriculoatrial 173
Venules 21
Verapamil 165
Vinca alkaloids 126
Visual analog scale 3
Visual analogue scales 17
Vital signs 5

W

Warfarin 164
Water excretion 21
Weaning 57
Weight gain 82, 80, 234
Well's criteria 9
Wolff-Parkinson-White syndrome 162, 169
Workup for
   infiltrative cardiomyopathy 357 (algorithm)
   ischemic cardiomyopathy 355 (algorithm)
   nonischemic cardiomyopathy 356 (algorithm)
Worsening
   dyspnea 156
   orthopnea 267
   status 252

X

Xanthine oxidase inhibitors 188